# Diagnostic Testing for Enteric Pathogens

*Editor*

ALEXANDER J. MCADAM

# CLINICS IN LABORATORY MEDICINE

www.labmed.theclinics.com

June 2015 • Volume 35 • Number 2

**ELSEVIER**

1600 John F. Kennedy Boulevard • Suite 1800 • Philadelphia, Pennsylvania, 19103-2899

http://www.theclinics.com

**CLINICS IN LABORATORY MEDICINE Volume 35, Number 2**
**June 2015 ISSN 0272-2712, ISBN-13: 978-0-323-38894-8**

Editor: Joanne Husovski
Developmental Editor: Colleen Viola

*Reprints.* For copies of 100 or more, of articles in this publication, please contact the Commercial Reprints Department, Elsevier Inc., 360 Park Avenue South, New York, New York 10010-1710. Tel. 212-633-3874, Fax: 212-633-3820, E-mail: reprints@elsevier.com.

*Clinics in Laboratory Medicine* (ISSN 0272-2712) is published quarterly by Elsevier Inc., 360 Park Avenue South, New York, NY 10010-1710. Months of issue are March, June, September, and December. Business and Editorial offices: 1600 John F. Kennedy Blvd., Suite 1800, Philadelphia, PA 19103-2899. Periodicals postage paid at NewYork, NY and additional mailing offices. Subscription prices are $250.00 per year (US individuals), $419.00 per year (US institutions), $135.00 per year (US students), $305.00 per year (Canadian individuals), $510.00 per year (Canadian institutions), $185.00 per year (Canadian students), $390.00 per year (international individuals), $510.00 per year (international institutions), $185.00 (international students). Foreign air speed delivery is included in all Clinics subscription prices. All prices are subject to change without notice. POSTMASTER: Send address changes to *Clinics in Laboratory Medicine*, Elsevier Health Sciences Division, Subscription Customer Service, 3251 Riverport Lane, Maryland Heights, MO 63043. **Customer Service: 1-800-654-2452 (US). From outside of the US and Canada, call 1-314-447-8871. Fax: 1-314-447-8029. E-mail: journalscustomerservice-usa@elsevier.com (for print support) or journalsonlinesuppor-t-usa@elsevier.com (for online support).**

*Clinics in Laboratory Medicine* is covered in *EMBASE/Exerpta Medica, MEDLINE/PubMed (Index Medicus), Cinahl, Current Contents/Clinical Medicine, BIOSIS* and *ISI/BIOMED.*

# Contributors

## EDITOR

**ALEXANDER J. McADAM, MD, PhD**
Department of Laboratory Medicine, Boston Children's Hospital, Boston, Massachusetts

## AUTHORS

**IBNE KARIM M. ALI, PhD**
Free-Living and Intestinal Amebas Laboratory, National Center for Emerging and Zoonotic Infectious Diseases, Centers for Disease Control and Prevention, Atlanta, Georgia

**CHERYL A. BOPP, MS**
Unit Chief, Epidemic Investigations Laboratory, Enteric Diseases Laboratory Branch, Division of Foodborne, Waterborne and Environmental Diseases, Centers for Disease Control and Prevention, Atlanta, Georgia

**ALLEN BRYAN, MD, PhD**
Clinical Fellow in Pathology, Division of Laboratory Medicine, Department of Pathology, Beth-Israel Deaconess Medical Center, Boston, Massachusetts

**CAREY-ANN D. BURNHAM, PhD**
Associate Professor, Department of Pathology and Immunology, Washington University School of Medicine, Washington University in St. Louis, St. Louis, Missouri

**VITALIANO A. CAMA, DVM, PhD**
Supervisory Microbiologist, Division of Parasitic Diseases and Malaria, Centers for Disease Control and Prevention, Atlanta, Georgia

**JOHN P. DEKKER, MD, PhD**
Medical Officer; Co-director of Bacteriology, Parasitology, and Molecular Epidemiology, Department of Laboratory Medicine, Clinical Center, National Institutes of Health, Bethesda, Maryland

**MATHEW D. ESONA, PhD**
Microbiologist, Division of Viral Diseases, Gastroenteritis and Respiratory Viruses Laboratory Branch, Centers for Disease Control and Prevention, Atlanta, Georgia

**ANDREW S. FIELD, MBBS(Hons), FRCPA, FIAC, DiplomaCytopathology(RCPA)**
Deputy Director and Senior Pathologist, Department of Anatomic Pathology, St Vincent's Hospital; Associate Professor, Notre Dame University Medical School, Sydney, New South Wales, Australia

**COLLETTE FITZGERALD, PhD**
Enteric Diseases Laboratory Branch, Division of Foodborne, Waterborne and Environmental Diseases, Centers for Disease Control and Prevention, Atlanta, Georgia

**KAREN M. FRANK, MD, PhD, D(ABMM)**
Supervisory Medical Officer; Chief of Microbiology, Department of Laboratory Medicine, Clinical Center, National Institutes of Health, Bethesda, Maryland

**RASHI GAUTAM, PhD**
Microbiologist, Division of Viral Diseases, Gastroenteritis and Respiratory Viruses Laboratory Branch, Centers for Disease Control and Prevention, Atlanta, Georgia

**PETER H. GILLIGAN, PhD, D(ABMM), F(AAM)**
Director, Clinical Microbiology-Immunology Laboratories, UNC HealthCare; Professor, Pathology-Laboratory Medicine and Microbiology-Immunology, UNC School of Medicine, Chapel Hill, North Carolina

**MARK D. GONZALEZ, PhD**
Division of Laboratory and Genomic Medicine, Department of Pathology and Immunology, Washington University School of Medicine, Washington University in St. Louis, St. Louis, Missouri

**ROMNEY M. HUMPHRIES, PhD, D(ABMM)**
Assistant Professor, Pathology and Laboratory Medicine, University of California Los Angeles, Los Angeles, California

**J. MICHAEL JANDA, PhD, D(ABMM)**
Director of Laboratory Services, Alameda County Public Health Laboratory, Oakland, California

**BONITA E. LEE, MD, MSc**
Associate Professor, Department of Pediatrics, University of Alberta, Edmonton, Alberta, Canada

**BLAINE A. MATHISON, BS**
Microbiologist, Division of Parasitic Diseases and Malaria, Centers for Disease Control and Prevention, Atlanta, Georgia

**ALEXANDER J. McADAM, MD, PhD**
Department of Laboratory Medicine, Boston Children's Hospital, Boston, Massachusetts

**DANNY A. MILNER Jr, MD, MSc, FCAP**
Associate Professor of Pathology and Pathologist, Brigham and Women's Hospital/ Harvard Medical School, Boston, Massachusetts

**SCOTT MORRISON, MSc**
Luminex Corporation, Austin, Texas

**ANNA E. NEWTON, MPH**
Surveillance Epidemiologist, Enteric Diseases Epidemiology Branch, Division of Foodborne, Waterborne and Environmental Diseases, Centers for Disease Control and Prevention, Atlanta, Georgia

**XIAOLI PANG, PhD**
Program Leader, Provincial Laboratory for Public Health, Walter Mackenzie Health Sciences Centre, University of Alberta Hospital; Professor, Department of Laboratory Medicine and Pathology, University of Alberta, Edmonton, Alberta, Canada

**AUDREY N. SCHUETZ, MD, MPH, D(ABMM)**
Associate Professor of Pathology and Laboratory Medicine, Weill Cornell Medical College/New York-Presbyterian Hospital, New York, New York

**YI-WEI TANG, MD, PhD**
Clinical Microbiology Service, Memorial Sloan-Kettering Cancer Center, Weill Cornell Medical College, Cornell University, New York, New York

**CRAIG B. WILEN, MD, PhD**
Department of Pathology and Immunology, Washington University School of Medicine, Washington University in St. Louis, St. Louis, Missouri

**ILAN YOUNGSTER, MD**
Clinical Fellow in Pediatrics, Division of Infectious Diseases, Boston Children's Hospital, Boston, Massachusetts

**HONGWEI ZHANG, MD, PhD**
Luminex Corporation, Austin, Texas

# Contents

> *Salmonella, Shigella,* and *Yersinia* cause a well-characterized spectrum of disease in humans, ranging from asymptomatic carriage to hemorrhagic colitis and fatal typhoidal fever. These pathogens are responsible for millions of cases of food-borne illness in the United States each year, with substantial costs measured in hospitalizations and lost productivity. In the developing world, illness caused by these pathogens is not only more prevalent but also associated with a greater case-fatality rate. Classic methods for identification rely on selective media and serology, but newer methods based on mass spectrometry and polymerase chain reaction show great promise for routine clinical testing.

> Shiga toxin–producing *Escherichia coli* (STEC) is among the common causes of foodborne gastroenteritis. STEC is defined by the production of specific toxins, but within this pathotype there is a diverse group of organisms. This diversity has important consequences for understanding the pathogenesis of the organism, as well as for selecting the optimum strategy for diagnostic testing in the clinical laboratory. This review includes discussions of the mechanisms of pathogenesis, the range of manifestations of infection, and the several different methods of laboratory detection of Shiga toxin–producing *E coli*.

> Vibriosis is a group of intestinal and extraintestinal infections caused by marine-dwelling bacteria of the genus *Vibrio*. Infections range from indolent illnesses to fulminant diseases, including cholera and necrotizing fasciitis. Most illnesses result from direct contact with the marine environment or consumption of shellfish, especially oysters. In the United States vibrio infections are increasing but are underreported because of lack of clinical recognition and appropriate detection in the microbiology laboratory. Recent advances to aid in the detection and identification of vibrio illnesses in the laboratory include rapid identification tests, new media, and molecular identification systems.

*Campylobacter* continues to be one of the most common bacterial causes of diarrheal illness in the United States and worldwide. Infection with *Campylobacter* causes a spectrum of diseases including acute enteritis, extraintestinal infections, and postinfectious complications. The most common species of *Campylobacter* associated with human illness is *Campylobacter jejuni*, but other *Campylobacter* species can also cause human infections. This comprehensive review includes discussion of the taxonomy, clinical manifestations of infection, epidemiology and the different methods of laboratory detection of *Campylobacter*.

The best laboratory diagnostic approach to detect *Clostridium difficile* infection (CDI) is the subject of ongoing debate. In the United States, nucleic acid amplification tests (NAAT) have become the most widely used tests for making this diagnosis. Detection of toxin in stool may be a better predictor of CDI disease and severity. Laboratories that have switched from toxin-based to NAAT-based methods have significantly higher CDI detection rates. The important issue is whether all NAAT-positive patients have CDI or at least some of those patients are excretors of the organism and do not have clinical disease.

Gastroenteritis due to enteric pathogens is generally a self-limiting disease for which antimicrobial treatment is not required. However, treatment should be considered for cases of severe or prolonged diarrhea, extraintestinal isolation of bacteria, or diarrhea in immunocompromised hosts, the elderly, and infants. Various resistance trends and current issues concerning antimicrobial susceptibility testing of enteric pathogens are reviewed in this article, including *Campylobacter, Salmonella, Shigella, Vibrio, Aeromonas, Plesiomonas*, and *Clostridium difficile*. Updated interpretive criteria from breakpoint-setting organizations are reviewed, along with explanations for recent changes in antimicrobial breakpoints.

Infectious diarrhea is a major cause of morbidity. A rapid and inexpensive assay for the diagnosis of infectious gastroenteritis would expedite appropriate therapy and prevent unnecessary and potentially invasive testing. This article summarizes assays for the diagnosis of infectious gastroenteritis based on the host response to bacterial, viral, or parasitic infection. This includes both systemic biomarkers (such as C-reactive protein, erythrocyte sedimentation rate, and serum cytokines) and fecal biomarkers (such as lactoferrin, fecal leukocyte analysis, and calprotectin). Although some of these assays have value as adjunct diagnostics, they lack sensitivity and specificity as stand-alone tests in this setting.

Norovirus is an important cause of gastroenteritis outbreaks globally and the most prevalent cause of sporadic gastroenteritis in many regions. Rapid and accurate identification of causative viral agents is critical for outbreak investigation, disease surveillance, and management. Because norovirus is not cultivable and has a highly diversified and variable genome, it is difficult to develop diagnostic assays. Detection methods have evolved from electron microscopy to conventional end-point reverse transcription polymerase chain reaction (RT-PCR), immunoassay, real-time RT-PCR, other molecular technologies, and nanotechnology array-based assays. The status and features of various testing methods are summarized in this review.

Group A rotavirus (RVA) is the major cause of acute gastroenteritis (AGE) in young children worldwide. Introduction of two live, attenuated rotavirus vaccines, Rotarix® and RotaTeq®, has dramatically reduced RVA-associated AGE and mortality. High-throughput, sensitive and specific techniques are required to rapidly diagnose and characterize rotavirus strains in stool samples for proper patient treatment and to monitor circulating vaccine and wild-type rotavirus strains. New molecular assays are rapidly developed that are more sensitive and specific than the conventional assays for detection, genotyping and full genome characterization of circulating rotavirus wild-type and vaccine (Rotarix® and RotaTeq®) strains causing AGE.

Among the *Entamoeba* species that infect humans, *Entamoeba histolytica* causes diseases, *Entamoeba dispar* is a harmless commensal, *Entamoeba moshkovskii* seems to be a pathogen, and the pathogenicity of *Entamoeba bangladeshi* remains to be investigated. Species-specific detection needed for treatment decisions and for understanding the epidemiology and pathogenicity of these amebae. Antigen-based detection methods are needed for *E dispar*, *E moshkovskii*, and *E bangladeshi*; and molecular diagnostic test capable of detecting *E histolytica*, *E dispar*, *E moshkovskii*, and *E bangladeshi* simultaneously in clinical samples. Next-generation sequencing of DNA from stool is needed to identify novel species of *Entamoeba*.

The coccidians *Cryptosporidium* spp, *Cyclospora cayetanensis*, and *Cystoisospora belli* and the flagellate *Giardia duodenalis* are pathogenic protozoa associated with gastrointestinal manifestations. Diagnosis relies heavily on microscopy, and although ova-and-parasite examinations can detect *Giardia* and *Cystoisospora, Cryptosporidium* and *Cyclospora* often require specific diagnostic requests. Approved non-microscopy methods are available for *Giardia* and *Cryptosporidium*, although negative results are frequently followed by microscopic assays. Polymerase chain reaction–based methods are not frequently used for diagnosis of *Giardia* and *Cryptosporidium* and have been used primarily for epidemiologic or outbreak investigations of *Giardia* and *Cryptosporidium*.

Infection by the ingested pathogens of microsporidia occur primarily in immunosuppressed patients (including untreated HIV/AIDS) and are diagnosed by stool examination, small bowel biopsy with special stains, or electron microscopy (for definitive speciation), or by various molecular techniques. Although electron microscopy has been the definitive diagnostic tool for speciation, genetic sequencing increasingly provides the definitive diagnosis for new species, such as *Anncaliia algerae*. Further genetic sequencing of the common pathogens may allow for the development of advanced molecular diagnostics providing high diagnostic sensitivity and throughput.

A wide range of enteric pathogens can cause infectious gastroenteritis. Conventional diagnostic algorithms are time-consuming and often lack sensitivity and specificity. Advances in molecular technology have provided new clinical diagnostic tools. Multiplex polymerase chain reaction (PCR)–based testing has been used in gastroenterology diagnostics in recent years. This article presents a review of recent laboratory-developed multiplex PCR tests and current commercial multiplex gastrointestinal pathogen tests. It focuses on two commercial syndromic multiplex tests: Luminex xTAG Gastrointestinal Pathogen Panel and BioFire FilmArray gastrointestinal test. Multiplex PCR tests have shown superior sensitivity to conventional methods for detection of most pathogens.

# Preface

# Diagnostic Testing for Enteric Pathogens

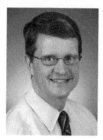

Alexander J. McAdam, MD, PhD
*Editor*

Enteric infections continue to be an important cause of morbidity and mortality worldwide. The suffering caused by these infections is greatest in the developing world, where gastrointestinal infections are thought to contribute to undernutrition in children and resulting deficits in cognitive and physical growth as well as childhood deaths.[1] Although the consequences are usually less severe in developed nations, the developed world is not spared from these infections. Foodborne illness associated with common pathogens is estimated to cause 9.4 million episodes of illness, including over 55,000 that require hospital admission and over a thousand deaths per year in the United States.[2] Traveler's diarrhea, often caused by enteric infections, occurs in 8% to 20% of travelers to some areas and causes a significant proportion of those travelers to change their plans.[3]

Diagnostic testing for pathogens that cause enteric infections is both important and interesting. The importance comes mainly from the utility of detecting a specific pathogen in guiding treatment, but these results are also useful for detection of outbreaks and other epidemiologic uses. This is an interesting area because of the clinical importance of the results, of course, but also because of the challenges of detecting pathogens in the background of abundant microbial flora found in stool and the range of methods and technologies used for this purpose. Microscopy (both conventional and electron), bacterial culture, immunoassays, and nucleic acid amplification tests all have important uses in testing for enteric pathogens and are discussed in this issue.

This issue includes articles on most of the major pathogens causing enteric infections as well as specialized articles on multiplex PCR tests, antibiotic susceptibility testing, and inflammatory markers. Each of the articles is meant to stand independently because many readers will pick and choose among them as suits their purpose. Since each article is comprehensive, there is a small amount of redundancy between the entries, but for those who read comprehensively, there is the opportunity to

Clin Lab Med 35 (2015) xi–xii
http://dx.doi.org/10.1016/j.cll.2015.03.002
0272-2712/15/$ – see front matter © 2015 Published by Elsevier Inc.

compare the opinions of multiple experts. I am very grateful to the authors for their excellent work and also to the editorial staff who have provided invaluable help in preparing this issue. I hope you will enjoy reading these articles as much as I have, and I am certain that you will find them very useful.

Alexander J. McAdam, MD, PhD
Department of Laboratory Medicine
Boston Children's Hospital
300 Longwood Avenue
Boston, MA 02115, USA

E-mail address:
alexander.mcadam@childrens.harvard.edu

### REFERENCES

1. MAL-ED Network Investigators. The MAL-ED study: a multinational and multidisciplinary approach to understand the relationship between enteric pathogens, malnutrition, gut physiology, physical growth, cognitive development, and immune responses in infants and children up to 2 years of age in resource-poor environments. Clin Infect Dis 2014;59(Suppl 4):S193–206.
2. Scallan E, Hoekstra RM, Angulo FJ, et al. Foodborne illness acquired in the United States—major pathogens. Emerg Infect Dis 2011;17(1):7–15.
3. Steffen R, Hill DR, DuPont HL. Traveler's diarrhea: a clinical review. JAMA 2015; 313(1):71–80.

# Salmonella, Shigella, and Yersinia

John P. Dekker, MD, PhD, Karen M. Frank, MD, PhD, D(ABMM)*

## KEYWORDS

• *Salmonella* • *Shigella* • *Yersinia* • Enteric • Gram-negative bacilli • Gastroenteritis

## KEY POINTS

- The global disease burden from *Salmonella/Shigella/Yersinia*, organisms reportable to public health departments, is quite high, with significant but fewer infections in the developed world.
- Although there is a broad spectrum of disease associated with these pathogens, infections are self-limiting in most cases. Antimicrobial therapy is ordinarily indicated only for severe gastrointestinal and systemic disease.
- Inactive strains of *Escherichia coli* can be difficult to distinguish from *Shigella* strains, using multiple laboratory methods.
- Molecular methods such as polymerase chain reaction and mass spectrometry are being used more routinely for identification of these organisms, but both methods have limitations.
- There is active investigation in the areas of vaccine development and characterization of virulence mechanisms.

## INTRODUCTION

In this review, the authors discuss 3 enteric pathogens: *Salmonella*, *Shigella*, and *Yersinia*. These important members of *Enterobacteriaceae* are responsible for significant morbidity and mortality, causing diarrhea and a spectrum of associated symptoms from mild to severe in most parts of the world. In this review, the authors cover infection and epidemiology; taxonomic classification; collection, transport, and storage of specimens; culture techniques; molecular detection methods; susceptibility testing; and treatment. Discussions that pertain to individual organisms are organized into individual sections starting with *Salmonella*, followed by *Shigella* and then *Yersinia*.

This work was supported by the intramural research program, NIH. The views expressed are those of the authors and do not necessarily reflect those of NIH or HHS.
Department of Laboratory Medicine, Clinical Center, National Institutes of Health, 10 Center Drive, MSC 1508, Bethesda, MD 20892-1508, USA
* Corresponding author.
*E-mail address:* karen.frank@nih.gov

Topics common to all 3 (such as collection, transport and storage of specimens, and molecular multiplex methods of detection) are discussed as they first occur, denoted as such in paragraph headings. Throughout, priority of discussion is placed on newer techniques and data, with less emphasis on details of classic methods available in reference textbooks.

### Salmonella Introduction

Members of the genus *Salmonella* cause a well-characterized spectrum of disease in humans, ranging from asymptomatic carriage to fatal typhoidal fever. In the developed world, food-borne acute gastroenteritis and enterocolitis are the most common forms of *Salmonella* infection, with an estimated 1.2 million annual cases of nontyphoidal Salmonellosis occurring in the United States.[1–3] Although relatively uncommon in the United States, typhoid, paratyphoid, and enteric fever constitute a very serious global public health problem, with 25 million new infections and greater than 200,000 deaths occurring annually.[4,5]

*Salmonella* is a member of the *Enterobacteriaceae*, originally characterized by the ability to metabolize citrate as a sole carbon source and lysine as a nitrogen source as well as the ability to produce hydrogen sulfide.[6] However, classic biochemical testing alone does not unambiguously distinguish key pathogenic members of this genus, and modern classification relies instead on serology and increasingly on molecular methods.

### Salmonella Disease Manifestations

Infection with *Salmonella* typically follows 2 very different disease courses, depending on whether the infecting *Salmonella* strain is a typhoidal or nontyphoidal serovar. Infection with nontyphoidal serovars ordinarily presents as diarrhea associated with fever and abdominal cramping 12 to 72 hours after infection.[7] In most cases in healthy individuals, this infection runs a self-limited course over 4 to 7 days; but, in susceptible hosts, certain nontyphoidal strains of *Salmonella* may spread systemically to other sites in the body. Although this is more common in those with compromised immune systems or underlying medical conditions (eg, sickle cell anemia), systemic spread of nontyphoidal *Salmonella* strains may also be seen in otherwise healthy individuals.

In contrast to infection with nontyphoidal *Salmonella*, infection with typhoidal strains (primarily serovars Typhi and Paratyphi) presents as a systemic, often serious, disease. After invading through intestinal mucosa, typhoidal strains disseminate through a transient primary bacteremia that may occur without diarrhea.[5] Following hematogenous dissemination, some individuals will develop typhoid fever, which involves high temperature (>39°C), vomiting, and headache, sometimes with complications that include neurologic involvement, intestinal perforation, and death.[5]

### Salmonella Taxonomic Classification

The classification of the salmonellae has a complicated history, resulting in part from multiple independent investigators using phenotypic, serologic, and genotypic methods to characterize phylogenetic relationships within the genus and in part from disagreements on nomenclature. The most recent consensus defines a classification scheme that recognizes 2 principal species of *Salmonella*: *S enterica* and *S bongori* (**Fig. 1**). In this scheme, *S enterica* is further classified into 6 subspecies: subspecies I or *S enterica* subsp *enterica*; subspecies II or *S enterica* subsp *salamae*; subspecies IIIa or *S enterica* subsp *arizonae*; subspecies IIIb or *S enterica* subsp *diarizonae*; subspecies IV or *S enterica* subsp *houtenae*; and subspecies VI or *S enterica* subsp *indica*.[8–10] Recent sequence analysis has shed light on the genetic

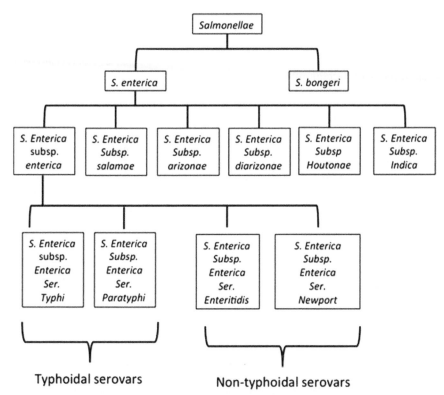

**Fig. 1.** Relationships within the *Salmonella* genus, including species, subspecies, and serovar designations, are illustrated. Note that serovars do not have official taxonomic status. Four representative serovars are shown for *S enterica* subsp *enterica*. Only the most common typhoidal serovars and representative nontyphoidal serovars are shown. There are greater than 2500 serovars in total, with the most common disease-causing serovars belonging to *S enterica* subsp *Enterica*.

relationships within this genus and has largely supported the aforementioned classification scheme.[4,11–20]

The 7 principal members of the *Salmonella* genus can be further subtyped by serologic methods, based on 3 antigens: O, H, and Vi. The serologic typing scheme identifies greater than 2500 serovars.[21] The resolution provided by serologic typing methods has proved valuable to epidemiologic tracking of isolates in outbreaks. Given that *S enterica* subsp *enterica* strains constitute most (as much as 99.5%) of the isolates cultured from humans and other warm-blooded animals, it is perhaps not surprising that most disease-causing serovars belong to this subspecies.[6,21] In contrast, *S bongori* and the other members of *S enterica* are more commonly isolated from cold-blooded animals and environmental sources; salmonellosis caused by serovars representing these other species is relatively rare, though infections do occur.

### Collection, Transport, and Storage of Specimens for Detection of Salmonella/Shigella/Yersinia

For laboratory diagnosis in cases of gastrointestinal (GI) disease, fecal specimens should be collected at the early stages of illness, ideally before antibiotics have been initiated.[6,22] Whole stools are the preferred specimen for culture, and examination of multiple specimens may improve the recovery of *Salmonella/Shigella/Yersinia*.[23] Consultation with the laboratory may be required where specimen rejection rules do not allow for serial cultures. Most commonly used pH-buffered stool transport media are compatible with recovery of *Salmonella/Shigella/Yersinia*, though Cary-Blair transport medium is preferred by many laboratories because of its compatibility with other common stool pathogens.[6,22]

Fecal specimens should be examined immediately on receipt or stored at 4°C if plating for culture or inoculation of broth will be delayed for greater than 1 to 2 hours following collection.[6,22] However, it should be noted that refrigeration of specimens containing *Shigella* in non–pH–buffered transport media may decrease recovery in culture.[22] In cases of suspected systemic spread, as with typhoidal *Salmonella*, cultures from other sources (blood, bone marrow, lymph node, and bone biopsy) that may be submitted should be collected and transported according to standard procedures appropriate to these specimen types.

### Salmonella Culture and Isolation

Stool culture is the most common source from which nontyphoidal serovars of *Salmonella* are recovered. Nontyphoidal strains of *Salmonella* may also be recovered from blood and tissue (lymph node, bone marrow, and so forth) in cases with systemic spread. Typhoidal strains may be more easily isolated from cultures of extraintestinal sites than from fecal cultures.[6]

*Salmonella* may be cultured on a variety of solid media. Typically, 2 selective and differential media, one of which is highly selective, are inoculated with the stool specimen. Hektoen and xylose-lysine-deoxycholate agars are highly selective and both detect hydrogen sulfide production, facilitating identification of *Salmonella* species. More highly selective agars, including Salmonella-Shigella, bismuth sulfite, and brilliant green agars may inhibit some strains of *Salmonella* sp, and thus are often used in combination with a less selective agar.[22] For this reason, a less selective differential enteric medium, such as MacConkey or eosin methylene blue, and a nonselective medium, such as 5% sheep blood agar may be inoculated in addition as part of the stool culture work up, depending on laboratory preference.[22] However, the growth of fecal flora on nonselective agars may obscure *Salmonella* colonies that are present in low numbers.

Stool may be inoculated into enrichment broths in addition to plated cultures. Enrichment broths serve to allow the growth of *Salmonella* while suppressing the growth of normal fecal flora and, thereby, improve the recovery yield. Two commonly used enrichment broths are tetrathionate broth and selenite broth.[22] Once isolated, *Salmonella* should be subcultured using standard techniques to obtain colonies for identification and susceptibility testing (if indicated) as well as for submission to the local public health laboratory.

### Identification Methods for Salmonella

Once *Salmonella* has been isolated in culture, there are a variety of methods available for identification and classification.[6] Definitive identification ordinarily relies on a combination of phenotypic and serologic methods. The widely used Kauffmann-White serologic typing scheme is based on the lipopolysaccharide O antigen, the H1 and H2 flagellar antigens, and the Vi antigen.[21] Although the O and H1 antigens are detectable in almost all strains of *Salmonella*, the H2 antigens are present only in certain strains, and the Vi antigen is found predominantly in typhoidal strains.[6] It should be noted that Vi, though useful for detection of serovar Typhi, may also be expressed in *Citrobacter* sp; therefore, the Vi antigen alone cannot be used for definitive identification.[6]

Serologic typing by the Kauffmann-White scheme yields greater than 2500 serovars, which may be designated by antigenic formulae expressed with the following convention: O antigen(s), Vi antigen if present: phase 1 H antigens(s):phase 2 H antigen(s) if present.[6,21] In the Kauffman-White scheme, the more than 1500 serovars from *S enterica* subsp *enterica* receive names; those from the other subspecies of *S enterica* and *S bongori* are referred to only by formulae.[21] By convention, serovar names are capitalized and not italicized; it is not necessary to include the *enterica* subspecies designation when referring to the serovar, as only subspecies *enterica* serovars are named. Thus both *S enterica* subsp *enterica* ser Enteritidis and *S enterica* ser Enteritidis are correct designations.[21] It is important to note that serovars do not have taxonomic status and should not be confused with species or subspecies of *Salmonella*.

As stated earlier, most of the identified serovars and most human pathogens belong to *S enterica* subsp *enterica*. Some serovars, such as Typhi and Paratyphi, are largely restricted to humans. Other serovars are generally restricted to particular zoonotic reservoirs and only occasionally cause human infection. However, infections caused by these serovars may be severe with systemic spread. These species include Derby and Choleraesuis (pig adapted), Saintpaul (poultry adapted), and Dublin (bovine adapted).[6] Yet other serovars, particularly Typhimurium and Enteritidis, pass between human and zoonotic reservoirs with ease, perhaps accounting for their high prevalence. The Centers for Disease Control and Prevention (CDC) survey data from 2011 suggests that the 3 most commonly reported serovars in the United States during the reporting period were Enteritidis, Typhimurium, and Newport.[24] Nontyphoidal salmonellosis was traditionally associated with meat and poultry products; but more recently, outbreaks have been caused increasingly by produce.[1–3]

Several techniques now exist for screening of primary specimens and enrichment broths before isolated colonies are available for the aforementioned methods. Selenite enrichment broth cultures may be screened by the Wellcolex Color *Salmonella* (Remel Inc, Lenexa, KS), a serologic agglutination-based method.[25] There are important limitations in sensitivity and specificity that one must be aware of with the Wellcolex test; in particular, expression of Vi antigen in *Citrobacter* sp and may lead to false positives with this assay, and not all *Salmonella* sp are identified by this test.[26]

### Antimicrobial Susceptibility Testing for Salmonella

The current guidelines from the Clinical Laboratory Standards Institute (CLSI)[27] state that routine susceptibility testing is indicated for typhoidal *Salmonella* serovars (Typhi and Paratyphi A–C) from all sites and for nontyphoidal serovars from extraintestinal sites. Fecal isolates should be tested for susceptibility to ampicillin, a fluoroquinolone, and trimethoprim-sulfamethoxazole. For extraintestinal isolates of *Salmonella*, a third-generation cephalosporin should be tested and reported additionally; chloramphenicol may be tested and reported if requested. It should be noted that first- and second-generation cephalosporins, cephamycins, and aminoglycosides may seem active in vitro against *Salmonella* but are not effective clinically and should not be reported as susceptible.[27]

The current CLSI breakpoints for ciprofloxacin and levofloxacin for *Salmonella* are less than for other *Enterobacteriaceae*.[27] The CLSI recommends that laboratories unable to implement the current (lowered) minimal inhibitory concentration breakpoints for fluoroquinolone testing should use nalidixic acid to test for reduced fluoroquinolone susceptibility. Strains resistant to nalidixic acid may be associated with clinical fluoroquinolone failures. *Salmonella* strains producing extended spectrum beta-lactamases and New Dehli metallo-beta-lactamase-1–type carbapenemases have been reported, as well as S enterica ser Typhi isolates with chromosomally integrated multidrug resistance islands.[28–30] It is, therefore, important for the laboratory and clinicians to be aware of the possibility of multidrug- and carbapenem-resistant isolates.

### Identification of Salmonella/Shigella/Yersinia by Mass Spectrometry

Molecular methods, including mass spectrometry and polymerase chain reaction (PCR)–based multiplex panels have been developed for the detection of enteric bacteria, and some laboratories are beginning to incorporate these techniques. These newer methods have the potential to improve our ability to provide rapid and accurate bacterial identification, but they have limitations that are important to understand. Commercial matrix-assisted laser desorption ionization–time-of-flight mass spectrometry (MALDI-TOF MS) instruments can provide rapid identifications of Salmonella and Yersinia and limited identification of Shigella.[31,32] Both the Biotyper (Bruker Daltonics, Inc., Billerica, MA, USA) and Vitek MALDI-TOF MS (bioMerieux, Inc., Durham, NC, USA) systems are approved by the Food and Drug Administration (FDA) for in vitro diagnostic use to identify cultured isolates of Y enterocolitica and Y pseudotuberculosis (species-level identification) and Salmonella (genus-level identification) but not Shigella. The Biomerieux Vitex MS system carries a manufacturer's note that confirmatory testing is recommended when identifications of Salmonella are made. Neither system is FDA approved for species-level or serovar-level classifications of Salmonella. However, recent literature suggests that MALDI-TOF mass spectrometry-based systems may have the power to distinguish among subspecies and some Salmonella serovars.[33] As this technology is new and experience is still relatively limited, caution is appropriate, as illustrated by a recent report of a patient with both bacteremia and GI symptoms for whom an isolate of Y pseudotuberculosis was misidentified as Y pestis using a MALDI-TOF MS method. This finding highlights the need for comprehensive MALDI-TOF MS spectral databases in combination with careful validations and appropriate additional confirmatory testing for this group of less commonly seen bacteria.[34]

Pulsed-field gel electrophoresis (PFGE) has been used extensively for epidemiologic typing of strains of Salmonella. Recently, a variety of molecular methods have been developed for distinguishing among strains of Salmonella/Shigella/Yersinia, including multi-locus sequence typing approaches, and PCR-based approaches.[35–42] Whole-genome sequencing–based approaches have also been used, facilitated by published reference genomes.[13,14,43–45]

### Polymerase Chain Reaction–Based Molecular Methods to Detect Salmonella/Shigella/Yersinia

Recently, several PCR-based multiplex GI pathogen identification panels have been marketed for use with primary stool specimens. These panels include the Filmarray system (bioFire Diagnostics, Inc., Salt Lake City, UT, USA),[46] BD MAX system (Becton, Dickinson & Co., Franklin Lakes, NJ, USA),[47] xTAG system (Luminex, Austin, TX, USA),[48,49] Gastrointestinal Infection Panel (Savyon Diagnostics, Ashdod, Israel),[48] and EasyScreen system (Genetic Signatures, Darlinghurst, Australia).[50] These panels allow rapid identification of Salmonella, Shigella, and Yersinia from primary stool specimens and offer substantially improved turnaround time on primary laboratory diagnosis compared with culture-based methods. Recovery of isolates from culture is still required for taxonomic classification and susceptibility testing. It should be noted that none of the commercially available multiplex PCR panels include Y pseudotuberculosis in the target list.

Although experience with these new panels is still relatively limited, several recent publications have begun to shed light on their performance. Wessels and colleagues[51] found that in comparison with conventional diagnostic methods, the Luminex xTAG panel reported almost twice as many pathogen identifications. However, not all of these positive results were confirmed by independent PCR assays, including one *Shigella* sp and 4 *Salmonella* sp out of a total of 83 positives reported by the instrument. The investigators, therefore, recommended that confirmatory testing be performed before reporting *Salmonella* with this method. A study of Luminex xTAG analyte specific reagents demonstrated sensitivity for *Salmonella* of 92% and for *Shigella* of 93%.[52] Conclusions regarding the sensitivity of this assay for detecting *Yersinia* sp were limited by the inclusion of only 3 isolates.[52] A study comparing the Biofire FilmArray and Luminex xTAG systems demonstrated a higher positivity rate with both assays compared with routine methods; however, presumed false positives were observed, consistent with other studies.[46] The EasyScreen system (Genetic Signatures, Darlinghurst, Australia) tested in Australia showed very good correlation of results between conventional and molecular methods for *Salmonella*, but evaluation of performance for the detection of *Shigella* and *Yersinia* was limited by the small numbers of isolates of these genera included in the study.[50] Adequate validation of these multiplexed panels can be quite difficult because of the number of pathogens that must be tested and the need to verify all presumed false positives with another equivalently sensitive method. Significant testing and experience should be accumulated before a laboratory considers replacing traditional methods with a single molecular method.

Another approach under investigation is PCR electrospray ionization MS (PCR-ESI-MS). Pierce and colleagues[53] evaluated a PCR-ESI-MS–based assay for testing of enteric pathogens in food samples that used broad-range oligonucleotide primers targeted to highly conserved regions in the genomes of target organisms. *Salmonella* was detected in samples tested by this method with high sensitivity, but *Shigella* was detected in only 81% of cases. As with MALDI-TOF MS–based methods, PCR-ESI-MS–based assays depend very much on the completeness of the database. In this study, identification of bacteria from food samples required the use of selective enrichment media and additional incubation time. Further work is needed to incorporate this method into routine use by food safety investigators.[53]

### *Shigella Epidemiology, Disease Manifestations, and Treatment*

Symptoms of *Shigella* infection include fever, malaise, watery diarrhea, cramping abdominal pain, and myalgia. The incubation period is 1 to 4 days, and the illness often resolves in 5 to 7 days. After 2 to 3 days, the volume and frequency of diarrhea may decrease to be replaced with blood and mucus in feces (dysentery), along with straining. Some individuals may not have symptoms but can still transmit the bacteria to others.[54] Although not as frequent as GI disease, there are multiple reports of bacteremia and other extraintestinal infections.[55–57] Complications of *Shigella* infection include hemolytic uremic syndrome and reactive arthritis.[58]

The worldwide incidence of shigellosis has been reported to be approximately 165 million cases, but the mortality has decreased substantially over the past 3 decades.[59–61] Although the causes of this decrease in shigellosis-associated mortality are likely to be multifactorial, it has occurred along with a decrease in prevalence of *S dysenteriae* type 1.[61] Infection with *S dysenteriae* type 1 carries relatively high mortality in the developing world, as demonstrated by the case fatality rate of 5% to 15% in Africa and Central America. There are an estimated 500,000 cases of shigellosis per year in the United States with 38 deaths.[62]

The only known natural reservoirs of *Shigella* are humans and large primates. Shigellosis is highly infectious, with a minimum inoculum of only 10 to 100 organisms required to cause disease.[63] Outbreaks often occur in the summer months. Transmission is through the fecal-oral route, with spread occurring person to person and through consumption of water or food contaminated with feces from infected individuals. Not surprisingly, shigellosis is seen more commonly under conditions that facilitate the spread of bacteria through the fecal-oral route, such as in daycare centers or in areas without indoor plumbing. Outbreaks have additionally been described among people in custodial institutions, orthodox Jews, international travelers, and men who have sex with men.[64–68] Asymptomatic infection is associated with the spread of disease and prolongation of outbreaks caused by silent transmission. Severe intestinal and extraintestinal manifestations can occur with all 4 species of *Shigella* but are most common with *S dysenteriae* type 1 partly because of the production of Shiga toxin.[69] Infections caused by *S dysenteriae* are often acquired by international travel and are often multidrug resistant.[70] Shigellosis caused by *S boydii* is uncommon and limited to the Indian subcontinent.[71] *S sonnei* is endemic in the United States and other developed countries. Infections associated with *S sonnei* tend to be mild or asymptomatic.

Antimicrobial therapy has been demonstrated to decrease the duration, transmission, and severity of symptoms. A decision to treat is based on the severity of symptoms and on the desire to reduce spread, balanced against the goal to reduce the development of more resistant isolates. In the United States, shigellosis is reportable to state-level public health laboratories; *Shigella* resistance is tracked by the National Antimicrobial Resistance Monitoring System for Enteric Bacteria, a collaboration of multiple US government agencies.

### Shigella Laboratory Identification

*Shigella*, a member of the *Enterobacteriaceae* family, is classified into 4 serologic subgroups: *S dysenteriae* (group A), *S flexneri* (group B), *S boydii* (group C), and *S sonnei* (group D). Although many investigators have treated these subgroups of *Shigella* as distinct taxonomic species, *Escherichia coli* and *Shigella* are very similar genetically (80%–90%); and the argument has been made that almost all *Shigella* strains could be considered a biotype of *E coli*.[72] *S boydii* 13 is the exception and has been reclassified as *Escherichia albertii*.[73,74] Because of their substantial genetic similarity, distinguishing *Shigella* from *E coli* often presents a challenge for the clinical microbiology laboratory. However, though they are genetically similar, *Shigella* and non-Shiga toxin-producing strains of *E coli* demonstrate different clinical behavior; their distinction in the microbiology laboratory facilitates their continued epidemiologic tracking as distinct entities.

To optimize the detection of *Shigella* in stool, samples should be plated on MacConkey and xylose-lysine-deoxycholate, Hektoen enteric, or deoxycholate citrate agar. Colonies are bluish-green on Hektoen agar and do not have the black center seen with *Salmonella*, as *Shigella* do not produce hydrogen sulfide. *Shigella* do not ferment lactose and xylose and are relatively inert biochemically. Some strains of *S sonnei* are exceptions and may ferment lactose. Most isolates do not produce gas, except some *S flexneri*.[6,75] Appropriate colonies can be characterized further using Kligler iron or triple sugar iron agar. Lysine decarboxylase tests are typically negative for *Shigella*. Groups A, B, and C have similar biochemical characteristics; but *S sonnei* has ornithine decarboxylase activity and beta-galactosidase activity.[75]

Serologic typing should be performed on *Shigella* isolates. Subgroup A (*S dysenteriae*) has 17 serotypes; subgroup B (*S flexneri*) has 14 serotypes further divided into subserotypes; subgroup C (*S boydii*) has 19 serotypes; and subgroup D (*S sonnei*) is a single serotype.[76,77] Confirmation of identification and serotype should be performed at a reference laboratory or public health laboratory for isolates from extraintestinal infections or when the primary laboratory does not have full serotyping capabilities. Enteroinvasive *E coli* (EIEC) are evolutionary intermediates between *E coli* and *Shigella*.[78] Some of the EIEC may cross-react with *Shigella* antisera. It should be noted that serologic testing of the serum of an infected individual is generally not useful for diagnosis.

Active or typical *E coli* strains can be distinguished from *Shigella* by several tests, including lysine decarboxylase, motility, gas production, acetate utilization, and mucate and lactose fermentation. However, inactive strains of *E coli* can have overlapping reactions with *Shigella*. Inactive strains of *E coli* that are nonmotile, anaerogenic biotypes are called Alkalescens-Dispar bioserotypes. In order to address this issue, different laboratories have developed different algorithms for the work-up of *E coli* and *Shigella* in stool specimens; however, many laboratories do not use procedures to distinguish *E coli* from *Shigella* when isolated from other body sites.

Given that *E coli* is a much more common isolate to recover from most sterile site cultures than *Shigella*, and given that many laboratories restrict procedures to distinguish *Shigella* from *E coli* to stool specimens, a *Shigella* occurring in a sterile site specimen may be misidentified as an *E coli*. This scenario is especially likely if identification depends on an automated system, as commercial systems, such as the Vitek 2 (bioMerieux, Inc., Durham, NC, USA), have a high rate of misidentification.[79] There are several reports examining API20E strips (bioMerieux Inc., Durham, NC, USA) for the identification of *Shigella*, with varying reports of accuracy.[80–83] If a *Shigella* isolate from an extraintestinal site were misidentified as an *E coli*, the reflex susceptibility performed and reported would be that appropriate for an *E coli* isolate. However, the CLSI guidelines differ for the two organisms, with first- and second-generation cephalosporins, cephamycins, and aminoglycosides excluded from testing for *Shigella* isolates, as false in vitro susceptibility my occur.[27] As a consequence, a *Shigella* misidentified from a site such as blood could mistakenly be treated with an ineffective agent (eg, aminoglycoside), with possible clinical failure. Furthermore, such a case could be missed in the tracking of *Shigella* incidence, unless *Shigella* was isolated from a concurrent stool specimen. An algorithm to distinguish *E coli* and *Shigella* is presented in **Fig. 2**.[72]

Given the long-standing difficulty in distinguishing *Shigella* from *E coli*, some newer methods have been evaluated. Khot and Fisher[84] applied ClinProTools software (Bruker Daltonics, Inc., Billerica, MA, USA) to develop an algorithm to distinguish *Shigella* from *E coli* using MALDI-TOF MS. The 3% rate of misidentification these investigators achieved is better than that seen with automated biochemical instruments. However, given the still significant error rate, such an approach does not obviate traditional biochemical approaches.[84]

Guidelines have been written to test all stool of all patients with acute, community-acquired diarrhea for Shiga-toxin producing *E coli*, because selective testing strategies, such as testing only bloody stool, or stool from children, or during summer months, fail to detect all positive samples.[85] Because of the low prevalence, not all hospitals have chosen to test all such stool samples. The Shiga toxin produced by *S dysenteriae* type 1 is very similar to the Shiga toxin 1 produced by some enterohemorrhagic *E coli*, so some rapid assays may detect the toxin from either *E coli* or this specific *Shigella* species.[86–88] *Shigella*s that do not produce the toxin should not be detected with those assays. It should be noted that Shiga toxin-encoding genes

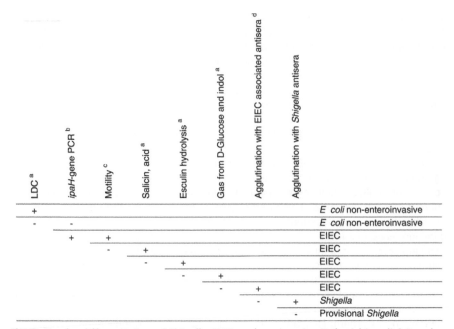

**Fig. 2.** Key for differentiation of *Shigella*, EIEC, and noninvasive *Escherichia coli*. [a] Based on *Edwards and Ewing's Identification of Enterobacteriaceae*. 4th edition. 1986 and/or *Cowan and Steel's Manual for the Identification of Medical Bacteria*. 3rd edition. 1993. [b] Performed with a standard PCR protocol, with primers designed to amplify a part of the conserved region of $ipaH_{7,8}$, as described by Buysse and colleagues. Microb Pathog. 19(5):335–49. [c] Incubated for 24 hours in brain heart infusion-medium at 37°C. [d] Known O:H serotypes of EIEC according to *Bergey's Manual of Systematic Bacteriology*. 2nd edition. volume 2. The *Proteobacteria*, Part B The *Gammaproteobacteria*. LDC, lysine decarboxylase. (*From* van den Beld MJ, Reubsaet FA. Differentiation between Shigella, enteroinvasive Escherichia coli (EIEC) and noninvasive Escherichia coli. Eur J Clin Microbiol Infect Dis 2012;31(6):902; with permission.)

can be detected in healthy volunteers by PCR of fecal samples, so correlation with clinical symptoms and culture of an isolate are essential for diagnosis when using this type of molecular assay.[89]

## Shigella Susceptibility Testing

*Shigella* isolates should be tested against ampicillin, a fluoroquinolone, and trimethoprim-sulfamethoxazole.[27] There is significant resistance to ampicillin and trimethoprim-sulfamethoxazole.[68,90] In Asia, resistance has been reported to ciprofloxacin, pivmecillinam, and azithromycin, with some emerging resistance to third-generation cephalosporins and additional drugs.[91–96] A recent report from studies in Bangladesh shows an increase in resistance to ciprofloxacin from 0% in 2004% to 44% in 2010.[97]

## Shigella Virulence Mechanism

*Shigella* pathogenesis involves translocation through ileal and colonic M cells, uptake by macrophages, basolateral invasion of epithelial cells, and dissemination within the mucosa.[98,99] *Shigella* has a large virulence plasmid, encoding a type III–secretion system and a set of secreted proteins. The system results in the injection of virulence factors into host colonic epithelial cells, leading to damage to the epithelial lining as well as proteins that antagonize the adaptive and innate immune response.[98,100] *Shigella* virulence is enhanced by the presence of enterotoxins, which is separate from the Shiga toxin produced in limited strains.[101] The genes encoding the Shiga toxin genes are located in the genome of heterogeneous lambdoid prophages. These are highly mobile genetic elements that play a role in horizontal gene transfer and genome diversification.[102] Shiga toxin is made by the *Shigella dysenteriae* type I strains and *E coli* O157:H7 among other *E coli* Shiga toxin–producing strains. Shigalike toxin II, also seen in some *E coli* strains, is 56% homologous with Shiga toxin (or Shigalike toxin I).[103]

### Shigella Vaccine

The declining incidence of shigellosis with increasing age suggests that natural immunity develops, implying that vaccines eliciting this natural response may be effective. There is currently no licensed *Shigella* vaccine; but there are multiple vaccines that are in preclinical stages or clinical trials, including live attenuated, killed whole-cell, conjugate, and subunit vaccines.[104] Vaccines have been designed against the O antigens, and also conjugate vaccines have been developed using several different conserved antigenic molecules.[101] Data are limited regarding the immune parameter that correlates with protective immunity.[77] More studies are needed before we will know if a *Shigella* vaccine will prove effective (**Box 1**).

### Yersinia Epidemiology and Disease Manifestations

*Yersinia* are zoonotic agents distributed worldwide, and there are both pathogenic and nonpathogenic strains.[105] *Yersinia* species associated with human disease include *Y pseudotuberculosis*, *Y enterocolitica*, and *Y pestis*. Of these clinically significant species, the authors only discuss *Y enterocolitica* and *Y pseudotuberculosis*, as this review is focused on enteric pathogens. Disease caused by *Y enterocolitica* manifests as terminal ileitis, lymphadenitis, and acute enterocolitis caused by ingestion of contaminated food or water. Symptoms typically develop 4 to 7 days after exposure and may last 1 to 3 weeks. Complications include skin rash, joint pains, and bacteremia.[106] Right-sided abdominal pain in some cases of *Y enterocolitica* infection may be confused with appendicitis. Illness may include erythema nodosum, polyarthritis, and less commonly septicemia or endocarditis.[107–110] Reactive arthritis is an uncommon complication but may be seen especially in immunocompromised patients and those with the HLA-B27 allele. Associated disorders also include inflammatory

---

**Box 1**
**Barriers to development of a *Shigella* vaccine**

- We have a limited understanding of protective immunity for *Shigella*.
- There are many serotypes of *Shigella*.
- There is a lack of an adequate animal model.
- There are concerns of producing reactive arthritis in vaccine trial recipients.
- There are concerns of gastrointestinal tract side effects or chronic conditions.
- There are challenges in the manufacturing process.
- Some individuals promote funding for clean water and sanitation over vaccine studies.

*Adapted from* Barry EM, Pasetti MF, Sztein MB, et al. Progress and pitfalls in Shigella vaccine research. Nat Rev Gastroenterol Hepatol 2013;10(4):246; with permission.

bowel disease and autoimmune thyroid disorders. Iron overload caused by underlying conditions, such as hereditary hemochromatosis or beta thalassemia, or treatment with deferoxamine, leads to an increased susceptibility to septicemia manifestations.[105,111]

Infections with *Y enterocolitica* are more common in the winter months and often seen in young children. There is one culture-confirmed case of *Y enterocolitica* per 100,000 individuals each year in the United States. The CDC tracks foodborne disease with the surveillance network FoodNet. The source of infection can include contaminated prepackaged deli meats, undercooked pork, unpasteurized milk, or untreated water. Preparation of chitterlings (large intestines of pigs), a dish for holiday meals, has been associated with multiple cases of infection in infants because of caregivers handling the contaminated food.[112–117] This organism is able to multiply at refrigerated temperatures, contributing to its role in food products and transfusion-related infections (**Box 2**).[118]

*Y pseudotuberculosis* is endemic in a variety of animals, including fowl. *Y pseudotuberculosis* usually produces a self-limited disease. The infection can manifest as mesenteric lymphadenitis and may also be confused with appendicitis.[119] Septicemic illness is rare and, if seen, would most likely occur in someone with underlying disorders that increase susceptibility to severe infection.[120–122] *Y pseudotuberculosis* has been reported as a foodborne pathogen.[123,124]

### Yersinia Laboratory Identification

*Yersinia* is a gram-negative bacillus in the Enterobacteriaceae family. There are 11 species of *Yersinia*, but only 3 are clearly human pathogens.[75] Genome sequencing reveals that *Y pestis* and *Y pseudotuberculosis* are closely related but significantly different than *Y enterocolitica*.[125] *Yersinia* can appear small and coccobacillary in gram-stained smears. It exhibits bipolar staining described as a safety pin shape on Giemsa staining. *Yersinia* grow on blood, chocolate, and MacConkey agar but may be overgrown by other organisms because of slow growth. *Yersinia* can form pinpoint colonies on both blood agar and MacConkey agar in 24 hours, particularly *Y pseudotuberculosis*. *Yersinia* are catalase positive, oxidase negative, and ferment glucose. *Yersinia* species have an alkaline over acid pattern on Kligler iron agar and are nonmotile at 36°C but motile at 22°C. Optimal growth is observed at 25°C to 32°C. Longer incubation reveals grey-white, 1- to 2-mm, convex colonies. *Y enterocolitica* appears

---

**Box 2**
**Prevention of *Yersinia* infections**

- Avoid raw or undercooked pork.
- Avoid unpasteurized milk and milk products.
- Wash hands with soap and water before preparing food or eating and after contact with animals or raw meat.
- Avoid contact with young children while preparing raw chitterlings.
- Clean all kitchen boards and utensils after preparing raw meat.
- Dispose of animal feces in a sanitary manner.

*From* Yersinia. National Center for Emerging and Zoonotic Infectious Diseases. Centers for Disease Control and Prevention (CDC). Available at: http://www.cdc.gov/nczved/divisions/dfbmd/diseases/yersinia/. Accessed November 22, 2014.

as small, lactose-negative colonies on MacConkey in 48 hours. Selective media, such as cefsulodin-irgasan-novobiocin (CIN), and incubation at lower temperatures can enhance detection. Colonies appear as a bull's eye with a red center on CIN agar, although some other bacteria will also give this appearance. Use of eosin methylene blue agar and triple-sugar iron agar may not result in a clear distinction from other co-liforms. *Y enterocolitica* incubated at room temperature will be more biochemically active; better identification at this temperature may be obtained with some systems, such as the API 20E (bioMerieux Inc., Durham, NC, USA), because commercial systems, such as Vitek 2 (bioMerieux Inc., Durham, NC, USA), may fail to identify these organisms under routine conditions.[126,127]

*Y pseudotuberculosis* is a pleomorphic gram-negative bacillus that can grow at temperatures ranging from 4°C to 43°C, with optimal temperatures between 25°C and 28°C.[128] Enteric *Yersinia* species can be distinguished biochemically; ornithine decarboxylase, sucrose, and sorbitol are all positive for *Y enterocolitica* and negative for *Y pseudotuberculosis*. Enzyme-linked immunosorbent assays and lateral-flow assays exist but are not commonly used for routine laboratory tests, instead being used primarily in research.

### Yersinia Serogroups

Of the 6 biovars of *Y enterocolitica* (1A, 1B, 2, 3, 4), 5 are pathogenic for humans.[129] It has been proposed that biotype 1A strains may represent a potential group of emerging pathogens. They can be identified in clinical specimens, but clear association with human disease has not been established.[130] Serology has been used in investigations of plague infections caused by *Y pestis* in cases when an organism was not recovered in culture. However, serology for *Y enterocolitica* and *Y pseudotuberculosis* is somewhat limited by cross-reactions caused by infections with other bacterial species and human exposure to nonpathogenic *Yersinia* species.

### Yersinia Virulence

One virulence factors of *Yersinia* is yersiniabactin, a siderophore iron uptake system present in virulent *Yersinia*, including *Y pestis*, *Y pseudotuberculosis*, and *Y enterocolitica* biotype 1B. The genes involved in the biosynthesis, transport, and regulation of yersiniabactin are located on a mobile genetic element, the high-pathogenicity island. This mobile element has contributed to the horizontal spread of yersiniabactin genes into other Enterobacteriaceae. In addition, *Yersinia* species contain alternative iron siderophore scavenging systems, with some strains containing all 3 systems, yersiniabactin, pseudochelin, and yersiniachelin.[131]

*Y pseudotuberculosis* has a virulence plasmid, pYV, that carries a type III secretion system that forms a needle structure on the bacterial surface for the injection of *Yersinia* outer proteins (Yops) into target host cells. This system results in disruption of both the innate and adaptive immune response, inhibiting phagocytosis.[128]

### Yersinia Susceptibility Testing

Some *Y enterocolitica* have chromosomally encoded beta lactamases, conferring resistance to ampicillin, cephalothin, and carbenicillin. Treatment of *Y enterocolitica* may include an aminoglycoside, doxycycline, trimethoprim-sulfamethoxazole, a third-generation cephalosporin, or a fluoroquinolone.[106] There is significant resistance to fluoroquinolones in some regions caused by mutation of the DNA gyrase gyr A gene and efflux mechanisms.[132] *Y pseudotuberculosis* infections do not usually require treatment; but bacteremia may be treated with ampicillin, tetracycline, or streptomycin. The organism is usually susceptible to extended-spectrum cephalosporins, aminoglycosides, chloramphenicol, tetracycline, and trimethoprim-sulfamethoxazole.[133]

### Chronic Disease Associated with Salmonella/Shigella/Yersinia Infections

An examination of cases of gastroenteritis caused by *Salmonella*, *Campylobacter*, *Shigella*, or *Yersinia* in US military personnel led to a report of a higher incidence of chronic health sequelae than some previous reports.[134] Pathogen-specific increases were observed with associated increased risk of irritable bowel disease, dyspepsia, constipation, and gastroesophageal reflux disease, with a relative risk of 13.1 for inflammatory bowel disease following *Yersinia* infection. Three separate meta-analyses have shown a significantly increased risk of irritable bowel syndrome following gastroenteritis caused by *Shigella*.[135–137]

### SELF-ASSESSMENT

1. Which of the following statements is true regarding *Salmonella*?
   a. *S bongori* is a common cause of salmonellosis in humans.
   b. Typhus is caused by a serovar of *S enterica* subsp *Indica*.
   c. Serovars of *Salmonella* have official taxonomic status similar to the named *Salmonella* subspecies.
   d. Typhoidal strains of *Salmonella* are more likely to cause systemic disease than nontyphoidal strains.
   e. Unpasteurized milk products are the most common source of human *Salmonella* infection in the United States

2. Which of the following statements is true regarding *Shigella*?
   a. Diarrhea from *Shigella* infection is almost always bloody.
   b. All patients with *Shigella* infection should receive antibiotics promptly to avoid sequelae.
   c. The black-centered colony on Hektoen agar is characteristic for *Shigella*.
   d. Two of the 4 groups of *Shigella* species typically carry the Shiga toxin gene.
   e. Inactive strains of *E coli* are very difficult to distinguish from *Shigella* with multiple laboratory identification systems.

3. Which of the following statements is true regarding *Yersinia*?
   a. *Y pestis*, *Y enterocolitica*, and *Y pseudotuberculosis* all have equally similar genomes.
   b. It is common for patients with *Y enterocolitica* to have bacteremia as a complication.
   c. There is currently no role for MALDI-TOF MS in the identification of *Yersinia* because of the poor performance in published studies.
   d. There are multiple reports of chronic GI diseases as sequelae of *Yersinia* infections.
   e. There are 50 serotypes of *Yersinia* known to be pathogenic in humans.

ANSWERS
Answer 1. d
Answer 2. e
Answer 3. d

### REFERENCES

1. Patrick ME, Adcock PM, Gomez TM, et al. Salmonella enteritidis infections, United States, 1985–1999. Emerg Infect Dis 2004;10(1):1–7.

2. Braden CR. Salmonella enterica serotype Enteritidis and eggs: a national epidemic in the United States. Clin Infect Dis 2006;43(4):512–7.

3. Hanning IB, Nutt JD, Ricke SC. Salmonellosis outbreaks in the United States due to fresh produce: sources and potential intervention measures. Foodborne Pathog Dis 2009;6(6):635–48.

4. Holt KE, Thomson NR, Wain J, et al. Pseudogene accumulation in the evolutionary histories of Salmonella enterica serovars Paratyphi A and Typhi. BMC Genomics 2009;10:36.

5. Dougan G, Baker S. Salmonella enterica serovar Typhi and the pathogenesis of typhoid fever. Annu Rev Microbiol 2014;68:317–36.

6. Nataro JP, Bopp CA, Fields PI, et al. Escherichia, Shigella, and Salmonella. In: Versalovic J, Carroll KC, Funke G, et al, editors. Manual of clinical microbiology, vol. 1, 10th edition. Washington, DC: ASM Press; 2011. p. 603–26.

7. Available at: www.cdc.gov/salmonella/general/. Accessed November 22, 2014.

8. Le Minor L, Popoff MY. Designation of Salmonella enterica sp. nov., nom. rev., as the type and only species of the genus Salmonella. Int J Syst Bacteriol 1987; 37(4):465–8.

9. Euzeby JP. Revised Salmonella nomenclature: designation of Salmonella enterica (ex Kauffmann and Edwards 1952) Le Minor and Popoff 1987 sp. nov., nom. rev. as the neotype species of the genus Salmonella Lignieres 1900 (approved lists 1980), rejection of the name Salmonella choleraesuis (Smith 1894) Weldin 1927 (approved lists 1980), and conservation of the name Salmonella typhi (Schroeter 1886) Warren and Scott 1930 (approved lists 1980). Request for an opinion. Int J Syst Bacteriol 1999;49(Pt 2):927–30.

10. Tindall BJ, Grimont PA, Garrity GM, et al. Nomenclature and taxonomy of the genus Salmonella. Int J Syst Evol Microbiol 2005;55(Pt 1):521–4.

11. Reeves MW, Evins GM, Heiba AA, et al. Clonal nature of Salmonella typhi and its genetic relatedness to other salmonellae as shown by multilocus enzyme electrophoresis, and proposal of Salmonella bongori comb. nov. J Clin Microbiol 1989;27(2):313–20.

12. Edwards RA, Olsen GJ, Maloy SR. Comparative genomics of closely related salmonellae. Trends Microbiol 2002;10(2):94–9.

13. McClelland M, Sanderson KE, Spieth J, et al. Complete genome sequence of Salmonella enterica serovar Typhimurium LT2. Nature 2001;413(6858):852–6.

14. Parkhill J, Dougan G, James KD, et al. Complete genome sequence of a multiple drug resistant Salmonella enterica serovar Typhi CT18. Nature 2001; 413(6858):848–52.

15. Porwollik S, McClelland M. Lateral gene transfer in Salmonella. Microbes Infect 2003;5(11):977–89.

16. Chiu CH, Tang P, Chu C, et al. The genome sequence of Salmonella enterica serovar Choleraesuis, a highly invasive and resistant zoonotic pathogen. Nucleic Acids Res 2005;33(5):1690–8.

17. Baker S, Dougan G. The genome of Salmonella enterica serovar Typhi. Clin Infect Dis 2007;45(Suppl 1):S29–33.

18. Litrup E, Torpdahl M, Malorny B, et al. Association between phylogeny, virulence potential and serovars of Salmonella enterica. Infect Genet Evol 2010;10(7): 1132–9.

19. Lan R, Reeves PR, Octavia S. Population structure, origins and evolution of major Salmonella enterica clones. Infect Genet Evol 2009;9(5):996–1005.

20. Jacobsen A, Hendriksen RS, Aaresturp FM, et al. The Salmonella enterica pangenome. Microb Ecol 2011;62(3):487–504.

21. Grimont PA, Weill FX. Antigenic formulae of the Salmonella serovars. 9th edition. Paris, France: WHO Collaborating Centre for Reference and Research on Salmonella; 2007. p. 1–166.

22. Gilligan PH, Janda JM, Karmali MA, et al. Laboratory diagnosis of bacterial diarrhea. Cumitech 1992;12A:1–28.

23. Ethelberg S, Olsen KE, Gerner-Smidt P, et al. The significance of the number of submitted samples and patient-related factors for faecal bacterial diagnostics. Clin Microbiol Infect 2007;13(11):1095–9.

24. Available at: www.cdc.gov/ncezid/dfwed/pdfs/salmonella-annual-report-2011-508c.pdf. Accessed November 22, 2014.

25. Bouvet PJ, Jeanjean S. Evaluation of two colored latex kits, the Wellcolex Colour Salmonella Test and the Wellcolex Colour Shigella Test, for serological grouping of Salmonella and Shigella species. J Clin Microbiol 1992;30(8):2184–6.

26. Scientific T. Wellcolex Color Salmonella rapid latex agglutination test [Package Insert]. Available at: http://www.thermoscientific.com/en/product/wellcolex-color-salmonella-rapid-latex-agglutination-test-kit.html. Accessed November 22, 2014.

27. CLSI. M100-S24: Performance standards for antimicrobial susceptibility testing; twenty-fourth informational supplement. 2014; M100–S24.

28. Gonzalez-Lopez JJ, Piedra-Carrasco N, Salvador F, et al. ESBL-producing salmonella enterica serovar typhi in traveler returning from Guatemala to Spain. Emerg Infect Dis 2014;20(11):1918–20.

29. Irfan S, Khan E, Jabeen K, et al. Clinical isolates of Salmonella enterica serovar Agona producing NDM-1 metallo-beta-lactamase: first report from Pakistan. J Clin Microbiol 2015;53:346–8.

30. Chiou CS, Alam M, Kuo JC, et al. Chromosome-mediated multidrug resistance in Salmonella enterica serovar Typhi. Antimicrob Agents Chemother 2015;59: 721–3.

31. Deng J, Fu L, Wang R, et al. Comparison of MALDI-TOF MS, gene sequencing and the Vitek 2 for identification of seventy-three clinical isolates of enteropathogens. J Thorac Dis 2014;6(5):539–44.

32. Sparbier K, Weller U, Boogen C, et al. Rapid detection of Salmonella sp. by means of a combination of selective enrichment broth and MALDI-TOF MS. Eur J Clin Microbiol Infect Dis 2012;31(5):767–73.

33. Martiny D, Busson L, Wybo I, et al. Comparison of the Microflex LT and Vitek MS systems for routine identification of bacteria by matrix-assisted laser desorption ionization-time of flight mass spectrometry. J Clin Microbiol 2012;50(4): 1313–25.

34. Gerome P, Le Fleche P, Blouin Y, et al. Yersinia pseudotuberculosis ST42 (O:1) strain misidentified as Yersinia pestis by mass spectrometry analysis. Genome Announc 2014;2(3). pii:e00435-14.

35. Pugliese N, Circella E, Pazzani C, et al. Validation of a seminested PCR approach for rapid detection of Salmonella enterica subsp. enterica serovar Gallinarum. J Microbiol Methods 2011;85(1):22–7.

36. Akiba M, Kusumoto M, Iwata T. Rapid identification of Salmonella enterica serovars, typhimurium, choleraesuis, Infantis, Hadar, enteritidis, Dublin and Gallinarum, by multiplex PCR. J Microbiol Methods 2011;85(1):9–15.

37. Tankouo-Sandjong B, Sessitsch A, Liebana E, et al. MLST-v, multilocus sequence typing based on virulence genes, for molecular typing of Salmonella enterica subsp. enterica serovars. J Microbiol Methods 2007;69(1): 23–36.

38. Duan R, Liang J, Shi G, et al. Homology analysis of pathogenic Yersinia species Yersinia enterocolitica, Yersinia pseudotuberculosis, and Yersinia pestis based on multilocus sequence typing. J Clin Microbiol 2014;52(1):20–9.
39. Mallik S, Virdi JS. Genetic relationships between clinical and non-clinical strains of Yersinia enterocolitica biovar 1A as revealed by multilocus enzyme electrophoresis and multilocus restriction typing. BMC Microbiol 2010;10: 158.
40. Ruekit S, Wangchuk S, Dorji T, et al. Molecular characterization and PCR-based replicon typing of multidrug resistant Shigella sonnei isolates from an outbreak in Thimphu, Bhutan. BMC Res Notes 2014;7:95.
41. Voskresenskaya E, Savin C, Leclercq A, et al. Typing and clustering of Yersinia pseudotuberculosis isolates by restriction fragment length polymorphism analysis using insertion sequences. J Clin Microbiol 2014;52(6):1978–89.
42. Wang YW, Watanabe H, Phung DC, et al. Multilocus variable-number tandem repeat analysis for molecular typing and phylogenetic analysis of Shigella flexneri. BMC Microbiol 2009;9:278.
43. Deng X, Shariat N, Driebe EM, et al. Comparative analysis of subtyping methods against a whole genome sequencing standard in Salmonella enterica serotype Enteritidis. J Clin Microbiol 2014;53:212–8.
44. McDonnell J, Dallman T, Atkin S, et al. Retrospective analysis of whole genome sequencing compared to prospective typing data in further informing the epidemiological investigation of an outbreak of Shigella sonnei in the UK. Epidemiol Infect 2013;141(12):2568–75.
45. Sangal V, Holt KE, Yuan J, et al. Global phylogeny of Shigella sonnei strains from limited single nucleotide polymorphisms (SNPs) and devolopment of a rapid and cost-effective SNP-typing scheme for strain identification by high-resolution melting analysis. J Clin Microbiol 2013;51(1):303–5.
46. Khare R, Espy MJ, Cebelinski E, et al. Comparative evaluation of two commercial multiplex panels for detection of gastrointestinal pathogens by use of clinical stool specimens. J Clin Microbiol 2014;52(10):3667–73.
47. Anderson NW, Buchan BW, Ledeboer NA. Comparison of the BD MAX enteric bacterial panel to routine culture methods for detection of Campylobacter, enterohemorrhagic Escherichia coli (O157), Salmonella, and Shigella isolates in preserved stool specimens. J Clin Microbiol 2014;52(4):1222–4.
48. Perry MD, Corden SA, Howe RA. Evaluation of the Luminex xTAG Gastrointestinal Pathogen Panel and the Savyon Diagnostics Gastrointestinal Infection Panel for the detection of enteric pathogens in clinical samples. J Med Microbiol 2014;63(Pt 11):1419–26.
49. Dunbar SA, Ritchie VB, Hoffmeyer MR, et al. Luminex (R) multiplex bead suspension arrays for the detection and serotyping of Salmonella spp. Methods Mol Biol 2015;1225:1–27.
50. Siah SP, Merif J, Kaur K, et al. Improved detection of gastrointestinal pathogens using generalised sample processing and amplification panels. Pathology 2014;46(1):53–9.
51. Wessels E, Rusman LG, van Bussel MJ, et al. Added value of multiplex Luminex Gastrointestinal Pathogen Panel (xTAG (R) GPP) testing in the diagnosis of infectious gastroenteritis. Clin Microbiol Infect 2014;20(3):O182–7.
52. Navidad JF, Griswold DJ, Gradus MS, et al. Evaluation of Luminex xTAG gastrointestinal pathogen analyte-specific reagents for high-throughput, simultaneous detection of bacteria, viruses, and parasites of clinical and public health importance. J Clin Microbiol 2013;51(9):3018–24.

53. Pierce SE, Bell RL, Hellberg RS, et al. Detection and identification of Salmonella enterica, Escherichia coli, and Shigella spp. via PCR-electrospray ionization mass spectrometry: isolate testing and analysis of food samples. Appl Environ Microbiol 2012;78(23):8403–11.

54. Shigella: CDC website. Available at: http://wwwcdcgov/shigella/; http://wwwcdcgov/pulsenet/pathogens/shigellahtml. Accessed November 22, 2014.

55. Papasian CJ, Enna-Kifer S, Garrison B. Symptomatic Shigella sonnei urinary tract infection. J Clin Microbiol 1995;33(8):2222–3.

56. Appannanavar SB, Goyal K, Garg R, et al. Shigellemia in a post renal transplant patient: a case report and literature review. J Infect Dev Ctries 2014;8(2):237–9.

57. Markham KB, Backes C Jr, Samuels P. Bacteremia and intrauterine infection with Shigella sonnei in a pregnant woman with AIDS. Arch Gynecol Obstet 2012; 286(3):799–801.

58. Acheson DW, Keusch GT. Shigella and enteroinvasive Escherichia coli. In: Blaser MJ, Smith PD, Ravdin JI, et al, editors. Infections of the gastrointestinal tract. New York: Raven Press; 1995. p. 763–84.

59. Kotloff KL, Winickoff JP, Ivanoff B, et al. Global burden of Shigella infections: implications for vaccine development and implementation of control strategies. Bull World Health Organ 1999;77(8):651–66.

60. Bardhan P, Faruque AS, Naheed A, et al. Decrease in shigellosis-related deaths without Shigella spp.-specific interventions, Asia. Emerg Infect Dis 2010;16(11): 1718–23.

61. Van de Verg LL, Venkatesan MM. Editorial commentary: a Shigella vaccine against prevalent serotypes. Clin Infect Dis 2014;59(7):942–3.

62. Scallan E, Hoekstra RM, Angulo FJ, et al. Foodborne illness acquired in the United States–major pathogens. Emerg Infect Dis 2011;17(1):7–15.

63. DuPont HL, Levine MM, Hornick RB, et al. Inoculum size in shigellosis and implications for expected mode of transmission. J Infect Dis 1989;159(6): 1126–8.

64. Centers for Disease Control and Prevention (CDC). Shigella sonnei outbreak among men who have sex with men–San Francisco, California, 2000–2001. MMWR Morbidity Mortality Weekly Rep 2001;50(42):922–6.

65. Centers for Disease Control and Prevention (CDC). Day care-related outbreaks of rhamnose-negative Shigella sonnei–six states, June 2001–March 2003. MMWR Morbidity Mortality Weekly Rep 2004;53(3):60–3.

66. Centers for Disease Control and Prevention (CDC). Outbreaks of multidrug-resistant Shigella sonnei gastroenteritis associated with day care centers–Kansas, Kentucky, and Missouri, 2005. MMWR Morbidity Mortality Weekly Rep 2006;55(39):1068–71.

67. Arvelo W, Hinkle CJ, Nguyen TA, et al. Transmission risk factors and treatment of pediatric shigellosis during a large daycare center-associated outbreak of multidrug resistant Shigella sonnei: implications for the management of shigellosis outbreaks among children. Pediatr Infect Dis J 2009;28(11):976–80.

68. Daskalakis DC, Blaser MJ. Another perfect storm: Shigella, men who have sex with men, and HIV. Clin Infect Dis 2007;44(3):335–7.

69. Khan WA, Griffiths JK, Bennish ML. Gastrointestinal and extra-intestinal manifestations of childhood shigellosis in a region where all four species of Shigella are endemic. PLoS One 2013;8(5):e64097.

70. Tauxe RV, Puhr ND, Wells JG, et al. Antimicrobial resistance of Shigella isolates in the USA: the importance of international travelers. J Infect Dis 1990;162(5): 1107–11.

71. von Seidlein L, Kim DR, Ali M, et al. A multicentre study of Shigella diarrhoea in six Asian countries: disease burden, clinical manifestations, and microbiology. PLoS Med 2006;3(9):e353.
72. van den Beld MJ, Reubsaet FA. Differentiation between Shigella, enteroinvasive Escherichia coli (EIEC) and noninvasive Escherichia coli. Eur J Clin Microbiol Infect Dis 2012;31(6):899–904.
73. Huys G, Cnockaert M, Janda JM, et al. Escherichia albertii sp. nov., a diarrhoea-genic species isolated from stool specimens of Bangladeshi children. Int J Syst Evol Microbiol 2003;53(Pt 3):807–10.
74. Hyma KE, Lacher DW, Nelson AM, et al. Evolutionary genetics of a new patho-genic Escherichia species: Escherichia albertii and related Shigella boydii strains. J Bacteriol 2005;187(2):619–28.
75. Winn WC Jr, Allen SD, Janda WM, et al. The enterobacteriacae. Koneman's color atlas and textbook of diagnostic microbiology. 6th edition. Baltimore (MD): Lippincott, Williams, & Wilkins; 2006. p. 211–302.
76. Lindberg AA, Karnell A, Weintraub A. The lipopolysaccharide of Shigella bacteria as a virulence factor. Rev Infect Dis 1991;13(Suppl 4):S279–84.
77. Porter CK, Thura N, Ranallo RT, et al. The Shigella human challenge model. Epidemiol Infect 2013;141(2):223–32.
78. Campilongo R, Di Martino ML, Marcocci L, et al. Molecular and functional profiling of the polyamine content in enteroinvasive E. coli: looking into the gap between commensal E. coli and harmful Shigella. PLoS One 2014;9(9): e106589.
79. Carroll KC, Borek AP, Burger C, et al. Evaluation of the BD Phoenix automated microbiology system for identification and antimicrobial susceptibility testing of staphylococci and enterococci. J Clin Microbiol 2006;44(6):2072–7.
80. Aldridge KE, Gardner BB, Clark SJ, et al. Comparison of micro-ID, API 20E, and conventional media systems in identification of Enterobacteriaceae. J Clin Microbiol 1978;7(6):507–13.
81. O'Hara CM, Rhoden DL, Miller JM. Reevaluation of the API 20E identification system versus conventional biochemicals for identification of members of the family Enterobacteriaceae: a new look at an old product. J Clin Microbiol 1992;30(1):123–5.
82. Peele D, Bradfield J, Pryor W, et al. Comparison of identifications of human and animal source gram-negative bacteria by API 20E and crystal E/NF systems. J Clin Microbiol 1997;35(1):213–6.
83. Robinson A, McCarter YS, Tetreault J. Comparison of Crystal Enteric/Nonfer-menter system, API 20E system, and Vitek AutoMicrobic system for identification of gram-negative bacilli. J Clin Microbiol 1995;33(2):364–70.
84. Khot PD, Fisher MA. Novel approach for differentiating Shigella species and Escherichia coli by matrix-assisted laser desorption ionization-time of flight mass spectrometry. J Clin Microbiol 2013;51(11):3711–6.
85. Gould LH, Bopp C, Strockbine N, et al. Recommendations for diagnosis of shiga toxin–producing Escherichia coli infections by clinical laboratories. MMWR Recomm Rep 2009;58(RR-12):1–14.
86. Gavin PJ, Peterson LR, Pasquariello AC, et al. Evaluation of performance and potential clinical impact of ProSpecT Shiga toxin Escherichia coli microplate assay for detection of Shiga Toxin-producing E. coli in stool samples. J Clin Microbiol 2004;42(4):1652–6.
87. Mackenzie AM, Lebel P, Orrbine E, et al. Sensitivities and specificities of premier E. coli O157 and premier EHEC enzyme immunoassays for diagnosis of

infection with verotxin (Shiga-like toxin)-producing Escherichia coli. The SYN-SORB Pk Study investigators. J Clin Microbiol 1998;36(6):1608–11.

88. He X, Patfield S, Hnasko R, et al. A polyclonal antibody based immunoassay detects seven subtypes of Shiga toxin 2 produced by Escherichia coli in human and environmental samples. PLoS One 2013;8(10):e76368.

89. Urdahl AM, Solheim HT, Vold L, et al. Shiga toxin-encoding genes (stx genes) in human faecal samples. APMIS 2013;121(3):202–10.

90. Ashkenazi S, Levy I, Kazaronovski V, et al. Growing antimicrobial resistance of Shigella isolates. J Antimicrob Chemother 2003;51(2):427–9.

91. Khatun F, Faruque AS, Koeck JL, et al. Changing species distribution and antimicrobial susceptibility pattern of Shigella over a 29-year period (1980–2008). Epidemiol Infect 2011;139(3):446–52.

92. Taneja N, Mewara A, Kumar A, et al. Cephalosporin-resistant Shigella flexneri over 9 years (2001–09) in India. J Antimicrob Chemother 2012;67(6):1347–53.

93. Vinh H, Nhu NT, Nga TV, et al. A changing picture of shigellosis in southern Vietnam: shifting species dominance, antimicrobial susceptibility and clinical presentation. BMC Infect Dis 2009;9:204.

94. Zhang W, Luo Y, Li J, et al. Wide dissemination of multidrug-resistant Shigella isolates in China. J Antimicrob Chemother 2011;66(11):2527–35.

95. Ghosh S, Pazhani GP, Chowdhury G, et al. Genetic characteristics and changing antimicrobial resistance among Shigella spp. isolated from hospitalized diarrhoeal patients in Kolkata, India. J Med Microbiol 2011;60(Pt 10):1460–6.

96. Jain S, Sharma M, Gupta R, et al. Multidrug resistant Shigella flexneri: a rare case of septicemia in an infant. J Clin Diagn Res 2014;8(6):DD03–4.

97. Azmi IJ, Khajanchi BK, Akter F, et al. Fluoroquinolone resistance mechanisms of Shigella flexneri isolated in Bangladesh. PLoS One 2014;9(7):e102533.

98. Phalipon A, Sansonetti PJ. Shigella's ways of manipulating the host intestinal innate and adaptive immune system: a tool box for survival? Immunol Cell Biol 2007;85(2):119–29.

99. Schroeder GN, Hilbi H. Molecular pathogenesis of Shigella spp.: controlling host cell signaling, invasion, and death by type III secretion. Clin Microbiol Rev 2008; 21(1):134–56.

100. Ogawa M, Handa Y, Ashida H, et al. The versatility of Shigella effectors. Nat Rev Microbiol 2008;6(1):11–6.

101. Barry EM, Pasetti MF, Sztein MB, et al. Progress and pitfalls in Shigella vaccine research. Nat Rev Gastroenterol Hepatol 2013;10(4):245–55.

102. Herold S, Karch H, Schmidt H. Shiga toxin-encoding bacteriophages–genomes in motion. Int J Med Microbiol 2004;294(2–3):115–21.

103. Donohue-Rolfe A, Acheson DW, Keusch GT. Shiga toxin: purification, structure, and function. Rev Infect Dis 1991;13(Suppl 4):S293–7.

104. Kim YJ, Yeo SG, Park JH, et al. Shigella vaccine development: prospective animal models and current status. Curr Pharm Biotechnol 2013;14(10):903–12.

105. Bottone EJ. Yersinia enterocolitica: the charisma continues. Clin Microbiol Rev 1997;10(2):257–76.

106. Yersinia: CDC Website. Available at: http://wwwcdcgov/nczved/divisions/dfbmd/diseases/yersinia/. Accessed November 22, 2014.

107. Cover TL, Aber RC. Yersinia enterocolitica. N Engl J Med 1989;321(1):16–24.

108. Foberg U, Fryden A, Kihlstrom E, et al. Yersinia enterocolitica septicemia: clinical and microbiological aspects. Scand J Infect Dis 1986;18(4):269–79.

109. Giamarellou H, Antoniadou A, Kanavos K, et al. Yersinia enterocolitica endocarditis: case report and literature review. Eur J Clin Microbiol Infect Dis 1995;14(2):126–30.

110. van der Heijden IM, Res PC, Wilbrink B, et al. Yersinia enterocolitica: a cause of chronic polyarthritis. Clin Infect Dis 1997;25(4):831–7.
111. Adamkiewicz TV, Berkovitch M, Krishnan C, et al. Infection due to Yersinia enterocolitica in a series of patients with beta-thalassemia: incidence and predisposing factors. Clin Infect Dis 1998;27(6):1362–6.
112. Centers for Disease Control and Prevention (CDC). Yersinia enterocolitica gastroenteritis among infants exposed to chitterlings–Chicago, Illinois, 2002. MMWR Morbidity Mortality Weekly Rep 2003;52(40):956–8.
113. Abdel-Haq NM, Asmar BI, Abuhammour WM, et al. Yersinia enterocolitica infection in children. Pediatr Infect Dis J 2000;19(10):954–8.
114. Fredriksson-Ahomaa M, Stolle A, Korkeala H. Molecular epidemiology of Yersinia enterocolitica infections. FEMS Immunol Med Microbiol 2006;47(3):315–29.
115. Jones TF. From pig to pacifier: chitterling-associated yersiniosis outbreak among black infants. Emerg Infect Dis 2003;9(8):1007–9.
116. Lee LA, Gerber AR, Lonsway DR, et al. Yersinia enterocolitica O: 3 infections in infants and children, associated with the household preparation of chitterlings. N Engl J Med 1990;322(14):984–7.
117. Lee LA, Taylor J, Carter GP, et al. Yersinia enterocolitica O:3: an emerging cause of pediatric gastroenteritis in the United States. The Yersinia enterocolitica Collaborative Study Group. J Infect Dis 1991;163(3):660–3.
118. Wagner SJ, Friedman LI, Dodd RY. Transfusion-associated bacterial sepsis. Clin Microbiol Rev 1994;7(3):290–302.
119. Tertti R, Vuento R, Mikkola P, et al. Clinical manifestations of Yersinia pseudotuberculosis infection in children. Eur J Clin Microbiol Infect Dis 1989;8(7):587–91.
120. Crchova V, Grondin C. Urinary infection due to Yersinia pseudotuberculosis. Vie Med Can Fr 1973;2(1):3–5.
121. Ljungberg P, Valtonen M, Harjola VP, et al. Report of four cases of Yersinia pseudotuberculosis septicemia and a literature review. Eur J Clin Microbiol Infect Dis 1995;14(9):804–10.
122. Naiel B, Raul R. Chronic prostatitis due to Yersinia pseudotuberculosis. J Clin Microbiol 1998;36(3):856.
123. Nuorti JP, Niskanen T, Hallanvuo S, et al. A widespread outbreak of Yersinia pseudotuberculosis O:3 infection from iceberg lettuce. J Infect Dis 2004; 189(5):766–74.
124. Jalava K, Hakkinen M, Valkonen M, et al. An outbreak of gastrointestinal illness and erythema nodosum from grated carrots contaminated with Yersinia pseudotuberculosis. J Infect Dis 2006;194(9):1209–16.
125. Reuter S, Connor TR, Barquist L, et al. Parallel independent evolution of pathogenicity within the genus Yersinia. Proc Natl Acad Sci U S A 2014;111(18):6768–73.
126. Archer JR, Schell RF, Pennell DR, et al. Identification of Yersinia spp. with the API 20E system. J Clin Microbiol 1987;25(12):2398–9.
127. Sharma NK, Doyle PW, Gerbasi SA, et al. Identification of Yersinia species by the API 20E. J Clin Microbiol 1990;28(6):1443–4.
128. Wunderink HF, Oostvogel PM, Frenay IH, et al. Difficulties in diagnosing terminal ileitis due to Yersinia pseudotuberculosis. Eur J Clin Microbiol Infect Dis 2014; 33(2):197–200.
129. Singhal N, Kumar M, Virdi JS. Molecular analysis of beta-lactamase genes to understand their differential expression in strains of Yersinia enterocolitica biotype 1A. Sci Rep 2014;4:5270.
130. Batzilla J, Heesemann J, Rakin A. The pathogenic potential of Yersinia enterocolitica 1A. Int J Med Microbiol 2011;301(7):556–61.

131. Rakin A, Schneider L, Podladchikova O. Hunger for iron: the alternative sidero-phore iron scavenging systems in highly virulent Yersinia. Front Cell Infect Micro-biol 2012;2:151.

132. Capilla S, Ruiz J, Goni P, et al. Characterization of the molecular mechanisms of quinolone resistance in Yersinia enterocolitica O:3 clinical isolates. J Antimicrob Chemother 2004;53(6):1068–71.

133. Pham JN, Bell SM, Martin L, et al. The beta-lactamases and beta-lactam antibi-otic susceptibility of Yersinia enterocolitica. J Antimicrob Chemother 2000;46(6): 951–7.

134. Porter CK, Choi D, Cash B, et al. Pathogen-specific risk of chronic gastrointes-tinal disorders following bacterial causes of foodborne illness. BMC Gastroen-terol 2013;13:46.

135. Dizdar V, Gilja OH, Hausken T. Increased visceral sensitivity in Giardia-induced postinfectious irritable bowel syndrome and functional dyspepsia. Ef-fect of the 5HT3-antagonist ondansetron. Neurogastroenterol Motil 2007; 19(12):977–82.

136. Falth-Magnusson K, Franzen L, Jansson G, et al. Infant feeding history shows distinct differences between Swedish celiac and reference children. Pediatr Al-lergy Immunol 1996;7(1):1–5.

137. Verdu EF, Mauro M, Bourgeois J, et al. Clinical onset of celiac disease after an episode of Campylobacter jejuni enteritis. Can J Gastroenterol 2007;21(7): 453–5.

# Shiga Toxin Producing *Escherichia coli*

Allen Bryan, MD, PhD[a], Ilan Youngster, MD[b], Alexander J. McAdam, MD, PhD[c],*

## KEYWORDS

- Shiga toxin–producing *Escherichia coli* • Enterohemorrhagic *Escherichia coli*
- *Escherichia coli* O157 • Gastroenteritis

## KEY POINTS

- Infection with Shiga toxin–producing *Escherichia coli* (STEC) causes a range of manifestations, from asymptomatic carriage to hemorrhagic colitis and hemolytic uremic syndrome.
- The primary mechanism by which STEC damages humans is production of Shiga toxins, which inhibit protein synthesis.
- The main reservoir for STEC is the intestinal tract of cattle; transmission usually occurs by ingestion of contaminated foods.
- The most common serotype of STEC is O157:H7, but other serotypes also commonly cause human infections.
- Diagnostic testing for STEC can be performed by culture, immunoassays, and molecular assays; these tests differ in their sensitivities and specificities, and in their ability to detect all STEC or only those of the O157:H7 serotype.

## INTRODUCTION

Enteropathogenic *Escherichia coli* are commonly classified pathotypically, by the patterns of manifestations observed in infection (**Table 1**). However, these descriptively useful terms can be subject to confusion, both from differences in exact case definitions, and from horizontal gene transfer between strains, which produces organisms causing infections with features fitting multiple classifications. Shiga toxin–producing *E coli* (STEC) is usually classified pathotypically as enterohemorrhagic *E coli* (EHEC). STEC is by far the most common type of EHEC, and so the 2 terms are sometimes used synonymously. This should be avoided, as Shiga toxins 1 and 2 (Stx1 and Stx2) can also be produced in strains with other characteristics consistent with enteroaggregative *E coli* (EAEC).[1–3] In this review, we briefly discuss the pathogenesis,

[a] Division of Laboratory Medicine, Department of Pathology, Beth-Israel Deaconess Medical Center, 330 Brookline Avenue, Boston, MA 02215, USA; [b] Division of Infectious Diseases, Boston Children's Hospital, 300 Longwood Avenue, Boston, MA 02115, USA; [c] Department of Laboratory Medicine, Boston Children's Hospital, 300 Longwood Avenue, Boston, MA 02115, USA
* Corresponding author.
*E-mail address:* alexander.mcadam@childrens.harvard.edu

Clin Lab Med 35 (2015) 247–272
http://dx.doi.org/10.1016/j.cll.2015.02.004
0272-2712/15/$ – see front matter © 2015 Elsevier Inc. All rights reserved.

**Table 1**
**Common pathotype classifications of *Escherichia coli* according to symptoms and infection site**

| Pathotype | Disease and Symptoms | Infection Site | Virulence Factors |
|---|---|---|---|
| Enterohaemorrhagic *E coli* | Watery diarrhea<br>Hemorrhagic colitis<br>Hemolytic-uremic syndrome | Distal ileum<br>Colon | *stx* |
| Enteropathogenic *E coli* | Profuse watery diarrhea | Small intestine | *eae, bfp* |
| Enteroaggregative *E coli* | Watery diarrhea, traveler's diarrhea, endemic infection of children | Intestines | *aat* family |
| Enteroinvasive *E coli* (and *Shigella*) | Shigellosis/bacterial dysentery | Colon | *tpaH, ial* |
| Enterotoxigenic *E coli* | Watery diarrhea, traveler's diarrhea | Small intestine | Labile toxin, stable toxin |
| Diffusely adherent *E coli* | Diffuse, persistent watery diarrhea | Intestine | ? |

The strength of the associations between the pathotypes and the disease or symptoms varies.

clinical manifestations, and epidemiology of STEC, and then focus on the laboratory detection of STEC in more depth.

## MICROBIOLOGY AND PATHOGENESIS
### Terminology

The defining characteristic of STEC is the production of 1 or more of the extracellular toxins known as Stx1 and Stx2, Shiga-like toxins,[4] or simply Shiga toxins. An alternate name for these toxins is verocytotoxins,[5] derived from the reaction of Vero monkey kidney cells to the toxins.[6] Although it is placed in a separate genus, *Shigella* species are phylogenetically within the clade *E coli*.[7] The high relatedness of these organisms is believed to have facilitated transfer of the genes for Stx1 from *Shigella* species to *E coli* via lambda or related phages.[8,9]

### Shiga Toxins

Stx1 is nearly identical to the *Shigella dysenteriae* toxin, differing by a single amino acid.[10,11] Stx2 was originally distinguished from Stx1 by neutralization by a separate antiserum.[12,13] Stx2 is exclusive to *E coli* and is found in numerous variants with only minor differences in amino acid sequence. All Shiga toxins are produced via a single operon containing at minimum the 2 genes *stxA* and *stxB*, and at least 1 promoter. The Shiga toxin operon(s) are embedded within the genomes of integrated lambdoid prophages.[14] They may be acquired by horizontal transmission via phage as well as by direct inheritance.[15]

Shiga toxins are AB5 toxins, meaning they are composed of a single copy of the ~32 kDa A component (produced by stxA), which bears the enzymatic activity of the toxin, and 5 copies of the ~8 kDa B component (produced by stxB), each of which bears 3 binding sites for the Shiga toxin receptor (**Fig. 1**).[16,17] The AB5 family additionally includes pertussis toxin, cholera toxin, and the labile enterotoxin of enterotoxigenic *E coli*.[18]

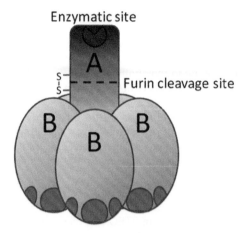

Enzymatic site

Furin cleavage site

Gb3 receptor binding sites (15 in all)

**Fig. 1.** Schematic diagram of the Shiga toxin (Stx) or Shiga-like toxin, showing the multiple binding (*B*) domains with a single catalytic, active (*A*) domain.

The mechanisms by which Stx1 and Stx2 are produced and released by STEC have not been explored fully. However, the production and release of Shiga toxins in STEC strains is known to be linked to the promoters and associated genes of the lambda prophage genomes in which they are embedded. For instance, most strains producing Stx1 and/or Stx2 are known to be induced by different environmental triggers, including low environmental iron,[19] environmental stressors,[20] and most critically, antibiotics, particularly antibiotics that target DNA synthesis.[21] The operon promoters mediating these responses to the environment are embedded within the prophage genome; they may regulate only Shiga toxin production, or be part of the overall regulation of the prophage. Given the strong linkage with the phage reproductive cycle and regulatory mechanism, it was assumed for many years that lysis was the only method of toxin release. Some evidence has suggested that Shiga toxin can be delivered without cell lysis, via outer membrane vesicles.[22,23] However, it is known that Stx1 and Stx2 may be delivered to the extracellular space by different mechanisms,[24] so the complete picture of non–lysis-mediated Shiga toxin release remains unclear.

AB5 toxins use a carbohydrate moiety for endocytotic transport into their target cells. The receptor for Stx1 and Stx2 is the cell membrane component globotriaosyl-ceramide (Gb3).[25] Interestingly, human intestinal epithelium cells do not express Gb3.[26] However, the Paneth cells, critical first responders for the innate immune defense of the intestinal lumen, do express Gb3,[27] and Stx1 and Stx2 may also bind to neutrophils traversing the endothelium and at other sites.[28,29] Recent reviews have also delineated potential additional means of Stx to transcytose across the epithelium, possibly by inducing changes in transport during mucosal inflammation.[30] Once across the luminal barrier, Stx finds its way to a variety of downstream tissues, most notably renal cortical tissue.[31] Gb3 recognition triggers endocytosis of the Stx1 and Stx2 and transport to the Golgi apparatus and endoplasmic reticulum.[32]

Once transported to sites of protein synthesis, the A component of the toxin acts as an *N*-glycosidase to inhibit protein synthesis in the cell. The enzymatic center of the A component is activated intracellularly by cleavage by the membrane-bound trypsin family protease furin, yielding A1 and A2 components that remain linked by a disulfide bond. Cleavage renders the A1 component up to 20 times more active than intact A component.[33] The target of the Shiga toxin is an adenine within the 28S rRNA of the 60S eukaryotic ribosome subunit.[34] The cleavage of this adenine leads to activation of apoptosis through several stress response pathways.[35]

Aside from Shiga toxin, many other virulence factors may be present in various STEC strains and contribute to their pathogenicity. These include adherence factors, such as intimin/eae,[36] an "effacement/adherence" factor. Eae forms part of the conserved "locus of enterocyte effacement" (LEE).[37] The LEE encodes a series of proteins inducing cytoskeletal changes in the eukaryotic target cell that enhance attachment and effacement of the bacterium, and a type III secretion system to deliver them.[38] The LEE system increases virulence of STEC, but it is not found in all STEC strains[39]; other adhesive agents are known but are not as well-characterized.[40,41]

### Case Study: The European O104:H4 Shiga Toxin–Producing Escherichia coli Outbreak (2011)

In the spring of 2011, a new strain of STEC was discovered during a clinical outbreak originating near Hamburg, Germany.[3,42] The epidemiology and clinical manifestations of this outbreak are discussed herein. Owing to the unexpected virulence and morbidity of the strain, an unprecedented effort was made to identify rapidly and understand the origins and virulence of the new strain.

This was the first outbreak for which rapid whole-genome sequencing was used to produce near-real-time analysis of an emerging pathogenic E coli strain. Leveraging the new next-generation sequencing capabilities, strains could now be completely sequenced within 1 week of receipt. Use of the public genomic databases such as the National Center for Biotechnology Information (NCBI) GeneBank and EMBL, aided bioinformaticians in rapidly analyzing and comparing sections of the genome of the new O104:H4 strain with those of previously studied strains.[43–46] Unbound by traditional restrictions on in vitro molecular experimentation, genome sequence data could be compared rapidly with all available strain genomes, not just those with the most similar clinical phenotype. Collaboration was facilitated over the Internet via Wikis and open-source data-sharing principles.

The results were not only striking in their speed and depth, but in the implications for understanding the evolution and epidemiology of STEC strains. The O104:H4 strain bore not only a lysogenic stx2-bearing lambdoid phage, but additional plasmids and insertions carrying EAEC adhesion virulence factors and multidrug resistance cassettes (**Fig. 2**).[46] These elements were found to be highly similar to genomic fragments from recently isolated EAEC strains in different parts of the world, implying a recent spread of virulence elements via horizontal gene transfer. Indeed, comparative analysis of different samples within the outbreak suggested that infection by an stx2-bearing lambdoid phage was the most recent gene transfer, endowing the strain with EHEC properties.[47] Rapid characterization permitted equally rapid development of molecular assays specific for the epidemic strain, first from the pathogen genes themselves, then from unique DNA sequences throughout the genome.[45]

### SEROTYPES OF SHIGA TOXIN–PRODUCING ESCHERICHIA COLI

Specific strains of E coli have long been described[48] and clinically defined by serotyping of specific surface antigens. The lipopolysaccharide somatic or O (Ohne) antigen and the flagellar or H (Hauch) antigen are used most frequently in serotyping of pathogenic E coli, because they have the best correlation with virulence factors.[49] A full serotyping of a strain may also involve additional antigens, such as the capsular or K (Kapsule) antigen.

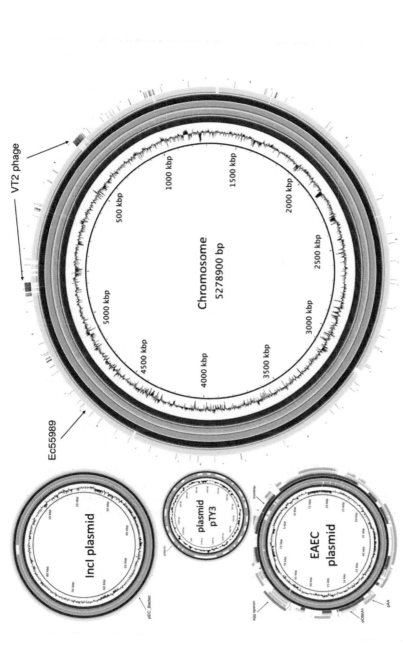

**Fig. 2.** A sample comparative analysis of the Shiga toxin producing *Escherichia coli* (STEC) 104:H4 TY2482 strain, produced June 18, 2011, by the Beijing Genomics Institute from a strain isolated in the last week of May. At right is the main chromosome of *E coli*; the native sections of the TY2482 strain are shown in yellow, those inserted via lambdoid stx-bearing phage are in red, and other colors indicate matches to additional outbreak genomes sequenced at other laboratories. At left are the plasmids of the strain; of particular note is the inclusion of the enteroaggregative *E coli* (EAEC) plasmid with adhesion virulence factors formerly not found in enterohemorrhagic *E coli* (EHEC) strains. This level of highly detailed analysis was made possible by rapid sequencing and worldwide cooperation, permitting in-depth understanding of virulence patterns, even while the outbreak was still ongoing. (*Courtesy of* Dr Kathryn Holt, PhD, University of Melbourne.)

The most common serotype of STEC detected in North America and portions of Europe is O157:H7 (abbreviated at O157).[50,51] O157 was the first STEC-associated serotype to be identified, after the linkage of a cytotoxic effect on Vero cells[52] to clinical symptoms[53] led to demonstrations that the Vero cytotoxin, the Shiga-like toxin, and the O157 toxin were identical.[54] This finding facilitated the identification of O157 as the pathogen responsible for enterohemorrhagic infections.[55] O157 is but the most common serotype of STEC. An increasing number of non-O157 cases have been noted by US Centers for Disease Control and Prevention (CDC) monitoring.[56,57] By 2010, O157 only caused 50% of confirmed STEC cases in the United States and its incidence varies around the globe (**Table 2**).[58] Therefore, although tests specific for O157 bear prominence in screening for cases in the United States, it is important to test for non-O157 STEC in all effected populations.

## CLINICAL SHIGA TOXIN–PRODUCING *ESCHERICHIA COLI* INFECTION
### Range of Manifestations

STEC infections cause a spectrum of diseases ranging in severity from asymptomatic carriage to hemorrhagic colitis and hemolytic uremic syndrome (HUS). After ingestion of as few as 100 organisms followed by an incubation period of 3 to 4 days, almost all infected patients develop watery diarrhea accompanied by significant abdominal cramping. In 80% to 90% of culture-proven cases, the diarrhea becomes grossly bloody 2 to 3 days after onset of loose stools. This phase of hemorrhagic diarrhea lasts on average 2 to 5 days before symptomatic resolution.[59,60] Hospitalization is required in 23% to 47% of symptomatic patients with acute diarrhea owing to STEC, with a median hospital stay of 6 to 14 days. Although the majority of patients recover uneventfully from uncomplicated diarrheal disease within 1 week, an estimated 6% to 25% of patients with STEC-related hemorrhagic colitis develop HUS, which is characterized by thrombocytopenia, microangiopathic hemolytic anemia, and acute renal injury with up to 50% requiring renal dialysis during the acute phase.[59–62] This number is likely greater in pediatric populations, where about two-thirds of cases are oligoanuric and will require dialysis. HUS generally complicates 6% to 9% of STEC infections overall and about 15% of infections in children under age 10; however, in outbreak situations these numbers can be as high as 15% to 25%.[63] Among patients who develop HUS, up to 50% require dialysis during the acute phase; mortality is 3% to 5%. Neurologic manifestations, including seizures and altered mentation, are not infrequently described, resembling thrombotic thrombocytopenic purpura.

The very young and the elderly are most susceptible to complications and death from STEC infection. This bacterial infection is the leading cause of acute kidney

| Table 2 | | |
| --- | --- | --- |
| Most common serotypes of Shiga toxin producing *Escherichia coli* isolated from outbreaks in humans from different locations, ordered by incidence | | |
| United States, 1983–2002 | Germany, 1999–2004 | Shizuoka, Japan, 2003–2007 |
| O157 | O157 | O26 |
| O26 | O103 | O103 |
| O111 | O26 | O111 |
| O103 | O941 | O157 |
| O121 | O145 | O165 |

Differing locations show variation in more common serotypes.
*Data from* Refs.[156–158]

failure in otherwise healthy children in developed countries. Children younger than 5 years are more likely to develop complications requiring hospitalization and kidney dialysis, and those older than 60 years are more likely to die regardless of the clinical complications.[64]

Long-term complications after HUS are encountered frequently, including chronic renal insufficiency, neurologic disorders, hypertension, and other cardiovascular diseases. Late gastrointestinal sequelae are common in patients with STEC infection even without HUS, and Marshall[65] described an incidence of 15% of irritable bowel syndrome symptoms 8 years after the acute infection.

### Significance of Shiga Toxins 1 and 2 in Disease Severity

Although both Stx1 and Stx2 are capable of causing HUS, Stx1 and Stx2 do not target the same tissues and organs. This is clear from animal models of disease where Stx2 was shown to be 400 times more potent than Stx1 in mice with the reverse being true in rabbits.[64,66] Stx2 is isolated most commonly from clinical isolates of STEC. In a recent review of 272 patients from Europe, Stx1 was present in 39%, Stx2 in 51%, and both genes in 9.6%. Of the patients with an STEC producing Stx1, 8.4% developed HUS; of those with Stx2, 74% developed HUS and among patients with a strain carrying both genes 53% developed HUS.[67] Although these numbers are biased by the fact that only hospitalized patients were included in the review, they illustrate the fact that Stx2 is more frequently associated with severe disease.

### Treatment

The treatment of STEC infection consists of supportive care and monitoring for the development of microangiopathic complications. Protection of renal function is achieved by intravenous volume expansion using isotonic crystalloids, especially if started early in the course of the disease.[59,68] It is important to remember that patients can seem to be deceptively well-hydrated while undergoing the initial phases of a severe prothrombotic process. Oral rehydration will not achieve the same beneficial effect on renal perfusion. Advanced supportive care in patients developing oligoanuric renal failure includes blood transfusions, peritoneal dialysis, and plasma exchange, although recent retrospective reports have questioned the utility of plasma exchange.[69] Antiperistaltic agents have been shown to increase the risk of systemic complications and should be avoided.[70,71]

Antimicrobial agents active against STEC are generally to be avoided during the acute phase of illness. Antibiotic treatment reduces the fecal bacterial burden of STEC but, with few exceptions, has been shown not to alter the duration of acute diarrheal illness[72,73] and, more important, to be associated with increased risk for development of HUS.[74–76] This detrimental effect is believed to be owing to either bacterial lysis or subsequent release of toxins, or direct induction of the bacteriophages by the antimicrobials.[77] Among the several reports that have shown correlation between antibiotic use and risk for HUS is a recent large prospective study.[75] Among 259 children younger than 10 years with *E coli* O157:H7 infection, HUS occurred more frequently in the 25 children who received antibiotics compared with those who did not receive (36% vs 12%). After adjustment for other variables, the absolute antibiotic-attributable risk increase for HUS incidence was 25%, corresponding with 1 case of HUS for every 4 children treated with antibiotics. However, some authors have challenged the dogma that antibiotics are contraindicated completely in patients with STEC infection, because azithromycin was shown not to increase expression of Stx in vitro.[78] Recent experience during the German O14:H4 outbreak suggests that treatment with azithromycin is beneficial in decolonizing patients who have recovered from the acute illness and are found to be long-term carriers of STEC (>28 days).[69,79,80]

In light of the difficulties treating this pathogen with standard approaches, several alternative experimental modalities have been evaluated. The anti–complement C5 monoclonal antibody eculizumab was used in refractory cases during the German outbreak. Despite an initial promising report of rapid clinical improvement in 3 pediatric cases treated with eculizumab,[81] preliminary findings in a larger cohort of patients showed no beneficial effect.[82] Other experimental treatments including anti-Stx antibodies and $Mn^{2+}$ have shown promise in animal models, but have yet to be evaluated in human trials.[66,83]

## EPIDEMIOLOGY OF SHIGA TOXIN–PRODUCING *ESCHERICHIA COLI*
### Sources and Significant Outbreaks

Disease caused by STEC has a global impact and has been reported from all 6 populated continents. Data on population-level incidence of sporadic STEC infections worldwide are scarce, but estimates range between 0.6 to 136 cases per 100,000 patient-years in different countries, with up to one-third of cases caused by O157 STEC. A recent systematic review by Majowicz and colleagues[84] estimated that STEC infection causes 2.8 million acute illnesses a year on a global scale.

Multiple large outbreaks have been recorded since 1982, mostly in industrialized countries. This might be a result of reporting bias owing to diagnostic resources and national reporting systems available in the developed world; however, other factors are contributing to this differential occurrence in outbreaks, including the large-scale centralized food production in industrialized countries that can serve as a widespread vector of dissemination in cases of food contamination.

The natural reservoir of STEC is the gastrointestinal tract of cattle and other ruminant animals such as sheep, goats, and deer. The pathogen does not cause disease in these animals that seem to lack receptors for Shiga-like toxins.[85]

The most common means of spread, particularly in outbreak situations, is ingestion of contaminated food products. Consumption of undercooked ground beef has been implicated in up to 40% of all major outbreaks[59,68] and was also the culprit in the first described major outbreak of *E coli* O157 in 1982, affecting 47 patients in the Pacific Northwest.[53] Other types of meat, unpasteurized dairy products, and leafy green vegetables are also commonly implicated as sources of outbreaks.[86–88] Almost any food product can be contaminated, as exemplified by outbreaks caused by apple juice, sprouts, and more recently, 77 patients in the United States who were infected through consumption of ready-to-bake cookie dough.[89] Foods typically are contaminated through the slaughter and processing of colonized animals, shedding of pathogens from colonized cattle into milk, and use of contaminated soil or contaminated irrigation water in produce production.

There are other sources of infection, although these cause fewer cases. Infection may be acquired through direct animal contact and petting zoos, farms, and even household pets have been implicated in transmission of STEC to humans.[90,91] Hale and colleagues[92] have estimated that 6% of O157 and 8% of non-O157 cases in the United States are acquired through contact with animals. Contaminated water can serve as a direct source of infection and outbreaks have been described after swimming in freshwater lakes and swimming pools.[93,94] Finally, person-to-person transmission through the fecal–oral route is well-documented, and can sustain transmission in a community after initial introduction of the pathogen. This has been shown in day care centers, nursing homes, and hospital settings.[68,95]

## Epidemiology of Shiga Toxin–Producing Escherichia coli in the United States

STEC is estimated to cause 265,000 illnesses each year in the United States, resulting in more than 3600 hospitalizations and 30 deaths.[92,96] The National Notifiable Diseases System of the CDC has been collecting data on laboratory-confirmed and probable cases of STEC O157 since 1990 and non-O157 STEC since 2000. The incidence rate of laboratory confirmed human STEC infections has been increasing steadily, with the 2011 data showing 1.8 cases per 100,000 population annually. About 41.1% of cases are caused by O157, with O26 and O103 each contributing another 10% of cases. The states with the highest incidence rates were Wisconsin (9.9), Utah (8.3), and Idaho (6.6), but cases were reported from all states. The highest incidence rates were reported in children younger than 5 years, with 3 times the rate of other age groups. Scallan and colleagues[97] estimated the annual number of illnesses caused by O157 in this age group at 8103, or 4.4 cases per 100,000, resulting in hospitalization of 724 children and 11 deaths.

## The O104:H4 Shiga Toxin–Producing Escherichia coli Outbreak

The outbreak of STEC O104:H4 in Northern Germany is among the most illustrative examples of the potential implications of STEC outbreak on public health in recent years. The virulence of this organism is discussed elsewhere in this article. During 55 days in May and June 2011, 3816 patients were diagnosed with O104:H4-related gastroenteritis, 845 patients developed HUS, and 54 patients died.[3,69,98,99] An additional 83 cases of hemorrhagic colitis and 54 cases of HUS were described in other European countries, and all had a history of travel in Northern Germany. This outbreak proved a major challenge to health professionals involved in patient care and public health. An extensive epidemiologic investigation identified sprouts from a single producer as the most likely cause; however, no microbiological confirmation was ever obtained. The outbreak was unusual in its extent and manifestations. The majority of patients were previously healthy adults, mostly middle-aged women. Of the patients, 22% developed HUS and there was an unusually high incidence of severe neurologic manifestations. The mean shedding was reported to be 34 days in patients not receiving antibiotics, with some individuals still actively shedding the pathogen 1 year after recovery.[69,99]

## LABORATORY TESTING FOR SHIGA TOXIN–PRODUCING ESCHERICHIA COLI INFECTION

There are several different methods available for detection of STEC in the clinical laboratory. These include culture, immunoassays for STEC-specific antigens, and molecular tests such as nucleic acid amplified tests. These are discussed in detail in subsequent sections in this article. The differences between these tests that are relevant to laboratory testing include those that are relevant to most clinical microbiology tests, namely, turnaround time, cost, sensitivity, and specificity. In addition, an important difference between these tests is that some of them detect only STEC O157, whereas others detect all STEC. The merits of detecting only STEC O157 and all STEC have been discussed and debated in great detail; however, the general consensus is that the test strategy should include detection of all STEC, even in areas where STEC O157 have been the primary pathogen in the past.[100–104]

## Culture Utility and Strategies

Non–culture-based methods can test for the presence of Stx1 and/or Stx2 by detection of specific DNA sequences or antigens; however, only isolation in pure culture of the pathogenic strain can permit a full phenotypic characterization of the organism for epidemiologic purposes. Furthermore, cultures may increase sensitivity by enriching the population of toxin-producing organisms, permitting detection in otherwise difficult circumstances. Cultures can be performed at sites with less equipment and training than molecular or serologic methods, impacting cost and time to diagnosis. Therefore, culture must be considered part of any thorough workup for STEC, especially in the outbreak setting.

Detection of STEC by culture is necessarily a multistep process. Detection of STEC in stool requires the use of selective and indicator (differential) media to differentiate STEC from the other organisms in the sample. Indicator media increase specificity and potentially increase sensitivity by introducing differential indicators for particular strains of STEC,[105–109] but are restricted by the biochemical means used to cause the chromogenic reactions. Finally, at least 1 confirmation step by an immunologic or molecular test must be made to confirm the diagnosis; this requirement is forced by the lack at present of agar-based selective or differential agents specific to the Shiga-like toxin itself. Indicator media are also relatively more expensive owing to the additional dyes and additives required.

Because O157 is the most common serotype of STEC in the United States, testing specifically for this strain may be useful for rapid clinical diagnosis in most cases. The 2009 CDC guidelines regarding STEC[100] recommend that "All stools submitted for testing from patients with acute community-acquired diarrhea (i.e., for detection of the enteric pathogens *Salmonella*, *Shigella*, and *Campylobacter*) should be cultured for O157 STEC on selective and differential agar." However, a negative result for O157 STEC does not rule out the presence of non-O157 STEC and so the guidelines continue, "These stools should be simultaneously assayed for non-O157 STEC with a test that detects the Shiga toxins or the genes including these toxins." These recommendations do not include strategies for limiting testing based on patient history or stool characteristics, because most cases were found not to fit the original case description: a majority of strains were found to cause primarily nonbloody diarrhea.[110]

### Sorbitol MacConkey Agar and derivatives

Sorbitol-MacConkey agar (SMAC) contains sorbitol in place of the lactose found in routine MacConkey agar, and also includes the same dye indicators to test for carbohydrate (sorbitol) fermentation. The addition of antibiotics, particularly cefixime, and specific inorganic salts such as tellurite, to SMAC[111–113] provides further selection for STEC. SMAC was used by the investigators of the first O157:H7 outbreak because the epidemic strain did not rapidly ferment sorbitol.[55] Further investigation showed that O157 STEC ferments sorbitol more slowly than 95% of naturally occurring *E coli* strains; the differential production was readily evident in recent cultures, but disappeared after extended incubation.[114] SMAC medium quickly became a common tool for detection of O157:H7 STEC.[115]

The genetic basis for slow sorbitol fermentation by O157 STEC has been investigated. The β-ᴅ-glucuronidase gene *uidA* controls the rate of sorbitol metabolism in *E coli*.[116] The original O157:H7 epidemic clone bears a double frame-shift mutation altering 6 amino acids in the UidA protein product, plus 6 additional amino acid point mutations, reducing the effectiveness of the enzyme.[117] Because the enzyme is not fully inactivated, however, it is vital to read plates within 24 to 48 hours of inoculation to prevent false negatives with this medium.

As convenient as SMAC plates proved for identification of the original and still common O157 strains of STEC, their operation depends on the linkage between the mutant *uidA* allele and the *stx* operon. Therefore, few non-O157 strains are detectable by this method. The utility of SMAC as a screening tool therefore depends on local epidemiology, and is suitable when O157 or closely related strains dominate clinical infections or when SMAC used in combination with methods that detect all serotypes of STEC.

SMAC is also available with selective agents, such as tellurite and cefixime.[118,119] The tellurite resistance gene cluster consists of 7 genes (terA-terF and terZ).[120] Tellurite resistance is highly linked to O157:H7 strains of STEC[121] with 1 study showing 98% presence among such strains, but it is variably present in other STEC.[122]

### Agars for specific detection of Shiga toxin–producing Escherichia coli

The full range of commercially available agars for clinical, veterinary, food science, and research applications is too broad to be described exhaustively herein. We succinctly describe several of the more common agars in use today as examples of the strategies used for selection, differentiation, and indication in these media.

Typical of the first wave of indicator agars was CHROMagar O157 (CHROMagar, Paris, France) that, like SMAC, is designed for detection of only O157 STEC.[105] CHROMagar O157 uses cefixime–tellurite as well as cefsulodin for selection, and multiple enzymatic reactions to produce the chromogenic indicators. CHROMagar O157 is designed to produce pink or mauve colonies when O157 is present, whereas other *E coli* and closely related enteric bacteria form blue colonies. CHROMagar O157 suffers from the same limitation as SMAC in failing to detect most non-O157 strains of STEC. One early study on CHROMagar O157[105] using a slate stock strains of STEC showed 98% sensitivity and 77% specificity for O157, and 94% specificity for non-O157, but only 19% sensitivity for non-O157. A more recent study in Calgary, Alberta,[106] using patient samples, compared CHROMagar O157 with SMAC and found them to be highly comparable, with only 1 discrepant result among 3090 negative samples and no discrepancies among 26 positive samples. However, only O157 strains of STEC were analyzed in this study.

Rainbow O157 agar (Biolog Inc, Hayward, CA) includes a mix of selective agents; depending on the background, a selection may be made of any or all of cefixime, tellurite, and novobiocin. Rainbow agars use chromogens to indicate the presence of bacterial enzymes. In the case of Rainbow O157, β-galactosidase acts to produce blue–black color, whereas β-glucuronidase reacts with a red-producing chromogen. This method depends on the presence of β-galactosidase production primarily in O157 strains and its absence in non-O157 strains. Most, but not all, nonpathogenic *E coli* strains produce β-glucuronidase, whereas most, but not all, O157 STEC strains do not. Interestingly, a minority of O157 strains and several non-O157 strains produce both enzymes at varying levels, producing colonies indicated in various shades of purple.

The O157:H7 ID or chromID agar (bioMerieux SA, Marcy-l'Etoile, France) likewise uses β-glucuronidase and β-galactosidase to activate its chromogenic indicators, but includes only sodium deoxycholate as a nonspecific Gram-negative selection medium. Cefixime–tellurite may be added as an additional selective agent by the laboratory at time of preparation.

The increasing prevalence and awareness of non-O157 STEC spurred the development of indicator agars for detection of both O157 and non-O157 STEC. As a result, additional chromogenic indicator agars have come to the market. CHROMagar STEC (CHROMagar) adds additional mechanisms to produce a mauve coloration for a wider range of STEC strains. A dye that fluoresces with ultraviolet light is additionally produced by non-O157 and some O157 strains. During the O104 outbreak, an O104-specific version of this plate was also marketed. A study in Paris, France,[108] of 329 clinical specimens showed 91% sensitivity and 84% specificity over all STEC samples tested with CHROMagar STEC. A similar study in Finland[107] with 264 samples indicated high detection sensitivities for O157 (85%), O26 (18/20 isolates), O111 (7 isolates), O121 (5 isolates), and O145 (26 isolates) while maintaining 98% specificity for STEC strains. In a study in Manitoba, Canada, where fewer than one-half of STEC strains isolated were O157, CHROMagar STEC was found to be just 86% sensitive for STEC detection.[106]

Perhaps the most comprehensive study to date of clinical and research STEC selective media[109] examined the growth of 96 STEC strains on 8 agar formulations: MacConkey; Rainbow O157 without selective additives; Rainbow O157 with novobiocin and tellurite; Rainbow O157 with cefixime, tellurite, and novobiocin; CHROMagar STEC; tryptone bile agar with cefixime and tellurite; tryptone bile with cefixime, tellurite, eosin Y, methylene blue, and lactose; and an experimental composite indicator agar.[123] Strains tested included 6 to 10 examples of serotypes O26, O45, O103, O111, O121, O145, and O157, as well as a selection of 31 additional less common serotypes. Commercial indicator agars had a higher tendency to inhibit the growth of rare strains, especially when additional selective additives were used, but with 1 exception (O111 on Rainbow–novobiocin–tellurite), 80% or more of each serotype among those listed would not be inhibited.

In summary, selection of a culture medium for screening for STEC infection requires consideration of the ease of use of the product, the selectivity and specificity of the agar, and the epidemiology that renders particular selective factors more or less useful in a specific laboratory. Efforts to improve the selectivity and specificity of STEC agars continue,[123,124] but unless a selective or differential medium mechanism tied directly to the Shiga toxin is available, there always remains the possibility of false-negative results from a rare or unexpected strain lacking the proper resistance, enzymatic, or indicative factors. These facts should be considered when selecting media for general screening, for reevaluating screening methods in the face of a potential STEC outbreak, and in choosing to proceed with alternate detection methodologies when clinical suspicion is high for STEC in the face of negative culture screening results.

### Immunoassays for Detection of Shiga Toxin–Producing Escherichia coli

There are a large number of immunoassays available for detection of STEC directly on stool or on selective cultures of stool. Most such tests detect Stx1 and Stx2, although one tests for the O157 antigen. This section discusses the use of these assays for initial detection of STEC. Reagents for serotyping of E coli isolated from stool for the O157 or H7 antigens will not be discussed.

#### Assays for detection of Shiga toxins 1 and 2

There are several immunoassays for Stx1 and Stx2 available and these are discussed individually in the subsequent sections and summarized in **Table 3**. Some general issues merit discussion before consideration of the individual tests. First, the acceptable specimens differ somewhat between the tests. Selective broth cultures of stool are generally acceptable specimens in these tests and use of this specimen results in the highest sensitivity in most studies, as well as in the manufacturer's package inserts. In some studies, samples for which the test does not have US Food and Drug Administration (FDA) approval have been included. Such use is permitted in the United States with extensive laboratory validation and so these studies are included in the discussion. Second, a variety of reference (gold) standards have been used to evaluate these assays. Selective culture (eg, SMAC), laboratory-developed polymerase chain reaction (PCR) tests and immunoassays (often including the immunoassay under evaluation) are combined commonly to form a composite

**Table 3**
**Performance characteristics of immunoassays for Shiga toxins 1 and 2 for detection of Shiga toxin–producing *Escherichia coli* in stool**

| Assay | Sample Tested | Sensitivity | Specificity | Gold Standard | Total Samples | Positives | Reference |
|---|---|---|---|---|---|---|---|
| Duopath Verotoxin (Stx 1/2) | Selective broth | 80/100 | 81.3/62.0 | PCR | 145 | 56 | 125 |
| Duopath Verotoxin | Colony sweep, selective agar | 100 | 100 | Premier EHEC | 291 | 43 | 126 |
| ImmunoCard STAT! EHEC | Selective broth | 19.0 | 100 | PCR and IA | 632 | 21 | 129 |
| ImmunoCard STAT! EHEC | Selective broth | 35.0 | 99.0 | PCR | 819 | 17 | 144 |
| Premier EHEC | Selective broth | 96.6 | 98.5 | PCR | 145 | 56 | 125 |
| Premier EHEC | Selective broth | 96.0 | 99.7 | Culture and IA | 5110 | 50 | 101 |
| Premier EHEC | Selective broth | 100 | 99.7 | Culture and IA | 974 | 15 | 128 |
| Premier EHEC | Selective broth | 28.5 | 100 | PCR and IA | 632 | 21 | 129 |
| ProSpecT STEC | Selective broth | 100 | 100 | Culture and IA | 2060 | 7 | 130 |

*Abbreviations:* EHEC, enterohemorrhagic *Escherichia coli*; IA, immunoassay; PCR, polymerase chain reaction.
*Data from* Refs.[101,125,126,128–130,144]

gold standard. For studies that use PCR tests or immunoassays in the reference standard, subsequent culture isolation is usually required for confirmation. It is important to note that, as more assays are included in the reference standard and if a sensitive PCR is included in the reference standard, this may reduce the apparent sensitivity of the immunoassay; thus, comparisons between studies should be made with care.

There are 2 lateral flow assays for detection and differentiation of Stx1 and Stx2, the Duopath Verotoxin test (Merck KGaA, Darmstadt, Germany) and ImmunoCard STAT! EHEC (Meridian Biosciences, Cincinnati, OH). The Duopath Verotoxin assay has been evaluated in 2 relatively large peer-reviewed studies, one of which used a selective broth culture and the other of which used colony growth from a selective agar.[125,126] The sensitivity of the assay was high in both studies. When the performances of the Stx1 and Stx2 tests are analyzed separately, the sensitivity of the Stx2 assay is greater, but the specificity is lower compared with the Stx1 assay. Of note, Duopath Verotoxin is FDA approved for use with culture isolates.[100] There is a single, relatively small study of the ImmunoCard STAT! EHEC assay.[127] In this study, the ImmunoCard STAT! EHEC had a modest sensitivity when used directly on unprocessed stool, but high sensitivity when used on selective broth culture of stool. The specificity of the assay was high with both specimen types.

There are 2 enzyme immunoassays (EIAs) for Stx1 and Stx2 available in the United States, the Premier EHEC (Meridian Biosciences) and the ProSpecT Shiga Toxin *E coli* Microplate Assay (Remel, Thermo Scientific, Lenexa, KS). Both of these can be performed directly on unprocessed stool or on enrichment broth cultures. Stool in transport media can be tested using Premier EHEC, and culture isolates can be tested using ProSpecT Shiga Toxin *E coli* Microplate Assay. The Premier EHEC test has been evaluated in 2 studies that included large numbers of positive specimens, both of which used the assay to test selective broth cultures.[101,125] Premier EHEC had sensitivities of greater than 95% and specificities of greater than 98% in both studies. Two smaller studies confirmed the high specificity of Premier EHEC, but one found the assay to be insensitive in comparison with a PCR assay.[128,129] A study including a small number of positive specimens and a large number of negative specimens found the ProSpecT Shiga Toxin *E coli* Microplate Assay to be both sensitive and specific.[130]

### Assays for detection of O157 antigen

The Immunocard STAT! *E coli* O157 Plus assay (Meridian Biosciences) is a rapid, lateral flow immunoassay for detection of STEC with the O157 antigen. The assay uses 2 antibodies, one that reacts to an unspecified epitope common to STEC, and a second to the O157 antigen. It can be used to test unprocessed stool, stool in Carey–Blair transport media or stool incubated overnight in MacConkey broth. There are no peer-reviewed evaluations of this product in the literature. An earlier product, ImmunoCard STAT! *E coli* O157:H7 that included an antibody to the H7 antigen as well as O157 antigen, performed well on specimens incubated with selective broth, but poorly when used directly on unprocessed stool.[127,131] Significant differences between the Immunocard STAT! *E coli* O157 Plus and Immunocard STAT! *E coli* O157 means that these results should not be expected to predict the performance of the Immunocard STAT! *E coli* O157 Plus test.

## MOLECULAR TESTING FOR SHIGA TOXIN–PRODUCING *ESCHERICHIA COLI*

Unlike culture-based or immunologic methods, molecular testing directly detects defining or characteristic genes of STEC. Unlike culture or serology, the presence of the *stx* genes causing EHEC symptomatology and the various virulence and resistance factors assisting pathogenicity can be directly detected and verified. Using real-time PCR cycling, extremely low detection limits may be achieved.[132,133]

The general drawback of targeted molecular testing is that one finds only what one seeks. Primers and probes are selected for specific known genetic sequences, and so they might not detect altered (mutated) forms of the genes and they will not detect phenotypic changes. Amplification targets must be chosen carefully to minimize exclusion of phenotypically pathologic strains. In addition, a narrow molecular primer or probe may not detect a particular strain with an unexpected mutation that prevents efficient amplification or detection. Because of these potential pitfalls, many tests, both commercial and laboratory developed, choose to amplify and/or probe multiple sites within a target locus and to probe for multiple virulence loci, in hopes of maximizing sensitivity or specificity.

### Targets of Amplification

The most common target of molecular testing for STEC is the *stx* operon itself. As described, 2 versions of *stx* exist, *stx1* and *stx2*. In addition to these detection targets, a positive control target, frequently an rRNA gene or a housekeeping gene, is used to verify the detection pipeline. Detection of each of these targets is the minimum for molecular detection of STEC.

Multiplex molecular tests allow detection of additional targets (pathogens) and improvement of assay performance through selection of multiple targets within a single pathogen (e.g., detection of *stx1* and *stx2* in STEC). Additional targets may be chosen from the virulence factors most associated with persistent disease. The β-D-glucuronidase gene *uidA*, discussed in the context of sorbitol and indicator agars, is a frequent target, as are the adhesion factor *eae* and the enterolysin *ehxA/hlyA*. The utility of these targets for verification of detection varies with the correlation of these genes with clinical symptoms, but may also have utility for epidemiologic tracking of an outbreak in progress and for distinguishing between clinical syndromes early in the course of an infection. Indeed, several efforts[134,135] have been made at developing multiplex assays distinguishing common genotypes associated with the pathotypes described in **Table 1**.

An additional application for molecular testing is detection of loci associated with a specific strain of STEC. This application was evaluated during the O104:H4 outbreak,[136,137] and a proof of concept for screening for common non-O157 strains with a PCR primer library has been demonstrated in both research[138] and clinical settings.[139] In the latter case, a stepwise and modular approach was taken to combine PCR serologic identification with Shiga toxin detection: the first round of primers tested for *stx1*, *stx2*, and *eae*, whereas the second round of primers was specific to 5 common serogroups of STEC. This method has been productive in laboratory tests for some time using either the *rfb* locus as the O-serotype target[140] or else a serotype-specific target (*wzx*, *wzy*, and *manC*, among others).[141]

### Laboratory-Developed Tests

Implementation of laboratory-developed tests in different settings illustrates simple and common methods of molecular testing for STEC.[142–144] In each case, 2 target sequences are selected each for the *stx1* and *stx2*, with the primers verified as unique against reference *E coli* sequences and the global NCBI sequence database using the publicly available sequence comparison algorithm BLASTN, provided on the NCBI website. Verification is undertaken against known positive and negative samples or isolates, as determined by serologic and immunologic methods. The specific primer design may be altered to permit alternate amplification methodologies, such as loop-mediated isothermal amplification (LAMP).[145]

Molecular methods can be used to directly test DNA extracts in stool for STEC or, alternatively, *E coli* cultured from stool can be tested to determine whether it is STEC. Detection of STEC from stool by molecular methods poses significant challenges stemming from the heterogenous and varied composition of stool. Specific challenges include the high levels of nucleic acids from the numerous other species of gut flora, and inhibitory substances that prevent the PCR reaction. It is therefore not only necessary to conduct DNA extraction, but it can be helpful to conduct additional purification before proceeding with a molecular test on DNA from stool. In contrast, detection from culture requires only extraction from the colony, and a much more standardized and controlled set of conditions pertains. Detection from culture has proven sufficiently reliable for it to be used as a "gold standard" in clinical trials of EIAs.[144] Direct testing of stool is also valuable, because some studies have suggested that direct stool testing is comparable or improves upon direct EIA testing.[132]

Sensitivity and specificity of molecular assays performed on cultured STEC are typically greater than 90%, although specific assays may perform better or worse with specific strains.[143] Performance is more varied with direct stool detection methods.[146] In a small-scale, head-to-head-to-head evaluation of PCR, EIA, and culture-based methods,[129] PCR outperformed 2 commercial EIAs and SMAC in sensitivity, limits of detection, and breadth of serotype detection.

### Commercial Assays

There are several commercial assays for detection of STEC, both for food product safety testing and for clinical and research use in humans. Not all assays are FDA approved for human diagnostic use, but FDA-approved assays have been available since 2007.[147] In addition, a number of research-use-only assays and assay components (probes, labels, etc) are available for in-house validation in PCR-based detection methods. Although few commercial reference laboratories offer PCR-based detection as yet, a number of commercial systems on the market offer detection either separately or, more frequently, as part of a panel of enteric or gastrointestinal molecular detection assays. FDA-approved multiplex panels that include detection of STEC are increasingly available.

Like the LDTs described, the targets of commercial assays for the specific detection of STEC are primarily the stx1 and stx2. As discussed, careful selection of probe locations is required if variants are not to be excluded. For example, it has been observed that most subtypes of stx1 and stx2 can be found admixed in patient populations, as demonstrated in 1 study in Brussels, Belgium.[148] Comparison of 7 commercially available PCR assays, all targeting stx1 and stx2, was made with strains containing the Stx1a, Stx1c, Stx1d, and Stx2a-g alleles, both singly and in a sparse selection of stx1/stx2 combinations.[149] Of these, only 1 detected all subtypes of stx1 and stx2. Stx2f, a rare subtype, was the most frequently undetected of the alleles, and all of the assays tested detected at least 75% of the variant strains submitted. Although individual assays have been reported in the literature as showing sensitivity and specificity favorable over enzymatic and culture-based methods,[150–155] there remains a relative dearth of publications directly comparing commercially available PCR-based methods in clinical contexts.

Whether additional loci other than the stx1 and stx2 operons are utilized by a commercial method depends on the scope of the test probes. Among assays attempting to detect many different species of enteric pathogens, no further probes are utilized specific to E coli with the EHEC phenotype. However, some assays attempt delineation of E coli pathotypes (see **Table 1**) by the presence of typical genes associated with these pathotypes. Some genes are shared between STEC and these pathotypes; eae, for instance, is held to be a prototypical gene in the EPEC pathotype, but is also found in most STEC strains. These probes may furnish additional verification of an STEC genotype.

**SELF-ASSESSMENT**

1. According to the 2009 CDC Guideline "Recommendations for Diagnosis of Shiga Toxin–Producing *Escherichia coli* Infections by Clinical Laboratories" stools tested for bacterial causes of acute community-acquired diarrhea should be tested for STEC by which of the following assays?
   a. Culture for O157 STEC, with no additional testing.
   b. A test for Shiga toxins or the genes encoding them, with no additional testing.
   c. Both culture for O157 STEC and a test for Shiga toxins or the genes encoding them.
   d. A test for intestinal inflammation, such as lactoferrin or leukocytes.
   e. Matrix-assisted laser desorption/ionization mass spectrometry.

2. Exposure to which of the following has been found NOT to induce increased production of Shiga toxins by STEC?
   a. Azithromycin.
   b. Antibiotics that target DNA synthesis.
   c. Low iron.
   d. Sorbitol.
   e. Tellurite.

3. Which of the following has been demonstrated to be important in determining the sensitivity of immunoassays for detection of Shiga toxins in stool?
   a. The serotype of STEC causing the infection.
   b. The severity of the manifestations of STEC infection.
   c. The method of extraction of the DNA from the stool specimen.
   d. Incubation of the stool in a selective broth before testing.
   e. Heat inactivation of the specimen before testing.

ANSWERS

Answer 1: c.

The CDC guideline calls for dual testing for O157 STEC and Shiga toxins to optimize the sensitivity of testing for STEC, the speed at which the organism is detected, and the speed at which the organism is available for serotyping at a reference (regional) laboratory for epidemiologic purposes such as outbreak detection.

Answer 2: a.

Exposure to specific stressors or conditions, including antibiotics that target DNA synthesis and low iron levels, has been shown to induce increased production of Shiga toxins by STEC; however, azithromycin does not have this effect. This has led to the controversial suggestion that azithromycin therapy might not be contraindicated in patients with STEC infection.

Answer 3: d.

Incubation of stool in a selective broth, such as MacConkey broth, before testing in immunoassays has been demonstrated to increase the sensitivity of testing.

**REFERENCES**

1. Iyoda S, Tamura K, Itoh K, et al. Inducible stx2 phages are lysogenized in the enteroaggregative and other phenotypic Escherichia coli O86:HNM isolated from patients. FEMS Microbiol Lett 2000;191(1):7–10.
2. Morabito S, Karch H, Mariani-Kurkdjian P, et al. Enteroaggregative, Shiga toxin-producing Escherichia coli O111:H2 associated with an outbreak of hemolytic-uremic syndrome. J Clin Microbiol 1998;36(3):840–2.
3. Frank C, Werber D, Cramer JP, et al. Epidemic profile of Shiga-toxin-producing Escherichia coli O104:H4 outbreak in Germany. N Engl J Med 2011;365(19):1771–80.
4. Barrett TJ, Kaper JB, Jerse AE, et al. Virulence factors in Shiga-like toxin-producing Escherichia coli isolated from humans and cattle. J Infect Dis 1992;165(5):979–80.
5. Karmali MA. Infection by verocytotoxin-producing Escherichia coli. Clin Microbiol Rev 1989;2(1):15–38.
6. Konowalchuk J, Speirs JI, Stavric S. Vero response to a cytotoxin of Escherichia coli. Infect Immun 1977;18(3):775–9.
7. Lan R, Alles MC, Donohoe K, et al. Molecular evolutionary relationships of enteroinvasive Escherichia coli and Shigella spp. Infect Immun 2004;72(9):5080–8.
8. Huang A, Friesen J, Brunton JL. Characterization of a bacteriophage that carries the genes for production of Shiga-like toxin 1 in Escherichia coli. J Bacteriol 1987;169(9):4308–12.

9. Datz M, Janetzki-Mittmann C, Franke S, et al. Analysis of the enterohemorrhagic Escherichia coli O157 DNA region containing lambdoid phage gene p and Shiga-like toxin structural genes. Appl Environ Microbiol 1996;62(3):791–7.

10. Strockbine NA, Jackson MP, Sung LM, et al. Cloning and sequencing of the genes for Shiga toxin from Shigella dysenteriae type 1. J Bacteriol 1988; 170(3):1116–22.

11. Seidah NG, Donohue-Rolfe A, Lazure C, et al. Complete amino acid sequence of Shigella toxin B-chain. A novel polypeptide containing 69 amino acids and one disulfide bridge. J Biol Chem 1986;261(30):13928–31.

12. Scotland SM, Smith HR, Rowe B. Two distinct toxins active on Vero cells from Escherichia coli O157. Lancet 1985;2(8460):885–6.

13. Strockbine NA, Marques LR, Newland JW, et al. Two toxin-converting phages from Escherichia coli O157:H7 strain 933 encode antigenically distinct toxins with similar biologic activities. Infect Immun 1986;53(1):135–40.

14. O'Brien AD, Newland JW, Miller SF, et al. Shiga-like toxin-converting phages from Escherichia coli strains that cause hemorrhagic colitis or infantile diarrhea. Science 1984;226(4675):694–6.

15. Smith HW, Green P, Parsell Z. Vero cell toxins in Escherichia coli and related bacteria: transfer by phage and conjugation and toxic action in laboratory animals, chickens and pigs. J Gen Microbiol 1983;129(10):3121–37.

16. Fraser ME, Chernaia MM, Kozlov YV, et al. Crystal structure of the holotoxin from Shigella dysenteriae at 2.5 A resolution. Nat Struct Biol 1994;1(1):59–64.

17. Fraser ME, Fujinaga M, Cherney MM, et al. Structure of Shiga toxin type 2 (Stx2) from Escherichia coli O157:H7. J Biol Chem 2004;279(26):27511–7.

18. Beddoe T, Paton AW, Le Nours J, et al. Structure, biological functions and applications of the AB5 toxins. Trends Biochem Sci 2010;35(7):411–8.

19. Calderwood SB, Mekalanos JJ. Iron regulation of Shiga-like toxin expression in Escherichia coli is mediated by the fur locus. J Bacteriol 1987;169(10): 4759–64.

20. Los JM, Los M, Wegrzyn G, et al. Differential efficiency of induction of various lambdoid prophages responsible for production of Shiga toxins in response to different induction agents. Microb Pathog 2009;47(6):289–98.

21. McGannon CM, Fuller CA, Weiss AA. Different classes of antibiotics differentially influence Shiga toxin production. Antimicrob Agents Chemother 2010;54(9): 3790–8.

22. Kolling GL, Matthews KR. Export of virulence genes and Shiga toxin by membrane vesicles of Escherichia coli O157:H7. Appl Environ Microbiol 1999; 65(5):1843–8.

23. Yokoyama K, Horii T, Yamashino T, et al. Production of Shiga toxin by Escherichia coli measured with reference to the membrane vesicle-associated toxins. FEMS Microbiol Lett 2000;192(1):139–44.

24. Shimizu T, Ohta Y, Noda M. Shiga toxin 2 is specifically released from bacterial cells by two different mechanisms. Infect Immun 2009;77(7):2813–23.

25. Jacewicz MS, Mobassaleh M, Gross SK, et al. Pathogenesis of Shigella diarrhea: XVII. A mammalian cell membrane glycolipid, Gb3, is required but not sufficient to confer sensitivity to Shiga toxin. J Infect Dis 1994;169(3):538–46.

26. Holgersson J, Jovall PA, Breimer ME. Glycosphingolipids of human large intestine: detailed structural characterization with special reference to blood group compounds and bacterial receptor structures. J Biochem 1991;110(1):120–31.

27. Schuller S, Heuschkel R, Torrente F, et al. Shiga toxin binding in normal and inflamed human intestinal mucosa. Microbes Infect 2007;9(1):35–9.

28. Brigotti M, Tazzari PL, Ravanelli E, et al. Clinical relevance of Shiga toxin concentrations in the blood of patients with hemolytic uremic syndrome. Pediatr Infect Dis J 2011;30(6):486–90.
29. Brigotti M, Carnicelli D, Arfilli V, et al. Identification of TLR4 as the receptor that recognizes Shiga toxins in human neutrophils. J Immunol 2013;191(9):4748–58.
30. Schuller S. Shiga toxin interaction with human intestinal epithelium. Toxins (Basel) 2011;3(6):626–39.
31. Boyd B, Lingwood C. Verotoxin receptor glycolipid in human renal tissue. Nephron 1989;51(2):207–10.
32. Sandvig K, van Deurs B. Endocytosis, intracellular transport, and cytotoxic action of Shiga toxin and ricin. Physiol Rev 1996;76(4):949–66.
33. Garred O, van Deurs B, Sandvig K. Furin-induced cleavage and activation of Shiga toxin. J Biol Chem 1995;270(18):10817–21.
34. Endo Y, Tsurugi K, Yutsudo T, et al. Site of action of a Vero toxin (VT2) from Escherichia coli O157:H7 and of Shiga toxin on eukaryotic ribosomes. RNA N-glycosidase activity of the toxins. Eur J Biochem 1988;171(1–2):45–50.
35. Smith WE, Kane AV, Campbell ST, et al. Shiga toxin 1 triggers a ribotoxic stress response leading to p38 and JNK activation and induction of apoptosis in intestinal epithelial cells. Infect Immun 2003;71(3):1497–504.
36. Beebakhee G, Louie M, De Azavedo J, et al. Cloning and nucleotide sequence of the eae gene homologue from enterohemorrhagic Escherichia coli serotype O157:H7. FEMS Microbiol Lett 1992;70(1):63–8.
37. McDaniel TK, Jarvis KG, Donnenberg MS, et al. A genetic locus of enterocyte effacement conserved among diverse enterobacterial pathogens. Proc Natl Acad Sci U S A 1995;92(5):1664–8.
38. Donnenberg MS, Kaper JB, Finlay BB. Interactions between enteropathogenic Escherichia coli and host epithelial cells. Trends Microbiol 1997;5(3):109–14.
39. Louie M, de Azavedo J, Clarke R, et al. Sequence heterogeneity of the eae gene and detection of verotoxin-producing Escherichia coli using serotype-specific primers. Epidemiol Infect 1994;112(3):449–61.
40. Doughty S, Sloan J, Bennett-Wood V, et al. Identification of a novel fimbrial gene cluster related to long polar fimbriae in locus of enterocyte effacement-negative strains of enterohemorrhagic Escherichia coli. Infect Immun 2002;70(12):6761–9.
41. Paton AW, Srimanote P, Woodrow MC, et al. Characterization of Saa, a novel autoagglutinating adhesin produced by locus of enterocyte effacement-negative Shiga-toxigenic Escherichia coli strains that are virulent for humans. Infect Immun 2001;69(11):6999–7009.
42. Centers for Disease Control and Prevention (CDC). Outbreak of Escherichia coli O104:H4 infections associated with sprout consumption - Europe and North America, May-July 2011. MMWR Morb Mortal Wkly Rep 2013;62(50):1029–31.
43. Bielaszewska M, Mellmann A, Zhang W, et al. Characterisation of the Escherichia coli strain associated with an outbreak of haemolytic uraemic syndrome in Germany, 2011: a microbiological study. Lancet Infect Dis 2011;11(9):671–6.
44. Brzuszkiewicz E, Thurmer A, Schuldes J, et al. Genome sequence analyses of two isolates from the recent Escherichia coli outbreak in Germany reveal the emergence of a new pathotype: Entero-Aggregative-Haemorrhagic Escherichia coli (EAHEC). Arch Microbiol 2011;193(12):883–91.
45. Ho CC, Yuen KY, Lau SK, et al. Rapid identification and validation of specific molecular targets for detection of Escherichia coli O104:H4 outbreak strain by use of high-throughput sequencing data from nine genomes. J Clin Microbiol 2011;49(10):3714–6.

46. Rohde H, Qin J, Cui Y, et al. Open-source genomic analysis of Shiga-toxin-producing E. coli O104:H4. N Engl J Med 2011;365(8):718–24.

47. Rasko DA, Webster DR, Sahl JW, et al. Origins of the E. coli strain causing an outbreak of hemolytic-uremic syndrome in Germany. N Engl J Med 2011; 365(8):709–17.

48. Kauffmann F. The serology of the coli group. J Immunol 1947;57(1):71–100.

49. Wolf MK. Occurrence, distribution, and associations of O and H serogroups, colonization factor antigens, and toxins of enterotoxigenic Escherichia coli. Clin Microbiol Rev 1997;10(4):569–84.

50. Rangel JM, Sparling PH, Crowe C, et al. Epidemiology of Escherichia coli O157:H7 outbreaks, United States, 1982–2002. Emerg Infect Dis 2005;11(4):603–9.

51. Byrne L, Vanstone GL, Perry NT, et al. Epidemiology and microbiology of Shiga toxin-producing Escherichia coli other than serogroup O157 in England, 2009–2013. J Med Microbiol 2014;63(Pt 9):1181–8.

52. Karmali MA, Steele BT, Petric M, et al. Sporadic cases of haemolytic-uraemic syndrome associated with faecal cytotoxin and cytotoxin-producing Escherichia coli in stools. Lancet 1983;1(8325):619–20.

53. Riley LW, Remis RS, Helgerson SD, et al. Hemorrhagic colitis associated with a rare Escherichia coli serotype. N Engl J Med 1983;308(12):681–5.

54. O'Brien AO, Lively TA, Chen ME, et al. Escherichia coli O157:H7 strains associated with haemorrhagic colitis in the United States produce a Shigella dysenteriae 1 (SHIGA) like cytotoxin. Lancet 1983;1(8326 Pt 1):702.

55. Wells JG, Davis BR, Wachsmuth IK, et al. Laboratory investigation of hemorrhagic colitis outbreaks associated with a rare Escherichia coli serotype. J Clin Microbiol 1983;18(3):512–20.

56. Centers for Disease Control and Prevention (CDC). Importance of culture confirmation of Shiga toxin-producing Escherichia coli infection as illustrated by outbreaks of gastroenteritis–New York and North Carolina, 2005. MMWR Morb Mortal Wkly Rep 2006;55(38):1042–5.

57. Centers for Disease Control and Prevention (CDC). Laboratory-confirmed non-O157 Shiga toxin-producing Escherichia coli–Connecticut, 2000–2005. MMWR Morb Mortal Wkly Rep 2007;56(2):29–31.

58. Centers for Disease Control and Prevention (CDC). Vital signs: incidence and trends of infection with pathogens transmitted commonly through food–food-borne diseases active surveillance network, 10 U.S. sites, 1996–2010. MMWR Morb Mortal Wkly Rep 2011;60(22):749–55.

59. Smith JL, Fratamico PM. Gunther NWt. Shiga toxin-producing Escherichia coli. Adv Appl Microbiol 2014;86:145–97.

60. Davis TK, McKee R, Schnadower D, et al. Treatment of Shiga toxin-producing Escherichia coli infections. Infect Dis Clin North Am 2013;27(3):577–97.

61. Tarr PI, Gordon CA, Chandler WL. Shiga-toxin-producing Escherichia coli and haemolytic uraemic syndrome. Lancet 2005;365(9464):1073–86.

62. Su C, Brandt LJ. Escherichia coli O157:H7 infection in humans. Ann Intern Med 1995;123(9):698–714.

63. Boyce TG, Swerdlow DL, Griffin PM. Escherichia coli O157:H7 and the hemolytic-uremic syndrome. N Engl J Med 1995;333(6):364–8.

64. Mayer CL, Leibowitz CS, Kurosawa S, et al. Shiga toxins and the pathophysiology of hemolytic uremic syndrome in humans and animals. Toxins (Basel) 2012;4(11):1261–87.

65. Marshall JK. Post-infectious irritable bowel syndrome following water contamination. Kidney Int Suppl 2009;(112):S42–3.

66. Ho NK, Henry AC, Johnson-Henry K, et al. Pathogenicity, host responses and implications for management of enterohemorrhagic Escherichia coli O157:H7 infection. Can J Gastroenterol 2013;27(5):281–5.

67. Bielaszewska M, Mellmann A, Bletz S, et al. Enterohemorrhagic Escherichia coli O26:H11/H-: a new virulent clone emerges in Europe. Clin Infect Dis 2013; 56(10):1373–81.

68. Rahal EA, Kazzi N, Nassar FJ, et al. Escherichia coli O157:H7-Clinical aspects and novel treatment approaches. Front Cell Infect Microbiol 2012;2:138.

69. Hauswaldt S, Nitschke M, Sayk F, et al. Lessons learned from outbreaks of Shiga toxin producing Escherichia coli. Curr Infect Dis Rep 2013;15(1):4–9.

70. Thielman NM, Guerrant RL. Clinical practice. Acute infectious diarrhea. N Engl J Med 2004;350(1):38–47.

71. Nelson JM, Griffin PM, Jones TF, et al. Antimicrobial and antimotility agent use in persons with Shiga toxin-producing Escherichia coli O157 infection in FoodNet Sites. Clin Infect Dis 2011;52(9):1130–2.

72. Bell BP, Griffin PM, Lozano P, et al. Predictors of hemolytic uremic syndrome in children during a large outbreak of Escherichia coli O157:H7 infections. Pediatrics 1997;100(1):E12.

73. Proulx F, Turgeon JP, Delage G, et al. Randomized, controlled trial of antibiotic therapy for Escherichia coli O157:H7 enteritis. J Pediatr 1992;121(2):299–303.

74. Smith KE, Wilker PR, Reiter PL, et al. Antibiotic treatment of Escherichia coli O157 infection and the risk of hemolytic uremic syndrome, Minnesota. Pediatr Infect Dis J 2012;31(1):37–41.

75. Wong CS, Mooney JC, Brandt JR, et al. Risk factors for the hemolytic uremic syndrome in children infected with Escherichia coli O157:H7: a multivariable analysis. Clin Infect Dis 2012;55(1):33–41.

76. Wong CS, Jelacic S, Habeeb RL, et al. The risk of the hemolytic-uremic syndrome after antibiotic treatment of Escherichia coli O157:H7 infections. N Engl J Med 2000;342(26):1930–6.

77. Kimmitt PT, Harwood CR, Barer MR. Toxin gene expression by Shiga toxin-producing Escherichia coli: the role of antibiotics and the bacterial SOS response. Emerg Infect Dis 2000;6(5):458–65.

78. Bielaszewska M, Idelevich EA, Zhang W, et al. Effects of antibiotics on Shiga toxin 2 production and bacteriophage induction by epidemic Escherichia coli O104:H4 strain. Antimicrob Agents Chemother 2012;56(6):3277–82.

79. Nitschke M, Sayk F, Hartel C, et al. Association between azithromycin therapy and duration of bacterial shedding among patients with Shiga toxin-producing enteroaggregative Escherichia coli O104:H4. JAMA 2012;307(10):1046–52.

80. Vonberg RP, Hohle M, Aepfelbacher M, et al. Duration of fecal shedding of Shiga toxin-producing Escherichia coli O104:H4 in patients infected during the 2011 outbreak in Germany: a multicenter study. Clin Infect Dis 2013;56(8):1132–40.

81. Lapeyraque AL, Malina M, Fremeaux-Bacchi V, et al. Eculizumab in severe Shiga-toxin-associated HUS. N Engl J Med 2011;364(26):2561–3.

82. Menne J, Nitschke M, Stingele R, et al. Validation of treatment strategies for enterohaemorrhagic Escherichia coli O104:H4 induced haemolytic uraemic syndrome: case-control study. BMJ 2012;345:e4565.

83. Mukhopadhyay S, Linstedt AD. Manganese blocks intracellular trafficking of Shiga toxin and protects against Shiga toxicosis. Science 2012;335(6066):332–5.

84. Majowicz SE, Scallan E, Jones-Bitton A, et al. Global incidence of human Shiga toxin-producing Escherichia coli infections and deaths: a systematic review and knowledge synthesis. Foodborne Pathog Dis 2014;11(6):447–55.

85. Pruimboom-Brees IM, Morgan TW, Ackermann MR, et al. Cattle lack vascular receptors for Escherichia coli O157:H7 Shiga toxins. Proc Natl Acad Sci U S A 2000;97(19):10325–9.

86. Conedera G, Mattiazzi E, Russo F, et al. A family outbreak of Escherichia coli O157 haemorrhagic colitis caused by pork meat salami. Epidemiol Infect 2007;135(2):311–4.

87. Ferguson DD, Scheftel J, Cronquist A, et al. Temporally distinct Escherichia coli O157 outbreaks associated with alfalfa sprouts linked to a common seed source–Colorado and Minnesota, 2003. Epidemiol Infect 2005;133(3):439–47.

88. Grant J, Wendelboe AM, Wendel A, et al. Spinach-associated Escherichia coli O157:H7 outbreak, Utah and New Mexico, 2006. Emerg Infect Dis 2008; 14(10):1633–6.

89. Neil KP, Biggerstaff G, MacDonald JK, et al. A novel vehicle for transmission of Escherichia coli O157:H7 to humans: multistate outbreak of E. coli O157:H7 infections associated with consumption of ready-to-bake commercial prepackaged cookie dough–United States, 2009. Clin Infect Dis 2012;54(4): 511–8.

90. Crump JA, Sulka AC, Langer AJ, et al. An outbreak of Escherichia coli O157:H7 infections among visitors to a dairy farm. N Engl J Med 2002;347(8):555–60.

91. Crump JA, Braden CR, Dey ME, et al. Outbreaks of Escherichia coli O157 infections at multiple county agricultural fairs: a hazard of mixing cattle, concession stands and children. Epidemiol Infect 2003;131(3):1055–62.

92. Hale CR, Scallan E, Cronquist AB, et al. Estimates of enteric illness attributable to contact with animals and their environments in the United States. Clin Infect Dis 2012;54(Suppl 5):S472–9.

93. Paunio M, Pebody R, Keskimaki M, et al. Swimming-associated outbreak of Escherichia coli O157:H7. Epidemiol Infect 1999;122(1):1–5.

94. Friedman MS, Roels T, Koehler JE, et al. Escherichia coli O157:H7 outbreak associated with an improperly chlorinated swimming pool. Clin Infect Dis 1999;29(2):298–303.

95. Panaro L, Cooke D, Borczyk A. Outbreak of Escherichia coli O157:H7 in a nursing home–Ontario. Can Dis Wkly Rep 1990;16(19):90–2.

96. Scallan E, Hoekstra RM, Angulo FJ, et al. Foodborne illness acquired in the United States–major pathogens. Emerg Infect Dis 2011;17(1):7–15.

97. Scallan E, Mahon BE, Hoekstra RM, et al. Estimates of illnesses, hospitalizations and deaths caused by major bacterial enteric pathogens in young children in the United States. Pediatr Infect Dis J 2013;32(3):217–21.

98. Buchholz U, Bernard H, Werber D, et al. German outbreak of Escherichia coli O104:H4 associated with sprouts. N Engl J Med 2011;365(19):1763–70.

99. Beutin L, Martin A. Outbreak of Shiga toxin-producing Escherichia coli (STEC) O104:H4 infection in Germany causes a paradigm shift with regard to human pathogenicity of STEC strains. J Food Prot 2012;75(2):408–18.

100. Gould LH, Bopp C, Strockbine N, et al. Recommendations for diagnosis of Shiga toxin–producing Escherichia coli infections by clinical laboratories. MMWR Recomm Rep 2009;58(RR-12):1–14.

101. Hermos CR, Janineh M, Han LL, et al. Shiga toxin-producing Escherichia coli in children: diagnosis and clinical manifestations of O157:H7 and non-O157:H7 infection. J Clin Microbiol 2011;49(3):955–9.

102. Schindler EI, Sellenriek P, Storch GA, et al. Shiga toxin-producing Escherichia coli: a single-center, 11-year pediatric experience. J Clin Microbiol 2014; 52(10):3647–53.

103. Marcon MJ. Point: should all stools be screened for Shiga toxin-producing Escherichia coli? J Clin Microbiol 2011;49(7):2390–4.

104. Kiska DL, Riddell SW. Counterpoint: should all stools be screened for Shiga toxin-producing Escherichia coli? J Clin Microbiol 2011;49(7):2394–7.

105. Bettelheim KA. Reliability of CHROMagar O157 for the detection of enterohaemorrhagic Escherichia coli (EHEC) O157 but not EHEC belonging to other serogroups. J Appl Microbiol 1998;85(3):425–8.

106. Church DL, Emshey D, Semeniuk H, et al. Evaluation of BBL CHROMagar O157 versus sorbitol-MacConkey medium for routine detection of Escherichia coli O157 in a centralized regional clinical microbiology laboratory. J Clin Microbiol 2007;45(9):3098–100.

107. Hirvonen JJ, Siitonen A, Kaukoranta SS. Usability and performance of CHROMagar STEC medium in detection of Shiga toxin-producing Escherichia coli strains. J Clin Microbiol 2012;50(11):3586–90.

108. Gouali M, Ruckly C, Carle I, et al. Evaluation of CHROMagar STEC and STEC O104 chromogenic agar media for detection of Shiga toxin-producing Escherichia coli in stool specimens. J Clin Microbiol 2013;51(3):894–900.

109. Gill A, Huszczynski G, Gauthier M, et al. Evaluation of eight agar media for the isolation of shiga toxin-Producing Escherichia coli. J Microbiol Methods 2014; 96:6–11.

110. Manning SD, Madera RT, Schneider W, et al. Surveillance for Shiga toxin-producing Escherichia coli, Michigan, 2001–2005. Emerg Infect Dis 2007; 13(2):318–21.

111. Zadik PM, Chapman PA, Siddons CA. Use of tellurite for the selection of verocytotoxigenic Escherichia coli O157. J Med Microbiol 1993;39(2):155–8.

112. Chapman PA, Siddons CA. A comparison of immunomagnetic separation and direct culture for the isolation of verocytotoxin-producing Escherichia coli O157 from cases of bloody diarrhoea, non-bloody diarrhoea and asymptomatic contacts. J Med Microbiol 1996;44(4):267–71.

113. Karch H, Janetzki-Mittmann C, Aleksic S, et al. Isolation of enterohemorrhagic Escherichia coli O157 strains from patients with hemolytic-uremic syndrome by using immunomagnetic separation, DNA-based methods, and direct culture. J Clin Microbiol 1996;34(3):516–9.

114. Farmer JJ 3rd, Davis BR. H7 antiserum-sorbitol fermentation medium: a single tube screening medium for detecting Escherichia coli O157:H7 associated with hemorrhagic colitis. J Clin Microbiol 1985;22(4):620–5.

115. March SB, Ratnam S. Sorbitol-MacConkey medium for detection of Escherichia coli O157:H7 associated with hemorrhagic colitis. J Clin Microbiol 1986;23(5): 869–72.

116. Feng P, Lum R, Chang GW. Identification of uidA gene sequences in beta-D-glucuronidase-negative Escherichia coli. Appl Environ Microbiol 1991;57(1):320–3.

117. Feng P, Lampel KA. Genetic analysis of uidA expression in enterohaemorrhagic Escherichia coli serotype O157:H7. Microbiology 1994;140(Pt 8):2101–7.

118. Onoue Y, Konuma H, Nakagawa H, et al. Collaborative evaluation of detection methods for Escherichia coli O157:H7 from radish sprouts and ground beef. Int J Food Microbiol 1999;46(1):27–36.

119. De Boer E, Heuvelink AE. Methods for the detection and isolation of Shiga toxin-producing Escherichia coli. Symp Ser Soc Appl Microbiol 2000;29:133S–43S.

120. Taylor DE. Bacterial tellurite resistance. Trends Microbiol 1999;7(3):111–5.

121. Bielaszewska M, Tarr PI, Karch H, et al. Phenotypic and molecular analysis of tellurite resistance among enterohemorrhagic Escherichia coli O157:H7 and

sorbitol-fermenting O157:NM clinical isolates. J Clin Microbiol 2005;43(1): 452–4.

122. Orth D, Grif K, Dierich MP, et al. Variability in tellurite resistance and the ter gene cluster among Shiga toxin-producing Escherichia coli isolated from humans, animals and food. Res Microbiol 2007;158(2):105–11.

123. Gill A, Martinez-Perez A, McIlwham S, et al. Development of a method for the detection of verotoxin-producing Escherichia coli in food. J Food Prot 2012; 75(5):827–37.

124. Teramura H, Sekiguchi J, Inoue K. A novel chromogenic screening medium for isolation of enterohemorrhagic Escherichia coli. Biocontrol Sci 2013;18(2):111–5.

125. Grif K, Orth D, Dierich MP, et al. Comparison of an immunochromatographic rapid test with enzyme-linked immunosorbent assay and polymerase chain reaction for the detection of Shiga toxins from human stool samples. Diagn Microbiol Infect Dis 2007;59(1):97–9.

126. Park CH, Kim HJ, Hixon DL, et al. Evaluation of the duopath verotoxin test for detection of shiga toxins in cultures of human stools. J Clin Microbiol 2003; 41(6):2650–3.

127. Stapp JR, Jelacic S, Yea YL, et al. Comparison of Escherichia coli O157:H7 antigen detection in stool and broth cultures to that in sorbitol-MacConkey agar stool cultures. J Clin Microbiol 2000;38(9):3404–6.

128. Kehl KS, Havens P, Behnke CE, et al. Evaluation of the premier EHEC assay for detection of Shiga toxin-producing Escherichia coli. J Clin Microbiol 1997;35(8):2051–4.

129. Vallieres E, Saint-Jean M, Rallu F. Comparison of three different methods for detection of Shiga toxin-producing Escherichia coli in a tertiary pediatric care center. J Clin Microbiol 2013;51(2):481–6.

130. Gavin PJ, Peterson LR, Pasquariello AC, et al. Evaluation of performance and potential clinical impact of ProSpecT Shiga toxin Escherichia coli microplate assay for detection of Shiga toxin-producing E. coli in stool samples. J Clin Microbiol 2004;42(4):1652–6.

131. Mackenzie A, Orrbine E, Hyde L, et al. Performance of the ImmunoCard STAT! E. coli O157:H7 test for detection of Escherichia coli O157:H7 in stools. J Clin Microbiol 2000;38(5):1866–8.

132. Gerritzen A, Wittke JW, Wolff D. Rapid and sensitive detection of Shiga toxin-producing Escherichia coli directly from stool samples by real-time PCR in comparison to culture, enzyme immunoassay and Vero cell cytotoxicity assay. Clin Lab 2011;57(11–12):993–8.

133. Chui L, Lee MC, Malejczyk K, et al. Prevalence of shiga toxin-producing Escherichia coli as detected by enzyme-linked immunoassays and real-time PCR during the summer months in northern Alberta, Canada. J Clin Microbiol 2011; 49(12):4307–10.

134. Botkin DJ, Galli L, Sankarapani V, et al. Development of a multiplex PCR assay for detection of Shiga toxin-producing Escherichia coli, enterohemorrhagic E. coli, and enteropathogenic E. coli strains. Front Cell Infect Microbiol 2012;2:8.

135. Barletta F, Ochoa TJ, Cleary TG. Multiplex real-time PCR (MRT-PCR) for diarrheagenic. Methods Mol Biol 2013;943:307–14.

136. Delannoy S, Beutin L, Burgos Y, et al. Specific detection of enteroaggregative hemorrhagic Escherichia coli O104:H4 strains by use of the CRISPR locus as a target for a diagnostic real-time PCR. J Clin Microbiol 2012;50(11):3485–92.

137. Zhang W, Bielaszewska M, Bauwens A, et al. Real-time multiplex PCR for detecting Shiga toxin 2-producing Escherichia coli O104:H4 in human stools. J Clin Microbiol 2012;50(5):1752–4.

138. Conrad CC, Gilroyed BH, McAllister TA, et al. Synthesis of O-serogroup specific positive controls and real-time PCR standards for nine clinically relevant non-O157 STECs. J Microbiol Methods 2012;91(1):52–6.

139. Kagkli DM, Weber TP, Van den Bulcke M, et al. Application of the modular approach to an in-house validation study of real-time PCR methods for the detection and serogroup determination of verocytotoxigenic Escherichia coli. Appl Environ Microbiol 2011;77(19):6954–63.

140. Paton AW, Paton JC. Detection and characterization of Shiga toxigenic Escherichia coli by using multiplex PCR assays for stx1, stx2, eaeA, enterohemorrhagic E. coli hlyA, rfbO111, and rfbO157. J Clin Microbiol 1998;36(2):598–602.

141. Anklam KS, Kanankege KS, Gonzales TK, et al. Rapid and reliable detection of Shiga toxin-producing Escherichia coli by real-time multiplex PCR. J Food Prot 2012;75(4):643–50.

142. Lefterova MI, Slater KA, Budvytiene I, et al. A sensitive multiplex, real-time PCR assay for prospective detection of Shiga toxin-producing Escherichia coli from stool samples reveals similar incidences but variable severities of non-O157 and O157 infections in northern California. J Clin Microbiol 2013; 51(9):3000–5.

143. Chui L, Couturier MR, Chiu T, et al. Comparison of Shiga toxin-producing Escherichia coli detection methods using clinical stool samples. J Mol Diagn 2010;12(4):469–75.

144. Chui L, Lee MC, Allen R, et al. Comparison between ImmunoCard STAT!((R)) and real-time PCR as screening tools for both O157:H7 and non-O157 Shiga toxin-producing Escherichia coli in Southern Alberta, Canada. Diagn Microbiol Infect Dis 2013;77(1):8–13.

145. Wang F, Jiang L, Ge B. Loop-mediated isothermal amplification assays for detecting shiga toxin-producing Escherichia coli in ground beef and human stools. J Clin Microbiol 2012;50(1):91–7.

146. Holland JL, Louie L, Simor AE, et al. PCR detection of Escherichia coli O157:H7 directly from stools: evaluation of commercial extraction methods for purifying fecal DNA. J Clin Microbiol 2000;38(11):4108–13.

147. Persson S, Olsen KE, Scheutz F, et al. A method for fast and simple detection of major diarrhoeagenic Escherichia coli in the routine diagnostic laboratory. Clin Microbiol Infect 2007;13(5):516–24.

148. Buvens G, De Gheldre Y, Dediste A, et al. Incidence and virulence determinants of verocytotoxin-producing Escherichia coli infections in the Brussels-Capital Region, Belgium, in 2008–2010. J Clin Microbiol 2012;50(4):1336–45.

149. Margot H, Cernela N, Iversen C, et al. Evaluation of seven different commercially available real-time PCR assays for detection of shiga toxin 1 and 2 gene subtypes. J Food Prot 2013;76(5):871–3.

150. Grys TE, Sloan LM, Rosenblatt JE, et al. Rapid and sensitive detection of Shiga toxin-producing Escherichia coli from nonenriched stool specimens by real-time PCR in comparison to enzyme immunoassay and culture. J Clin Microbiol 2009; 47(7):2008–12.

151. Buchan BW, Olson WJ, Pezewski M, et al. Clinical evaluation of a real-time PCR assay for identification of Salmonella, Shigella, Campylobacter (Campylobacter jejuni and C. coli), and shiga toxin-producing Escherichia coli isolates in stool specimens. J Clin Microbiol 2013;51(12):4001–7.

152. Koziel M, Kiely R, Blake L, et al. Improved detection of bacterial pathogens in patients presenting with gastroenteritis by use of the EntericBio real-time Gastro Panel I assay. J Clin Microbiol 2013;51(8):2679–85.

153. Koziel M, Corcoran D, O'Callaghan I, et al. Validation of the EntericBio Panel II(R) multiplex polymerase chain reaction system for detection of Campylobacter spp., Salmonella spp., Shigella spp., and verotoxigenic E. coli for use in a clinical diagnostic setting. Diagn Microbiol Infect Dis 2013;75(1):46–9.

154. Cremonesi P, Pisani LF, Lecchi C, et al. Development of 23 individual TaqMan(R) real-time PCR assays for identifying common foodborne pathogens using a single set of amplification conditions. Food Microbiol 2014;43:35–40.

155. Anderson NW, Buchan BW, Ledeboer NA. Comparison of the BD MAX enteric bacterial panel to routine culture methods for detection of Campylobacter, enterohemorrhagic Escherichia coli (O157), Salmonella, and Shigella isolates in preserved stool specimens. J Clin Microbiol 2014;52(4):1222–4.

156. Brooks JT, Sowers EG, Wells JG, et al. Non-O157 Shiga toxin-producing Escherichia coli infections in the United States, 1983–2002. J Infect Dis 2005;192(8): 1422–9.

157. Werber D, Beutin L, Pichner R, et al. Shiga toxin-producing Escherichia coli serogroups in food and patients, Germany. Emerg Infect Dis 2008;14(11):1803–6.

158. Hiroi M, Takahashi N, Harada T, et al. Serotype, Shiga toxin (Stx) type, and antimicrobial resistance of Stx-producing Escherichia coli isolated from humans in Shizuoka Prefecture, Japan (2003–2007). Jpn J Infect Dis 2012;65(3):198–202.

# Vibriosis

J. Michael Janda, PhD, D(ABMM)[a], Anna E. Newton, MPH[b],
Cheryl A. Bopp, MS[c],*

## KEYWORDS

- Vibriosis • *Vibrio* • Cholera • Marine • Aquatic • *V vulnificus* • Seafood

## KEY POINTS

- Vibrio infections are increasing in the United States.
- Chief risk factors associated with vibriosis include consumption of raw or undercooked seafood or shellfish, and trauma associated with the marine environment.
- A detailed medical history is necessary in order to suspect vibriosis, and this includes direct or indirect aquatic exposures.
- Two life-threatening vibrio infections are cholera and necrotizing fasciitis; septicemia can occasionally be observed as a primary infection or secondary complication of serious disease as well.
- Specialized media are necessary to isolate vibrios in cases of diarrheal disease.

## HISTORY AND GENERAL EPIDEMIOLOGY

Vibriosis is the general name for a group of clinical conditions of varying severity typically associated with the genus *Vibrio*, whose members are facultatively anaerobic, cytochrome oxidase–positive, gram-negative bacilli, many of which require salt for growth. These illnesses can range from mild cases of gastroenteritis to life-threatening situations such as septicemia and invasive skin and soft tissue infections (SSTI). In the past, all of these infections were attributed to species residing in the genus *Vibrio*, which were linked together by common phenotypes, habitats, modes of transmission, and disease syndromes (eg, gastroenteritis). However, with the introduction of polyphasic taxonomy, phylogenetic analysis assessing multiple house-keeping genes, and DNA-DNA hybridization, it is now known that several of these

Disclosures: The authors have no relevant financial or nonfinancial relationships with the products described in this article.
[a] Department of Public Health, Alameda County Public Health Laboratory, 1000 Broadway, Suite 500, Oakland, CA 94607, USA; [b] Enteric Diseases Epidemiology Branch, Division of Foodborne, Waterborne and Environmental Diseases, Centers for Disease Control and Prevention, 1600 Clifton Road, Atlanta, GA 30333, USA; [c] Enteric Diseases Laboratory Branch, Division of Foodborne, Waterborne and Environmental Diseases, Centers for Disease Control and Prevention, 1600 Clifton Road, Atlanta, GA 30333, USA
* Corresponding author.
*E-mail address:* cherylbopp@gmail.com

species traditionally thought to be *Vibrio* belong to genera distinct from core members including *Vibrio cholerae*. These taxa include *Grimontia* (*Vibrio*) *hollisae* and *Photobacterium* (*Vibrio*) *damselae*, which have already been reclassified to new or established genera, whereas still others, such as *Vibrio parahaemolyticus* and *Vibrio alginolyticus*, continue to reside in the genus *Vibrio* but merit consideration for transfer and reclassification to another genus based on phylogenetic evidence.[1]

Members of the genus *Vibrio*, which total more than 100 species, are predominantly associated with a variety of marine, estuarine, or other aquatic habitats.[2] The limited exception to this rule are the nonhalophilic, or non–salt-requiring, species *V cholerae* and *Vibrio mimicus*, which can be found in polluted to pristine freshwater environments. Most vibrios can exist in a variety of states in the marine environment, ranging from free-living forms to existing as commensals in association with various aquatic groups. Less than 15% of *Vibrio* species have been associated with human disease, with the remaining taxa designated as environmental species. **Table 1** lists the 13 Vibrionaceae species most frequently isolated from human infections in the United States. For some groups, fewer than 5 case reports have been published so knowledge regarding their disease spectrum is limited. In the case of cholera, which does not occur in the United States except for imported cases, the disease ranking mirrors global data accumulated by the World Health Organization.[3]

Surveillance data indicate that 97% of nonfoodborne vibrio infections (NFVI) originate from coastal regions of the United States, with the Gulf coast predominating (57%) followed by the Atlantic seaboard (24%).[4,5] Current estimates suggest that at least 8000 vibrio infections occur annually in the United States, with most (75%) illnesses being food associated.[5] However, modeling studies suggest that more than 50,000 domestically acquired foodborne vibrio infections may occur each year.[4] Epidemiologic data suggest that the incidence of foodborne vibriosis is increasing in the United States, with the latest figures reporting a 32% higher rate of 0.51 in 100,000 compared with 2010 to 2012 data.[6] Data from Florida also document the increasing incidence of vibrio infections (0.48 in 100,000) despite educational campaigns to reduce certain vibrio infections.[7]

Although the incidence of vibriosis varies by state (highest, Hawaii, 1.7; lowest, Oklahoma, 0.03) the 3 most common species involved in human illness in the United States are *V parahaemolyticus*, *Vibrio vulnificus*, and *V alginolyticus* (see **Table 1**) in decreasing order of frequency,[4,5] although some state-to-state variation exists as *V vulnificus* is the most common species reported in Florida.[7] Most of these vibrio infections involve cases of gastroenteritis or SSTI resulting from traumatized mucosal surfaces. **Table 2** lists frequency data of the most commonly isolated vibrios by anatomic site submitted to the US Centers for Disease Control and Prevention (CDC) from 2001 to 2009. Case fatality rates (CFRs) range from 8.2% to 4.7%, although some national studies of vibriosis report CFRs of greater than 30% in association with *V vulnificus* infection.[4] Florida has the highest CFR (10.0%), which is associated with the higher recovery rate of *V vulnificus* in culture in that state.[7]

## CLINICAL DIAGNOSIS

Although the overall incidence of vibriosis is low, the definitive diagnosis of such illnesses is critical because several species-associated disease syndromes, including cholera (toxigenic *V cholerae* O1) and necrotizing fasciitis (*V vulnificus*), are life-threatening events.[7] Current data suggest that various conditions associated with vibriosis are either misdiagnosed or not considered as part of the diagnosis during initial presentation with accompanying symptoms. These factors include that

**Table 1**

Disease spectrum and general epidemiology of *Vibrio* and *Vibrio*-like organisms causing human infections

| Organism | Group | Disease Associations | Epidemiology | | |
|---|---|---|---|---|---|
| | | | O | E | P |
| *V cholerae* O1, O139 | Nonhalophilic | Cholera>gastroenteritis | ● | ● | ● |
| *V cholerae* non-O1, O139 | Nonhalophilic | Gastroenteritis>wound infections>sepsis | ● | ● | ○ |
| *V mimicus* | Nonhalophilic | Gastroenteritis>>sepsis | ● | ○ | ○ |
| *V alginolyticus* | Halophilic | Otitis media>wounds infections>>sepsis | ○ | ○ | ○ |
| *V cincinnatiensis* | Halophilic | Meningitis (single case) | ○ | ○ | ○ |
| *V fluvialis* | Halophilic | Gastroenteritis>>otitis media>sepsis = peritonitis = biliary disease | ● | ○ | ○ |
| *V furnissii* | Halophilic | Sepsis (limited data) | ○ | ○ | ○ |
| *V harveyi* (*V carchariae*) | Halophilic | Wound infection = sepsis (limited data) | ○ | ○ | ○ |
| *V metschnikovii* | Halophilic | Wound infection>pneumonia, sepsis (limited data) | ○ | ○ | ○ |
| *V navarrensis* | Halophilic | Sepsis = wound infections>gastroenteritis | ○ | ○ | ○ |
| *V parahaemolyticus* | Halophilic | Gastroenteritis>>wound infections | ● | ● | ● |
| *V vulnificus* | Halophilic | Wound infections>gastroenteritis>sepsis | ● | ○ | ○ |
| *G hollisae* | Halophilic | Gastroenteritis>sepsis | ○ | ○ | ○ |
| *P damselae* | Halophilic | Wound infections>sepsis | ○ | ○ | ○ |

●: published data supporting this epidemiologic association; ○: no data at present supporting these epidemiologic associations.
*Abbreviations:* E, epidemic associated; O, outbreak associated; P, pandemic associated.

**Table 2**
Vibrio spp and site of isolation; Cholera and Other Vibrio Illness Surveillance (COVIS), United States, 2001–2009 (N = 5212)

| Species | Blood or Other Normally Sterile Site, n (%) | Gastrointestinal Site, n (%) | Skin or Soft Tissue Site, n (%) | Other, Nonsterile Site, n (%) | Multiple, n (%) | Unknown, n (%) |
|---|---|---|---|---|---|---|
| V alginolyticus (n = 694) | 33 (5) | 27 (4) | 572 (82) | 39 (6) | 2 (<1) | 21 (3) |
| Toxigenic V cholerae serogroups O1 and O139 (n = 54) | 0 (0) | 54 (100) | 0 (0) | 0 (0) | 0 (0) | 0 (0) |
| V cholerae (excluding toxigenic O1 and O139) (n = 514) | 108 (21) | 288 (56) | 61 (12) | 30 (6) | 6 (1) | 21 (4) |
| V cincinnatiensis (n = 3) | 1 (33) | 0 (0) | 1 (33) | 0 (0) | 0 (0) | 1 (33) |
| P damselae (n = 26) | 1 (4) | 1 (4) | 22 (85) | 2 (8) | 0 (0) | 0 (0) |
| V fluvialis (n = 268) | 15 (6) | 193 (72) | 30 (11) | 16 (6) | 2 (<1) | 12 (4) |
| V furnissii (n = 15) | 4 (27) | 5 (33) | 4 (27) | 2 (13) | 0 (0) | 0 (0) |
| V harveyi (n = 1) | 0 (0) | 0 (0) | 0 (0) | 1 (100) | 0 (0) | 0 (0) |
| G hollisae (n = 63) | 0 (0) | 53 (83) | 4 (6) | 2 (0) | 0 (0) | 4 (6) |
| V metschnikovii (n = 6) | 1 (17) | 2 (33) | 3 (50) | 0 (0) | 0 (0) | 0 (0) |
| V mimicus (n = 117) | 10 (9) | 81 (69) | 11 (9) | 8 (6) | 1 (<1) | 6 (5) |
| V parahaemolyticus (n = 2283) | 47 (2) | 1803 (79) | 283 (12) | 20 (<1) | 13 (<1) | 117 (5) |
| V vulnificus (n = 944) | 549 (58) | 32 (3) | 251 (27) | 12 (1) | 84 (9) | 15 (2) |
| Total | 793 (15) | 2585 (50) | 1332 (26) | 143 (3) | 121 (2) | 238 (5) |

(1) only 31% of patients with NFVI received appropriate antimicrobial treatment at any time during their illness and only 14% received appropriate therapy initially; (2) estimated vibriosis associated with foodborne disease was underdiagnosed by an estimated multiplier factor of 142, which was 5 to 70 times greater than almost all other enteric pathogens except non-O157 STEC and yersiniosis; (3) estimated numbers of vibrio infections are much higher than current laboratory-confirmed cases (80,000 vs 8000); and (4) delayed hospitalization of longer than 2 days and the failure to administer effective antibiotics was associated with poor outcomes.[4,5] These data suggest that clinicians are often not considering *Vibrio* species in their admitting or primary diagnosis, particularly with regard to extraintestinal infections.

There are 3 critical steps required to help establish the diagnosis of vibriosis either as the causative agent of a gastrointestinal or extraintestinal infection. The first of these is to obtain a medical history from the patient that suggests or is compatible with the possibility of vibriosis. **Table 3** lists some of the common associations that warrant suspicion of infections with 1 or more *Vibrio* species. The central underlying theme for all of these associations is direct or indirect contact with the marine environment, brackish waters, or their inhabitants, including fish, shellfish, and other invertebrate species. For the 2 nonhalophilic *Vibrio* species (*V cholerae*, *V mimicus*) this also includes freshwater sources, most often polluted but in rare instances unadulterated.[8] Approximately 70% of exposures seem to be associated with recreational activities, with 5% or less linked to occupational exposure.[5] However, in a large percentage of cases a connection between the illness and marinelike or aquatic ecosystems cannot be found either on initial presentation or on follow-up.

A second important step in the diagnosis of vibriosis is the recognition of species-specific disease syndromes that carry high mortalities or are of major public health importance. For instance, although cholera may be recognized quickly by clinicians in highly endemic areas such as India, Nigeria, Democratic Republic of the Congo, and Somalia, the immediate recognition of a case of cholera in the United States or other nations where cholera is rare or nonexistent may be problematic, delayed, or simply go unnoticed because of a lack of familiarity with classic symptoms, such as occurred in Haiti in 2010.[9,10]

In addition, information about a case of suspected vibriosis needs to be immediately communicated by the medical staff to the microbiology laboratory before the receipt and processing of anatomic samples because, regardless of body site, vibrio infections may require specialized processing and identification procedures to ensure a correct diagnosis.

## CLINICAL SYNDROMES
### Cholera

Cholera is a life-threatening gastrointestinal disease associated with toxigenic *V cholerae* serogroups O1 (biotypes Classical and El Tor; common serotypes Ogawa and Inaba) and O139. Both serogroups can cause epidemic cholera but serogroup O1 has been responsible for 7 global pandemics with the seventh beginning in 1961 in Indonesia and still ongoing. The ability of both O1 and O139 strains to produce classic cholera is linked to their unique possession of 2 virulence determinants, namely a cholera toxin and a toxin-coregulated pilus, which are absent in most isolates belonging to the more than 200 other non-O1, non-O139 serogroups within the species.

The World Health Organization estimates that the total cases of cholera in 2013 ranged between 1.4 million and 4.3 million cases, with an associated 28,000 to

**Table 3**
Epidemiologic and risk factors associated with vibrio infection

| Food | Occupation | Recreation | Trauma | Natural Disasters | Foreign Travel | Hobbies |
|---|---|---|---|---|---|---|
| • Crustacean shellfish<br>  ○ Shrimp<br>  ○ Crabs<br>  ○ Crayfish<br>  ○ Prawns<br>• Molluscan shellfish<br>  ○ Oysters<br>  ○ Clams (cockles)<br>• Other<br>  ○ Eel (raw)<br>  ○ Fish (raw, unspecified)<br>  ○ Turtle eggs<br>• Water<br>  ○ Freshwater (adulterated)<br>  ○ Well water | • Fishing<br>• Seafood handlers | • Boating<br>• Surfing<br>• Swimming<br>• Shore walking<br>• Water skiing | • Penetrating injuries or lacerations caused by:<br>  ○ Fish hook<br>  ○ Fish fin<br>  ○ Harpoon<br>  ○ Cleaning fish<br>  ○ Coral<br>• Open wound exposed to:<br>  ○ Fish<br>  ○ Boat keel (marine)<br>  ○ Seaweed dressing | • Flooding<br>• Tsunamis<br>• Hurricanes<br>• Cyclones | • Japan<br>• Southeast Asia<br>• Africa<br>• Haiti | • Ornamental aquariums |

142,000 deaths.[3] Almost half of all cases reported originated from the cholera epidemic that started in Haiti (>58,000) in 2010 and the Dominican Republic (~2000). In the United States most cases of cholera occurring between 2001 and 2010 were associated with foreign travel to Asia; whereas from 2010 to 2011 most cholera cases (>80%) involved travel to Haiti and the Dominican Republic.[11] The CFR for all 26 countries reporting cholera deaths was 2.43%, with Guinea (10.03%) and the Congo (13.61%) recording the highest individual rates overall.

Although gastrointestinal symptoms associated with O1 infection vary significantly based on the group at risk (endemic vs epidemic settings), patient demographics (age), genetic host factors (ABO blood group), and other factors, the cardinal clinical features associated with classic cholera are pathognomonic for the disease. In its most fulminant form (cholera gravis) the gastrointestinal syndrome is characterized by an unrelenting purging of bowel contents at rates approaching or slightly exceeding 1 L/h in the absence of appreciable pain or fever.[12] Vomiting is also common. The voluminous release of fluid can include shedding of the mucosal lining of the gastrointestinal tract, appearing as flecks of tissue often described as rice-water stools.[12] Furthermore, the voiding of such large quantities of gastrointestinal contents has 2 serious complications, namely severe dehydration and unbalanced potassium and calcium electrolyte levels.[12,13] If this condition remains unabated, without treatment, death can result within hours of onset from hypotensive shock and cardiac arrest. Many other sequelae are occasionally observed.[12,13] Antimicrobial therapy for moderate to severe cases of cholera (tetracyclines, fluoroquinolones, and macrolides) can help shorten the duration of diarrhea and reduce fecal shedding.

Infrequently, V cholerae non-O1, non-O139 strains carry the cholera toxin gene and produce gastrointestinal symptoms indistinguishable from cholera. Two serogroups recognized to produce such disease in the United States in the past decade or so are O75 and O141.[14,15] The clinical disease in these settings typically consists of an afebrile patient with profuse watery diarrhea (>10 evacuations per day), vomiting, and moderate dehydration. Cholera gravis has not been detected in any of these persons and electrolyte imbalance has been minimal. It is presently unclear whether toxigenic O75 and O141 isolates have the capacity to produce outbreaks or epidemic cholera. They are currently reportable as vibriosis, not cholera.

### Gastroenteritis

In the United States, the most common syndrome associated with *Vibrio* and *Vibrio*-like agents is secretory (watery) enteritis. The species most commonly isolated from noncholera gastroenteritis include *V parahaemolyticus*; non-O1, non-O139 *V cholerae*; *V vulnificus*; and *Vibrio fluvialis*. Because vibriosis enteritis is clinically indistinguishable from that caused by other gram-negative enteropathogens and the frequency of vibriosis in the United States is low, microbiology laboratories need to be alerted when medical histories suggest this as a likely diagnosis. The principal risk factor for these foodborne infections is the consumption of raw or undercooked seafood, particularly shellfish, and related products. Most of these illnesses are of mild to moderate severity with most persons recovering uneventfully without the need to seek medical attention.

*V parahaemolyticus* is the most common cause of foodborne vibriosis in the United States and is a leading cause of food-associated gastroenteritis in many countries, including Japan and Taiwan where culinary habits often involve the consumption of raw seafood or fish as part of the daily diet. The most common vehicles of infection include oysters, clams, and mussels, or local dishes in certain regions of the world, such as ceviche in Peru.[16] *V parahaemolyticus* typically presents as a secretory diarrhea accompanied by abdominal pain, vomiting, low-grade fever, headache, and chills.[16] Blood in the stool is almost always absent but the high percentage of vomiting (55%) is unusual among gram-negative bacteria causing diarrhea.[17]

Non-O1, non-O139 *V cholerae* gastrointestinal infections are common and are again associated with seafood ingestion. Recent CDC surveillance data from Cholera and Other Vibrio Illness Surveillance (COVIS) describes 697 non-O1, non-O139 infections over a 15-year period with 39.9% of individuals hospitalized and 5.0% mortality.[4] Most of these isolates comprising the other 200+ serogroups lack cholera toxin (>98%) and the toxin-coregulated pilus genes, although they may possess other cholera-associated virulence factors. Disease conditions range from asymptomatic colonization, to mild to moderate diarrhea (with or without blood), to frank severe gastroenteritis mimicking classic cholera. Traditional dogma has usually held that choleralike disease is typically restricted to rare non-O1, non-O139 strains carrying the cholera toxin gene and that severe gastroenteritis is normally found only with persons with other comorbid conditions. However, one recent study from India suggests that 70% of non-O1, non-O139 diarrheal infections resembled cholera, with severe dehydration noted in 22.5% of cases and 39.4% with abdominal pain.[18] All of these symptoms were present mostly in persons more than 5 years of age with monomicrobic infections caused by various serogroups lacking cholera toxin. Rare fatal infections associated with non-O1, non-O139 *V cholerae* gastroenteritis are reported more frequently nowadays. Two recent infections were described in persons with underlying renal problems and hematologic conditions. In one case, profuse diarrhea (20 episodes per day) continued for 3 days unabated before electrolyte replacement therapy was initiated. In both instances supportive medical interventions did not resolve the diarrheal episodes and patients succumbed to hypovolemic shock and cardiac arrest in 1 instance and extensive intestinal necrosis in the other.[19,20] In neither instance was the *V cholerae* strain recovered from any site other than stool.

Little information is presently available regarding *V vulnificus* gastroenteritis. Only a few cases have been published in the literature and most of these were simultaneously associated with other enteric pathogens or involved persons taking medications to reduce gastric acidity. Most persons had previously consumed oysters directly before the onset of disease. A recent reputed case of *V vulnificus* diarrhea involved an 18-month-old child with severe dehydration, respiratory infection, and pallor.[21] CDC reports that approximately 3% of the *V vulnificus* cases reported to COVIS had a gastrointestinal specimen site (see **Table 2**). Furthermore, between 1998 and 2007 the state of Florida reported that 28.6% of *V vulnificus* illnesses presented as gastroenteritis.[7] These data suggest that *V vulnificus* diarrhea does exist and may simply be overlooked. Whether these infections mostly occur in immunocompetent persons or can lead to invasive disease after primary infection is unknown.

*V fluvialis* is currently the fifth most common *Vibrio* species identified by the CDC and the state of Florida.[4,7] Since 2002 it has emerged as an important pathogen in India and has been linked to 1 large outbreak of diarrheal disease there in association with *Salmonella* in a dish containing minced meat, lamb, and beans.[22,23] The disease has most often been observed in adults (73%) as an afebrile, watery diarrhea (86%) without abdominal pain. Severe dehydration has been noted in 28% of patients.[23]

### Wound Infections

A second common clinical syndrome associated with *Vibrio* species involves SSTI. SSTIs involving marine vibrios are the direct result of traumas involving a penetrating injury or a preexisting open wound, abrasion, or laceration coming in direct contact with seawater or intimate contact with marine-associated products such as a fish fin, fish hook, or other nautical equipment, including ships or boats. The range of

SSTIs can vary from a mild to moderate cellulitis in normal individuals to fulminant invasive infections such as necrotizing fasciitis, found primarily in immunocompromised populations. Symptoms associated with vibrio infections include vesicle formation with edema and erythema that may rapidly progress to hemorrhagic bullae (**Fig. 1**).[24]

The most common pathogenic vibrios associated with SSTIs are *V vulnificus*; *V parahaemolyticus*; *V alginolyticus*; *P damselae*; and nontoxigenic, non-O1, non-O139 *V cholerae*.[24,25] *V vulnificus* is by far the most important member of this group both in frequency and as a cause of life-threatening illnesses. From the onset of infection, symptoms caused by *V vulnificus* can present in as little as 12 hours and death can result as early as 24 to 48 hours without appropriate diagnosis and medical treatment.[24,26] *V vulnificus* infections typically appear as frank cellulitis (88%) with bullae (88%), fever (65%), and chills (29%).[25] Persons with one of several immunologically compromised conditions, including malignancy, liver disease, diabetes, alcoholism, or those with iron overload conditions (hemochromatosis), are especially prone to developing a rapidly progressing cellulitis leading to destruction of subcutaneous tissues and fascial planes.[27] Fifty percent of all persons with underlying conditions and *V vulnificus* cellulitis go on to develop necrotizing fasciitis versus only 3% in healthy persons.[25] CFRs in various clinical series range from 7% to 24%.[28]

The second most important species in this group is *P damselae*. Although *P damselae* is much less common than *V vulnificus*, present evidence suggests that wound infections caused by this bacterium are extremely aggressive, have more serious complications, and a higher mortality than *V vulnificus*.[29] Some cases are so fulminant that antimicrobial therapy cannot control the eventually progressive fatal infection,[29,30] which makes the rapid laboratory diagnosis to species of *Vibrio*-associated wound infections especially critical in these instances.[24] Although other *Vibrio* species occasionally cause severe wound infections, their overall frequency relative to the 2 species mentioned earlier is much lower, as is the mortality.[31]

### Septicemia

The third syndromic disease associated with vibriosis is septicemia. Bloodborne infections have been attributed to all of the pathogenic species to date but *V vulnificus* is the preeminent pathogen of this group. *Vibrio*-associated bacteremia can often be distinguished from other gram-negative sepsis by the presence of metastatic skin lesions within 36 hours of onset.[32] In the case of *V vulnificus*, sepsis can occur as an extension

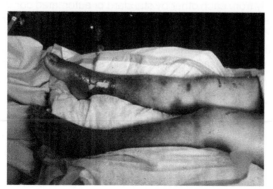

**Fig. 1.** *Vibrio* wound infection of the extremities with extensive hemorrhage and necrosis.

of invasive wound infection or can appear as a primary septicemia without preexisting disease. Primary *V vulnificus* septicemia almost invariably occurs in people with underlying medical conditions, most notably hepatic dysfunctions.[33] The most common source of infection in this group is the consumption of raw or undercooked oysters. Estimates suggest that between 90% and 96% of individuals presenting with primary sepsis previously consumed raw oysters within a week of the illness.[27,34] Symptoms include fever and chills (33%), hypotension (75%), and nausea and vomiting.[27,32] Diarrhea may or may not be present. The initial presentation can quickly extend from erythematous lesions to hemorrhagic bullae and necrotic ulcers. The disease is most often observed in men in their mid-50s.[33,34] Hospitalization rates exceed 85% and CFRs may approach 40% to 50%.[32–34]

Serious complications and mortalities caused by sepsis from other *Vibrio* species are much lower. When *V cholerae* causes sepsis it is almost always because of serogroups other than O1 or O139.

### Miscellaneous

Vibrios have been isolated from numerous anatomic sites, including the ear, eye, gallbladder, and sinuses, and from peritoneal fluid, urine, and so on. A recent study from Taiwan found that these other illnesses accounted for less than 5% of all noncholera infections.[35]

## LABORATORY DIAGNOSIS

The laboratory diagnosis of vibrio infections can be challenging because isolation by standard culture methods is difficult. Special enrichment and plating media may be required to recover the causal agent from fecal and gastrointestinal specimens. Furthermore, for some species, growth characteristics on standard enteric media may be unusual. For example, *G hollisae* fails to grow or grows poorly on selective media designed for vibrios, such as thiosulfate-citrate-bile salts-sucrose agar (TCBS) or on other enteric gram-negative agars, including MacConkey. These special culture issues demand the use of nonselective media like blood agar plate (BAP) to help recover vibrios from both sterile and nonsterile sites. BAP not only supports the plating efficiency of difficult-to-grow species but aids in colonial recognition of many hemolytic species. Rapid spot tests can also be performed (oxidase, indole) off BAP to rule in or rule out the possible presence of vibrios. In addition to these obstacles, several other genera that can inhabit marine ecosystems can produce symptoms similar to those produced by *Vibrio* spp and it may be difficult to separate these biochemically from each other by standard or automated commercial identification systems. These other gram-negative genera include *Aeromonas*, *Plesiomonas*, and *Shewanella*.[36,37]

It is hoped that culture-independent diagnostic tests and other molecular approaches will eventually lead to faster and more specific methods to identify vibrios and avoid the misidentifications that were common in the past.[38]

### Collection, Transport, and Enrichment

All specimens from patients suspected as possibly having vibriosis should ideally be collected as soon as possible postonset and this is especially true for fecal specimens. For cases of diarrhea, bulk or watery stool samples are preferable to rectal swabs because this optimizes the chance of recovering *Vibrio* species.[39] Cary-Blair is the preferred transport medium for stool samples, although others, such as Amies and Stuart, are also satisfactory. Buffered glycerol saline should be avoided because this is toxic to *V cholerae*. During cholera outbreaks in remote areas, liquid stool samples can be collected on gauze or blotting paper discs and transported in tightly sealed containers to the nearest laboratory for testing after adding several drops of saline to avoid desiccation.[39,40] Studies suggest this method detects ~80% of cholera cases versus those recovered using Cary-Blair.[40]

Special transport media or precautions are not typically necessary when vibrios are involved in extraintestinal infection but standard plating media for such sites should always include blood agar.

The standard enrichment broth for fecal samples suspected of harboring vibrios is alkaline peptone water (pH 8.6). This enrichment broth is useful in detecting vibrios either by standard plate culture or by rapid or molecular assays.

### Isolation

The standard selective medium for the isolation of *Vibrio* spp from diarrheal samples is TCBS, although others exist.[32,39] Growth on TCBS with the presence of sucrose fermentation (yellow colonies) or lack thereof (green colonies) helps to separate presumptive vibrios into different groups.[39] *V cholerae* and *V parahaemolyticus* can also be selectively isolated from feces and presumptively identified using chromID Vibrio (bioMérieux, Marcy l'Etoile, France). The former species appears blue-green on this medium, whereas the latter is pink.[41] Limited published data using fresh and seeded stools suggest that the sensitivity of chromID Vibrio is comparable with TCBS and perhaps superior in specificity.[41] Isolated colonies are then picked for confirmation using conventional, commercial, or molecular methods. For nonintestinal infections that may involve *Vibrio* species, multiple isolated colonies should be screened for oxidase and indole positivity, sensitivity to 2,4-diamino-6,7 diisopropylpteridine (O/129), and salt tolerance if needed.

### Rapid Diagnostic Tests

No rapid diagnostic tests (RDTs) for vibriosis have been approved by the US Food and Drug Administration (FDA) for clinical diagnosis. Because of the preeminent public health importance of *V cholerae* and its role in epidemic and pandemic cholera, commercial companies developed RDTs to screen for and detect the presence of O1 and later O139 strains in outbreak settings. One of the earliest marketed versions was the CHOLERA SMART test by New Horizons Diagnostics Corporation (Columbia, MD). The current version is CHOLERA SMART II, which is a lateral flow immunoassay that takes only 15 minutes to perform. The assay detects the A antigen of O1 lipopolysaccharide. Other assays include a latex agglutination assay that captures O1 antigen (Denka Seiken, Tokyo, Japan) and an immunochromatographic and colorimetric test to detect *V cholerae* O1 and O139 (Crystal VC Rapid Dipstick test, Span Diagnostics, Surat, India). None of these assays are FDA approved and they are sold for research use only (RUO).[39,42]

A troubling multicenter study from Bangladesh, the University of Maryland, and Japan suggests that both the culture and the dipstick methods are missing many cases of cholera. Even when additional assays are used, including direct fluorescent antibody, multiplex polymerase chain reaction (PCR), and lytic phage plaque assay, no single test is close to detecting all cases.[42] Thus no gold standard exists to detect cholera in the clinical laboratory.[42]

### Culture-independent Diagnostic Testing

Over the past several years commercial companies have developed diagnostic test systems to detect syndromic disease caused by several pathogenic bacteria and viruses. These systems center on nested multiplex PCR reactions and provide final identification results in a matter of minutes to several hours without the need to perform time-consuming conventional media-based testing.[38] Two gastrointestinal systems, Luminex xTAG Gastrointestinal Pathogen Panel (GPP) (Austin, TX) and the FilmArray Gastrointestinal Panel (BioFire Diagnostics Inc, Salt Lake City, UT) simultaneously detect 14 and 22 agents respectively. The FDA approved the *V cholerae* target on October 1, 2014, for the xTAG GPP and the FilmArray Panel was FDA approved to detect *V cholerae* on May 14, 2014. As this general technology gains acceptance in clinical microbiology laboratories it will require such facilities to retain stool samples until test results indicate that *V cholerae* O1 is not present. When this target is detected by either system the remaining stool sample must be forwarded immediately to a regional or state public health laboratory for culture confirmation of the molecular test results. The CDC can also be contacted regarding disposition and testing of remnant samples on *V cholerae* target–positive specimens. Neither system will eliminate the need for routine isolation of noncholera vibrios when vibriosis is suspected because these panels do not presently capture targets for *V mimicus*, *V fluvialis*, *V parahaemolyticus*, *V vulnificus*, and others. Multiplex PCR assays to detect vibrios such as *V cholerae*, *V parahaemolyticus*, and *V fluvialis* from stool specimens have been evaluated but are RUO at present.[43]

### Identification

Identification of vibrios in the clinical microbiology laboratory can be challenging. The issues with conventional testing are that it is media intensive, technically demanding, slow to yield a final identification, and typically available only in state or federal reference laboratories.[39] In addition to potential issues in their recovery from gastrointestinal specimens, many vibrios show phenotypic features similar to other clinically significant oxidase-positive genera, such as *Aeromonas*. Initial separation of isolates into appropriate genera often requires specialized tests that are not always available in all laboratories or on commercial panels. These specialized tests include sensitivity to the vibriostatic agent O/129 at 10 and 150 µg, string test, growth on TCBS, gas from glucose, salt tolerance, and ornithine decarboxylase (ODC) activity.[39] For at least 2 clinical settings (cholera, necrotizing fasciitis), the rapid and accurate detection and identification of *V cholerae*, *V vulnificus*, and *P damselae* can have serious public health consequences, as well as grave clinical consequences. All presumptive *V cholerae* isolates need to be immediately referred to state reference public health laboratories or the CDC for culture confirmation, serogroup and biotype analysis, and cholera toxin testing.

#### Commercial automated systems

Commercial identification systems are notoriously poor regarding the accurate identification of vibrios to species.[44] Many systems are highly inaccurate in the identification of important species such as *V cholerae*, *V vulnificus*, *V parahaemolyticus*, and *V alginolyticus*.[44] Second, many nonvibrios, such as aeromonads, are often (7%–16%) misidentified as pathogenic vibrios.[45] The single most common error these systems make is the misidentification of *Aeromonas hydrophila* as *V fluvialis* or vice versa because both organisms have essentially identical biotypes on commercial panels.[46] In addition, uncommon *Aeromonas* species that are ODC positive are often identified as vibrios.[37] Because of this, any presumptively identified *Vibrio* isolates that are judged to be clinically significant need to be confirmed by a second method (conventional, matrix-assisted laser desorption/ionization time-of-flight mass spectrometry [MALDI-TOF MS]).

## Molecular methods

The emergence of newer molecular technologies, such as 16S ribosomal DNA gene sequencing (16S), multilocus sequence analysis, and MALDI-TOF MS holds promise for identification of vibrios.[39] Although there are no definitive studies on the accuracy of 16S for *Vibrio* identification, 16S has been used to confirm *Vibrio* strains identified by commercial test systems or to identify strains with low probability scores or isolates showing atypical reactions.[46,47] Nucleotide sequence determination methods targeting various genes, including the *rpoB* gene sequencing and multilocus sequence analysis of other housekeeping genes, have been able to identify to the species level vibrios that were not identified by phenotypic methods.[1,48,49] MALDI-TOF MS has the potential to provide highly accurate and rapid identification results from isolated colonies as long as libraries are available with enough unique mass spectral peaks to provide recognition.[50] Wang and colleagues,[51] using the Vitek MS Axima Assurance mass spectrometer (bioMérieux, Durham, NC), found that the system correctly identified 3 strains of *V vulnificus* and 2 strains of *V parahaemolyticus* to species. In contrast, 2 strains of *Vibrio harveyi* could not be identified on the Microflex LT MS Biotyper (Bruker Daltonics, Bremen, Germany).[52] For 2 *V cholerae* strains the Vitek MS identified both to species, whereas the Biotyper could only identify each to genus level.[53] However, the Biotyper system was able to correctly identify *P damselae* and *V harveyi* causing a severe polymicrobic wound infection in a 64-year-old man.[54]

## SELF ASSESSMENT

1. Cholera is an often life-threatening diarrheal illness associated with pandemic spread and infection by:
   a. V parahaemolyticus
   b. Nontoxigenic V cholerae
   c. G hollisae
   d. V cholerae serogroups O1 or O139
   e. V vulnificus
2. A detailed medical history is necessary to suspect vibriosis and to guide laboratory testing, especially for gastroenteritis or diarrheal disease. Which of the following foods are most likely to be a vehicle for vibrio infection?
   a. Poultry
   b. Oysters
   c. Beef
   d. Leafy green vegetables
   e. Cheese
3. Necrotizing fasciitis is most often associated with which Vibrio species?
   a. V cholerae
   b. V alginolyticus
   c. V vulnificus
   d. V mimicus
   e. G hollisae

Answers
   Answer 1: d

   Refer to the text for details.

   Answer 2: b

Refer to **Table 3**.

Answer 3: c

Refer to the text for details.

## REFERENCES

1. Sawabe T, Ogura Y, Matsumura Y, et al. Updating the *Vibrio* clades defined by multilocus sequence phylogeny: proposal of eight new clades, and the description of *Vibrio tritonius* sp. nov. Front Microbiol 2013;4:414.
2. Takemura AF, Chien DM, Polz MF. Associations and dynamics of Vibrionaceae in the environment, from genus to the population level. Front Microbiol 2014;5:38.
3. Cholera, 2013. Wkly Epidemiol Rec 2014;89:345–55.
4. Newton A, Kendall M, Vugia DJ, et al. Increasing rates of vibriosis in the United States, 1996–2010: review of surveillance data from 2 systems. Clin Infect Dis 2012;54(S5):S391–5.
5. Dechet AM, Yu PA, Koram N, et al. Nonfoodborne *Vibrio* infections: an important cause of morbidity and mortality in the United States, 1997–2006. Clin Infect Dis 2008;46:970–6.
6. Crim SM, Iwamoto M, Huang JY, et al. Incidence and trends of infection with pathogens transmitted commonly through food – foodborne diseases active surveillance network, 10 U.S. sites, 2006–2013. MMWR Morb Mortal Wkly Rep 2014;63:328–32.
7. Weis KE, Hammond RM, Hutchinson R, et al. *Vibrio* illness in Florida, 1998–2007. Epidemiol Infect 2011;139:591–8.
8. Walker E, Carpenter J, Plemmons R, et al. Freshwater non-O1 *Vibrio cholerae* infection. South Med J 2010;103:1061–2.
9. Ivers LC, Walton DA. The "first" case of cholera in Haiti: lessons for global health. Am J Trop Med Hyg 2012;86:36–8.
10. Chin C-S, Sorenson J, Harris JB, et al. The origin of the Haitian cholera outbreak strain. N Engl J Med 2011;364:33–42.
11. Loharikar A, Newton AE, Stroika S, et al. Cholera in the United States, 2001 – 2011: a reflection of patterns of global epidemiology and travel. Epidemiol Infect 2015;143:695–703.
12. Waldor MK, Ryan ET. Vibrio cholerae. In: Bennett JE, Dolin RE, Blaser MJ, editors. Mandell, Douglas and Bennett's: principles and practices of infectious diseases. 8th edition. Philadelphia: Elsevier; 2014. p. 2471–9.
13. Reyes-Corcho A, Pinsker RW, Sarkar S, et al. *Cholera gravis* associated with acute renal failure in a traveler from Haiti to the United states. Travel Med Infect Dis 2012;10:236–9.
14. Tobin-D-Angelo M, Smith AR, Bulens SN, et al. Severe diarrhea caused by cholera toxin-producing *Vibrio cholerae* serogroup O75 infections acquired in the southeastern United States. Clin Infect Dis 2008;47:1035–40.
15. Crump JA, Bopp CA, Greene K, et al. Toxigenic *Vibrio cholerae* O141-associated cholera-like diarrhea and bloodstream infection in the United States. J Infect Dis 2003;187:866–8.
16. Yeung PS, Boor KI. Epidemiology, pathogenesis, and prevention of foodborne *Vibrio parahaemolyticus* infections. Foodborne Pathog Dis 2004;1:74–88.
17. Daniels NA, MacKinnon L, Bishop R, et al. *Vibrio parahaemolyticus* infections in the United States, 1973–1998. J Infect Dis 2000;181:1661–6.

18. Dutta D, Chowdhury G, Pazhani GP, et al. *Vibrio cholerae* non-O1, non-O139 serogroups and cholera-like diarrhea, Kolkata, India. Emerg Infect Dis 2013;19: 464–7.
19. Farina C, Marini F, Schiaffino E, et al. A fatal *Vibrio cholerae* O37 enteritis. J Med Microbiol 2010;59:1538–40.
20. Tamura S, Taniguchi F, Nakamoto C, et al. Fatal diarrheal disease caused by *Vibrio cholerae* O67 in a patient with myelodysplastic syndrome. Intern Med 2013;52:1635–9.
21. De A, Mathur M. *Vibrio vulnificus* diarrhea in a child with respiratory infection. J Glob Infect Dis 2011;3:300–2.
22. Chowdhury G, Pazhani G, Dutta D, et al. *Vibrio fluvialis* in patients with diarrhea, Kolkata, India. Emerg Infect Dis 2012;18:1868–71.
23. Chowdhury G, Sarkar A, Pazhani GP, et al. An outbreak of foodborne gastroenteritis caused by dual pathogens, *Salmonella enterica* serovar Weltevreden and *Vibrio fluvialis* in Kolkata, India. Foodborne Pathog Dis 2013;10:904–6.
24. Noonburg GE. Management of extremity trauma and related infections occurring in the aquatic environment. J Am Acad Orthop Surg 2005;13:243–53.
25. Oliver JD. Wound infections caused by *Vibrio vulnificus* and other marine bacteria. Epidemiol Infect 2005;133:383–91.
26. Finkelstein R, Oren I. Soft tissue infections caused by marine bacterial pathogens: epidemiology, diagnosis, and management. Curr Infect Dis Rep 2011;13: 470–7.
27. Bross MH, Soch K, Morales R, et al. *Vibrio vulnificus* infection: diagnosis and treatment. Am Fam Physician 2007;76:539–44.
28. Horseman MA, Surani S. A comprehensive review of *Vibrio vulnificus*: an important cause of severe sepsis and skin and soft-tissue infection. Int J Infect Dis 2011;15:e157–66.
29. Rivas AJ, Lemos ML, Osorio CR. *Photobacterium damselae* subsp. *damselae*, a bacterium pathogenic for marine animals and humans. Front Microbiol 2013; 4:283.
30. Goodell KH, Jordan MR, Graham R, et al. Rapidly advancing necrotizing fasciitis caused by *Photobacterium* (*Vibrio*) *damselae*: a hyperaggressive variant. Crit Care Med 2004;32:278–81.
31. Ottaviani D, Leoni F, Rocchegiani E, et al. Unusual case of necrotizing fasciitis caused by *Vibrio cholerae* O137. J Clin Microbiol 2011;49:757–9.
32. Neil MA, Carpenter CJ. Other pathogenic vibrios. In: Bennett JE, Dolin RE, Blaser MJ, editors. Mandell, Douglas and Bennett's: principles and practices of infectious diseases. 8th edition. Philadelphia: Elsevier; 2014. p. 2480–4.
33. Menon MP, Yu PA, Iwamoto M, et al. Pre-existing medical conditions associated with *Vibrio vulnificus* septicaemia. Epidemiol Infect 2014;142:878–81.
34. Daniels NA. *Vibrio vulnificus* oysters: pearls and perils. Clin Infect Dis 2011;52: 788–92.
35. Hou CC, Lai CC, Liu WL, et al. Clinical manifestation and prognostic factors of non-*cholerae Vibrio* infections. Eur J Clin Microbiol Infect Dis 2011;30:819–24.
36. Myung DS, Jung YS, Kang SJ, et al. Primary *Shewanella algae* bacteremia mimicking *Vibrio* septicemia. J Korean Med Sci 2009;24:1192–4.
37. Abbott SL, Seli LS, Catino M Jr, et al. Misidentification of unusual *Aeromonas* species as members of the genus *Vibrio*: a continuing problem. J Clin Microbiol 1998;36:1103–4.
38. Janda JM, Abbott SL. Culture-independent diagnostic testing: have we opened Pandora's box for good? Diagn Microbiol Infect Dis 2014;80:171–6.

39. Abbott SL, Janda JM, Farmer JJ III. *Vibrio* and related organisms. In: Versalovic J, Carroll KC, Funke G, et al, editors. Manual of clinical microbiology. 10th edition. Washington, DC: ASM Press; 2011. p. 666–76.

40. Page AL, Alberti KP, Guénolé A, et al. Use of filter paper as a transport medium for the laboratory diagnosis of cholera under field conditions. J Clin Microbiol 2011;49:3021–3.

41. Eddabra R, Piemont Y, Scheftel JM. Evaluation of a new chromogenic medium, chromID™ Vibrio, for the isolation and presumptive identification of *Vibrio cholerae* and *Vibrio parahaemolyticus* from human clinical specimens. Eur J Clin Microbiol Infect Dis 2011;30:733–7.

42. Page AL, Alberti KP, Mondonge V, et al. Evaluation of a rapid test for the diagnosis of cholera in the absence of a gold standard. PLoS ONE 2012;7(5):e37360.

43. Vinothkumar K, Bhardwaj AK, Ramamurthy T, et al. Triplex PCR assay for the rapid identification of 3 major *Vibrio* species, *Vibrio cholerae*, *Vibrio parahaemolyticus*, and *Vibrio fluvialis*. Diagn Microbiol Infect Dis 2013;76:526–8.

44. Saini A, Kaur H, Purwar S, et al. Discrepancies in identification of *Vibrio cholerae* strains as members of the Aeromonadaceae and Enterobacteriaceae by automated microbial identification systems. Lett Appl Microbiol 2012;55:22–6.

45. Lamy B, Laurent F, Verdier I, et al. Accuracy of 6 commercial systems for identifying clinical *Aeromonas* isolates. Diagn Microbiol Infect Dis 2010;67:9–14.

46. Ratnaraja N, Blackmore T, Byrne J, et al. *Vibrio fluvialis* peritonitis in a patient receiving continuous ambulatory peritoneal dialysis. J Clin Microbiol 2005;43:514–5.

47. Nagao M, Shimizu Y, Kawada Y, et al. Two cases of sucrose-fermenting *Vibrio vulnificus* infection in which 16S rDNA sequencing was useful. Jpn J Infect Dis 2006;59:108–10.

48. Gladney LM, Tarr CL. Molecular and phenotypic characterization of *Vibrio navarrensis* isolates associated with human illness. J Clin Microbiol 2014;52:4070–4.

49. Tarr CL, Patel JS, Puhr ND, et al. Identification of *Vibrio* isolates by a multiplex PCR assay and *rpoB* sequence determination. J Clin Microbiol 2007;45:134–40.

50. Dieckmann R, Strauch E, Alter T. Rapid identification and characterization of *Vibrio* species using whole-cell MALDI-TOF mass spectrometry. J Appl Microbiol 2010;109:199–211.

51. Wang W, Xi H, Huang M, et al. Performance of mass spectrometric identification of bacteria and yeasts routinely isolated in a clinical microbiology laboratory using MALDI-TOF MS. J Thorac Dis 2014;6:524–33.

52. Rodríguez-Sánchez B, Marín M, Sánchez-Carrillo C, et al. Improvement of matrix-assisted laser desorption/ionization time-of-flight mass spectrometry identification of difficult-to-identify bacteria and its impact in the workflow of a clinical microbiology laboratory. Diagn Microbiol Infect Dis 2014;79:1–6.

53. Martiny D, Busson L, Wybo I, et al. Comparison of the Microflex LT and Vitek MS systems for routine identification of bacteria by matrix-assisted laser desorption ionization-time of flight mass spectrometry. J Clin Microbiol 2012;50:1313–25.

54. Hundenborn J, Thurig S, Kommerell M, et al. Severe wound infection with *Photobacterium damselae* ssp. *damselae* and *Vibrio harveyi*, following a laceration injury in marine environment: a case report and review of the literature. Case Rep Med 2013;2013:610632.

# Campylobacter

Collette Fitzgerald, PhD

## KEYWORDS

- *Campylobacter* • *Campylobacter jejuni* • Gastroenteritis • Campylobacteriosis

## KEY POINTS

- Campylobacter continues to be a major public health problem.
- Infection with *Campylobacter* causes a spectrum of diseases, including acute enteritis, extraintestinal infections, and postinfectious complications.
- The gastrointestinal tracts of domestic and wild birds and animals are the main reservoirs for *Campylobacter*.
- The most common species of *Campylobacter* associated with human illness are *Campylobacter jejuni* and *Campylobacter coli*, but other *Campylobacter* species also can cause human infections.
- Diagnostic testing for *Campylobacter* can be performed by a variety of methods, including culture, stool antigen assays, and molecular assays; these tests differ in their sensitivities and specificities, and the nonculture methods detect but do not differentiate between *C jejuni* and *C coli* and other *Campylobacter* species.

## INTRODUCTION

*Campylobacter* is one of the most common causes of bacterial diarrheal illness in the United States and worldwide. Although there are many species within the genus *Campylobacter*, *Campylobacter jejuni* is the most commonly isolated from fecal specimens, with almost 90% of reported cases of *Campylobacter* infections caused by *C jejuni*. This review briefly discusses the taxonomy, clinical manifestations, epidemiology of *Campylobacter*, and then focuses on the laboratory detection of *Campylobacter* in more depth.

## CAMPYLOBACTER TAXONOMY

The *Campylobacter* genus consists of a large and diverse group of bacteria currently comprising 26 species (http://www.bacterio.cict.fr/c/campylobacter.html). **Table 1** highlights the known sources and human disease associations with each species.

Enteric Diseases Laboratory Branch, Division of Foodborne, Waterborne and Environmental Diseases, Centers for Disease Control and Prevention, 1600 Clifton Road, Atlanta, GA 30329, USA
E-mail address: chf3@cdc.gov

Clin Lab Med 35 (2015) 289–298
http://dx.doi.org/10.1016/j.cll.2015.03.001
0272-2712/15/$ – see front matter Published by Elsevier Inc.

labmed.theclinics.com

**Table 1**
**Currently described *Campylobacter* species**

| *Campylobacter* Species | Known Sources | Human Disease Associated |
|---|---|---|
| *C jejuni* subsp *jejuni* | Poultry, cattle, sheep, wild birds, pigs | Gastroenteritis, meningitis, septicemia, Guillain-Barre syndrome |
| *C jejuni* subsp *doylei* | Humans | Gastroenteritis, septicemia |
| *C coli* | Pigs, poultry, sheep, wild birds, cattle | Gastroenteritis, septicemia, meningitis |
| *C lari* subsp *lari* | Wild birds, poultry, dogs, cats | Gastroenteritis, septicemia |
| *C lari* subsp *concheus* | Shellfish | Gastroenteritis |
| *C fetus* subsp *fetus* | Cattle, sheep, reptiles | Gastroenteritis, septicemia |
| *C fetus* subsp *venerealis* | Cattle, sheep | Septicemia |
| *C fetus* subsp *testudium* | Reptiles | Gastroenteritis, cellulitis |
| *C upsaliensis* | Dogs, cats | Gastroenteritis, septicemia |
| *C helveticus* | Cats, dogs | Gastroenteritis |
| *C insulaenigrae* | Marine mammals | Gastroenteritis |
| *C peloridis* | Shellfish | Gastroenteritis |
| *C hyointestinalis* subsp *hyointestinalis* | Pigs, cattle | Gastroenteritis |
| *C hyointestinalis* subsp *lawsonii* | Pigs | None at present |
| *C lanienae* | Cattle, pigs | Gastroenteritis |
| *C sputorum* bv *sputorum* | Cattle, pigs | Abscesses, gastroenteritis |
| *C sputorum* bv *faecalis* | Sheep, bulls | None at present |
| *C sputorum* bv *paraureolyticus* | Cattle | Gastroenteritis |
| *C concisus* | Humans, domestic pets | Gastroenteritis, periodontal disease, abscesses |
| *C curvus* | Humans | Periodontal disease, gastroenteritis |
| *C rectus* | Humans | Periodontal disease, abscesses |
| *C showae* | Humans | Periodontal disease, abscesses |
| *C ureolyticus* | Humans | Gastroenteritis, septicemia, soft tissue abscesses |
| *C gracilis* | Humans | Periodontal disease, abscesses |
| *C hominis* | Humans | None at present |
| *C mucosalis* | Pigs | None at present |
| *C avium* | Poultry | None at present |
| *C canadensis* | Whooping cranes | None at present |
| *C cuniculorum* | Rabbits | None at present |
| *C subantarticus* | Gray-headed albatrosses, black-browed albatrosses, gentoo penguins | None at present |
| *C volucris* | Black-headed gulls | None at present |
| *C corcagiensis* | Lion-tailed macaques | None at present |
| *C iguaniorum* | Reptiles | None at present |

Although *C jejuni* and *Campylobacter coli* cause most human infections, 15 additional species have been detected or isolated from humans.[1] Current methods routinely used in clinical and public health laboratories were developed for and are biased toward the isolation of *C jejuni*. In addition, because campylobacters are difficult to differentiate phenotypically and many clinical laboratories do not identify *Campylobacter* isolates to the species level, the true clinical and public health importance of the other species remains to be determined.

*C jejuni*, *C coli*, *Campylobacter lari*, and *Campylobacter upsaliensis* form a genetically close group and are known as the thermotolerant campylobacters, because they grow optimally at 42°C.[2] The remaining *Campylobacter* species fall into 3 general groups: (1) species that infrequently cause disease in humans and are associated with livestock animals (eg, *Campylobacter fetus*, *Campylobacter sputorum*, and *Campylobacter hyointestinalis*); (2) species either implicated in periodontal disease or isolated from humans (eg, *Campylobacter curvus*, *Campylobacter rectus*, *Campylobacter showae*, *Campylobacter concisus*); and (3) species that have not been isolated from food or water and are not associated with human illness (eg, *Campylobacter insulaenigrae*, *Campylobacter canadensis*).[3] Despite differences in source and host association, members of the *Campylobacter* genus have several basic features in common. They are small, slightly curved or spiral gram-negative rods that may form a coccoid form in old cultures and under conditions of stress. They are usually motile and species are generally microaerobic; however, some strains grow anaerobically or aerobically. An atmosphere containing increased hydrogen is required by some species for microaerobic growth.[4]

## CAMPYLOBACTER DISEASE MANIFESTATION

*Campylobacter* infections cause a spectrum of diseases, including acute enteritis, extraintestinal infections (eg, bacteremia, abscess, meningitis) and postinfectious complications. *Campylobacter* generally causes a self-limited clinical illness that lasts 5 to 7 days; the infection resolves without antimicrobial treatment in the great majority of cases but 5% to 10% of patients relapse after their initial illness.[5] Symptoms of infection typically begin 2 to 5 days after ingesting the bacteria and include diarrhea with cramping, acute abdominal pain, often with fever, and some nausea and vomiting. In neonates and young infants, bloody diarrhea without fever can be the only manifestation of infection. Extraintestinal *Campylobacter* infections are rare in people in good health, but are more likely to occur in those who are immunocompromised, elderly, or pregnant. The most common type is bacteremia with or without diarrheal illness. Patients with *Campylobacter* infections are at increased risk for several postinfectious complications, including Guillain-Barre syndrome (GBS), reactive arthritis, and irritable bowel syndrome.[6]

*C jejuni* is the most commonly identified bacterial cause of GBS, preceding paralysis in 30% of patients with GBS.[7] Reactive arthritis is estimated to occur in 2% to 5% of patients and irritable bowel syndrome in 33% of patients following *Campylobacter* infection.[8,9]

## CAMPYLOBACTER EPIDEMIOLOGY

*Campylobacter* is the most common cause of diarrheal illness in the United States, estimated to cause 1.3 million illnesses, 13,240 hospitalizations, and 119 deaths each year.[10] The incidence for 10 US sentinel sites (Foodborne Diseases Active Surveillance Network, FoodNet) in 2014 was 13.7 per 100,000 people, which represents a statistically significant decline from the 2006–2008 baseline.[11] The highest incidence of infection is among persons younger than 5 years, although incidence among persons 60 years and older appears to be increasing. Among human *Campylobacter* isolates in FoodNet with species information, 89% are *C jejuni*, 8% are *C coli*, and the remaining 3% are other species. Most *Campylobacter* infections are acquired domestically, but *Campylobacter* is also a major cause of traveler's diarrhea.[12]

The gastrointestinal tracts of domestic and wild birds and animals are reservoirs of infection. Many farm animals and meat sources can harbor the organism, and pets (especially young animals), including dogs, cats, hamsters, and birds, are potential sources of infection. Transmission of *C jejuni* and *C coli* occurs by ingestion of contaminated food or water or by direct contact with fecal material from infected animals or people. Improperly cooked poultry, untreated water, and unpasteurized milk have been the main vehicles of transmission.

*Campylobacter* infections are usually sporadic; outbreaks are not detected often compared with other enteric pathogens. Although a variety of foods, including poultry, other meats, and produce have been linked to outbreaks in the United States, the most common single food implicated is unpasteurized milk.[13] Person-to-person transmission is uncommon for outbreaks of campylobacteriosis despite the low infectious dose of *C jejuni*.

## LABORATORY TESTING FOR *CAMPYLOBACTER* INFECTION
### Introduction

Laboratory diagnosis of *Campylobacter* infections can be challenging because the organism is difficult to isolate, grow, and identify. Recent reports describing clinical laboratory practices for *Campylobacter* diagnostics in Pennsylvania[14] and the Food-borne Diseases Active Surveillance Network (FoodNet) sites[15] highlight the wide range of testing practices in use; currently no best-practice clinical or public health laboratory guidelines exist for laboratory diagnosis of *Campylobacter* infections, yet they are needed. There are several different methods available for detection of *Campylobacter* in the clinical laboratory. These include culture, stool immunoassays for *Campylobacter*-specific antigen, and molecular tests, such as nucleic acid–amplified tests. These are discussed in detail in the sections that follow.

### Collection, Transport, and Storage of Specimens

For laboratory diagnosis of *Campylobacter* from patients with acute gastrointestinal symptoms, fecal specimens are preferred[16]; however, rectal swabs are acceptable in infants and young children when feces are otherwise difficult to obtain.[17,18] A stool specimen should be collected during the acute phase of the diarrheal illness and before antibiotic treatment is initiated.[19] For routine purposes, a single specimen is sufficient to recover *Campylobacter*, but 2 samples may be desirable depending on clinical circumstances.[16] Standard rejection criteria for bacterial stool samples apply for *Campylobacter*.[19] Unpreserved stool maintained at room temperature must be received in the laboratory within 2 hours. A transport medium such as modified Cary-Blair should be used when a delay of more than 2 hours is anticipated and for transporting rectal swabs. Specimens received in Cary-Blair should be stored at 4°C if processing is not performed immediately.[16]

*Campylobacter* can be occasionally isolated from routine anaerobic cultures of blood or wound specimens. Cultures from these other sources should be collected and transported according to standard procedures appropriate to these specimen types. If an isolate does not grow on subculture, it should be incubated in a microaerobic atmosphere at 37°C for possible *Campylobacter* isolation.

## Culture and Isolation

Isolation of *Campylobacter* from clinical specimens, primarily fecal samples, involves direct plating of the specimen (nonenriched) onto selective media, which prevents the overgrowth of other bacteria in the specimen and the use of a microaerobic (5% $O_2$, 10% $CO_2$, 85% $N_2$) environment. Most clinical laboratories routinely culture stool specimens for *Campylobacter* using conditions that were developed and favor isolation of *C jejuni* and *C coli*; no single culture method currently available will isolate all *Campylobacter* species.

### Campylobacter jejuni and Campylobacter coli

Given that *C jejuni* and *C coli are* the primary species isolated from fecal specimens in patients with *Campylobacter* gastroenteritis, clinical laboratories should focus on using appropriate methods for isolation of these 2 species. Although other *Campylobacter* species will occasionally be isolated using routine culture methods, an alternative method for isolation of species other than *C jejuni* or *C coli* also may be needed in the laboratory in some instances and is described in the following paragraph.

*C jejuni* and *C coli* can be isolated from fecal specimens by direct plating of the specimen on selective media and incubation in a microaerobic atmosphere at 42°C for 72 hours. A variety of blood-based and charcoal-based media are commercially available for the isolation of *C jejuni/coli* from human fecal specimens. These include the blood-based media, Campy-CVA (cefoperazone-vancomycin-amphotericinB), Skirrow agar, the charcoal-based media mCCDA (modified charcoal cefoperazone deoxycholate agar), and Karmali agar. To achieve the optimal yield of *Campylobacter* from stool specimens, the use of more than one type of selective media, with one being blood-free (mCCDA or Karmali), increases the yield from stools by as much as 15%.[20] Campy-CVA, mCCDA, or Karmali media is recommended if only a single medium is used.[16]

### Enrichment Culture

Several enrichment broths have been formulated to enhance recovery of *Campylobacter* from stool including Preston enrichment, *Campylobacter* enrichment broth, and Campy-thio.[21] Inclusion of an enrichment step may be beneficial in instances in which low numbers of organisms are expected, but the clinical advantage and cost-effectiveness of using enrichment as part of routine culture has not been studied adequately and it is not recommended for routine use.[16]

### Species Other Than Campylobacter jejuni/Campylobacter coli

A passive filtration technique that uses a nonselective plating medium and an incubation temperature of 37°C instead of 42°C,[22] is an effective approach to isolate species other than *C jejuni/C coli* that are susceptible to antibiotics present in commonly used *Campylobacter*-selective media. The method is based on the principle that campylobacters can pass through membrane filters (0.45–0.65 μm) because of their small size and motility, whereas other stool flora are retained during the short processing time.[16] Nonselective medium, such as tryptose blood agar, in combination with filtration incubated at 37°C under microaerobic conditions, preferably with an atmosphere containing increased hydrogen (5%–7% $H_2$) for at least 96 hours, will allow isolation of the non–*C jejuni/coli* species, including the hydrogen-requiring species.[23] This method should be used to complement direct culture to selective plating media, as the technique is not as sensitive as direct culture.[24]

## Culture-independent Diagnostic Tests

Culture-independent diagnostic tests (CIDTs) for detection of this fastidious organism, directly in stool specimens without the specialized media and equipment that are needed for *Campylobacter* culture, have emerged as an alternative to culture-based methods. Both stool antigen tests and nucleic acid amplification tests (NAATs) are now commercially available. CIDTs are rapid, and provide same-day results; however, they do not yield an isolate for antibiotic susceptibility testing or epidemiologic studies.[25]

## Stool Antigen Assays

There are 3 immunoassays cleared by the Food and Drug Administration (FDA) in the United States: the ProSpecT Campylobacter Microplate Assay (Remel, Lenexa, KS), the Premier CAMPY (Meridian Bioscience, Cincinnati, OH), and the Immuno*Card* STAT! CAMPY (Meridian Bioscience, Cincinnati, OH). Each of these immunoassays detects a common *Campylobacter* surface antigen that is shared by *C jejuni* and *C coli*, so the immunoassays detect both species of *Campylobacter* in stool specimens but cannot differentiate them. The immunoassays also have been reported to cross react with *Campylobacter upsaliensis*,[26,27] a recognized cause of gastrointestinal disease. Initial published evaluations of *Campylobacter* stool antigen CIDTs reported comparable or better sensitivities than conventional culture methods.[28–30] More recent evaluations[31,32] and clinical case investigations[33,34] have questioned the specificity of these assays.

## Nucleic Acid Amplification Tests

Laboratory-developed NAATs have been used to detect *Campylobacter* in stool specimens,[35–37] and they improve time to detection and identify to the species level, including identification of less common *Campylobacter* species missed by conventional culture.[16] Clinical laboratories considering the implementation of laboratory-developed NAAT for campylobacters must fully understand the steps needed to establish the performance characteristics of such assays as well as Clinical Laboratory Improvement Amendments regulatory requirements.

Several commercially available multiplex NAAT assays that detect *Campylobacter* species and other gastrointestinal pathogens, have received FDA clearance for use in the United States. These include the Luminex xTAG gastrointestinal pathogen panel (Luminex, Austin, TX),[38,39] the Hologic GenProbe Prodesse ProGastro panel (Hologic, Bedford, MA),[40] the BioMerieux Biofire Filmarray system (BioMerieux, Cambridge, MA),[41] and the Becton Dickinson BD MAX system (Becton Dickinson Diagnostics, Sparks, MD),[42] with other platforms also marketed for use on stool specimens, including the Savyon Diagnostics system (Savyon Diagnostics, Ashdod, Israel)[39] and Genetic Signatures system (Genetic Signatures, Darlington, Australia).[43] These panels provide a comprehensive, rapid, and streamlined alternative to culture for *Campylobacter* and other etiologic agents of infectious gastroenteritis. Recovery of isolates from culture is still required for susceptibility testing and public health surveillance purposes. Although these panels certainly look promising, there is at this time insufficient published validation data on the US products to assess the performance characteristics of these panels. These panels are discussed in detail elsewhere in this issue.

## Identification of Campylobacter

*Campylobacter jejuni* can be identified from primary selective media based on growth on selective plates at 42°C, Gram stain appearance, positive oxidase reaction, and rapid hippurate hydrolysis testing.[16] Strains with this phenotype can be reliably reported as *C jejuni*. Hippurate-negative, thermophilic strains can be further tested with indoxyl acetate and positive strains reported as *C jejuni/C coli*. For *Campylobacter* species other than *C jejuni/C coli*, phenotypic characterization alone will not provide definitive species-level identification. The use of additional molecular identification methods, such as species-specific PCR,[44,45] single-target gene sequencing (16S rRNA, rpoB),[46] and matrix-assisted laser desorption/ionization time-of-flight mass spectrometry[47–49] are recommended for these organisms.

## SELF-ASSESSMENT

1 Which of the following statements is true regarding *Campylobacter* organism or infection?
   a. Outbreaks of *Campylobacter* infections are common.
   b. Secondary transmission is common during a *Campylobacter* outbreak.
   c. Poultry is the most common food associated with *Campylobacter* outbreaks.
   d. Only *C jejuni* and *C coli* cause human disease.
   e. There are 26 species within the *Campylobacter* genus.
2. Which of the following statements is true regarding *Campylobacter*?
   a. *Campylobacter* is a gram-positive organism.
   b. *C jejuni* grows optimally at 25°C.
   c. Serotyping is a high-resolution subtyping tool useful for *Campylobacter*.
   d. *C jejuni* is hippurate positive.
   e. *Campylobacter* is isolated only from human stool and no other human source sites.
3. Which of the following statements is true regarding *Campylobacter* organism or infection?
   a. GBS is a postinfectious complication of a *Campylobacter* infection.
   b. Hektoen is a *Campylobacter*-selective media.
   c. CIDTs detect all *Campylobacter* species.
   d. NAAT assays take 3 days to run.
   e. Filtration is more sensitive than direct culture to selective plating media.

ANSWERS

Answer 1: E.
There are 26 species currently defined with the *Campylobacter* genus.

Answer 2: D.
*C jejuni* is positive in the hippurate phenotypic test. This test is a useful test to differentiate *C jejuni* from the other thermotolerant *Campylobacter* species.

Answer 3: A.
Patients with *Campylobacter* infections are at increased risk for several postinfectious complications, including GBS.

## REFERENCES

1. Man SM. The clinical importance of emerging *Campylobacter* species. Nature reviews. Gastroenterol Hepatol 2011;8(12):669–85.
2. On SL. Taxonomy of *Campylobacter, Arcobacter, Helicobacter* and related bacteria: current status, future prospects and immediate concerns. Symp Ser Soc Appl Microbiol 2001;1S–15S.

3. Miller WG, Parker CT. *Campylobacter* and *Arcobacter.* In: Fratamico P, Liu Y, Kathariou S, editors. Genomes of foodborne and waterborne pathogens. Washington, DC: ASM Press; 2011. p. 49–65.

4. Vandamme PF, Rossau R, Hoste B, et al. Revision of *Campylobacter, Helicobacter,* and *Wolinella* taxonomy: emendation of generic descriptions and proposal of *Arcobacter* gen. nov. Int J Syst Bacteriol 1991;41:88–103.

5. Blaser MJ. Epidemiologic and clinical features of *Campylobacter jejuni* infections. J Infect Dis 1997;176(Suppl 2):S103–5.

6. Skirrow MB, Blaser MJ. Clinical aspects of Campylobacter infection. 2nd edition. Washington, DC: ASM Press; 2000.

7. Yuki N, Hartung HP. Guillain-Barre syndrome. N Engl J Med 2012;366(24): 2294–304.

8. Pope JE, Krizova A, Garg AX, et al. Campylobacter reactive arthritis: a systematic review. Semin Arthritis Rheum 2007;37(1):48–55.

9. Marshall JK. Post-infectious irritable bowel syndrome following water contamination. Kidney Int Suppl 2009;(112):S42–3.

10. Scallan E, Hoekstra RM, Angulo FJ, et al. Foodborne illness acquired in the United States–major pathogens. Emerg Infect Dis 2011;17(1):7–15.

11. Crim SM, Iwamoto M, Huang JY, et al, Centers for Disease Control and Prevention (CDC). Incidence and trends of infection with pathogens transmitted commonly through food–Foodborne Diseases Active Surveillance Network, 10 U.S. sites, 2006-2013. MMWR Morb Mortal Wkly Rep 2014;63(15):328–32.

12. Kendall ME, Crim S, Fullerton K, et al. Travel-associated enteric infections diagnosed after return to the United States, Foodborne Diseases Active Surveillance Network (FoodNet), 2004-2009. Clin Infect Dis 2012;54(Suppl 5):S480–7.

13. Taylor EV, Herman KM, Ailes EC, et al. Common source outbreaks of *Campylobacter* infection in the USA, 1997-2008. Epidemiol Infect 2013;141(5):987–96.

14. M'Ikanatha NM, Dettinger LA, Perry A, et al. Culturing stool specimens for *Campylobacter* spp., Pennsylvania, USA. Emerg Infect Dis 2012;18(3): 484–7.

15. Hurd S, Patrick M, Hatch J, et al. Clinical laboratory practices for the isolation and identification of *Campylobacter* in Foodborne Diseases Active Surveillance Network (FoodNet) sites: baseline information for understanding changes in surveillance data. Clin Infect Dis 2012;54(Suppl 5):S440–5.

16. Fitzgerald C, Nachamkin I. Campylobacter and Arcobacter. 10th edition. Washington, DC: ASM Press; 2011. p. 885–9.

17. Buchino JJ, Suchy FJ, Snyder JW. Bacterial diarrhea in infants and children. Perspect Pediatr Pathol 1984;8(2):163–80.

18. Rishmawi N, Ghneim R, Kattan R, et al. Survival of fastidious and nonfastidious aerobic bacteria in three bacterial transport swab systems. J Clin Microbiol 2007;45(4):1278–83.

19. Gilligan PH, Janda JM, Karmali MA, et al. Laboratory diagnosis of bacterial diarrhea. Cumitech 12A. Washington, DC: ASM Press; 1992.

20. Endtz HP, Ruijs GJ, Zwinderman AH, et al. Comparison of six media, including a semisolid agar, for the isolation of various *Campylobacter* species from stool specimens. J Clin Microbiol 1991;29(5):1007–10.

21. Corry JE, Post DE, Colin P, et al. Culture media for the isolation of campylobacters. Int J Food Microbiol 1995;26(1):43–76.

22. Steele TW, McDermott SN. The use of membrane filters applied directly to the surface of agar plates for the isolation of *Campylobacter jejuni* from feces. Pathology 1984;16(3):263–5.

23. Vandenberg O, Dediste A, Houf K, et al. Arcobacter species in humans. Emerg Infect Dis 2004;10(10):1863–7.

24. Goossens H, Vlaes L, De Boeck M, et al. Is "*Campylobacter upsaliensis*" an unrecognised cause of human diarrhoea? Lancet 1990;335(8689):584–6.

25. Cronquist AB, Mody RK, Atkinson R, et al. Impacts of culture-independent diagnostic practices on public health surveillance for bacterial enteric pathogens. Clin Infect Dis 2012;54(Suppl 5):S432–9.

26. Couturier BA, Couturier MR, Kalp KJ, et al. Detection of non-*jejuni* and -*coli Campylobacter* species from stool specimens with an immunochromatographic antigen detection assay. J Clin Microbiol 2013;51(6):1935–7.

27. Hindiyeh M, Jense S, Hohmann S, et al. Rapid detection of *Campylobacter jejuni* in stool specimens by an enzyme immunoassay and surveillance for *Campylobacter upsaliensis* in the greater Salt Lake City area. J Clin Microbiol 2000; 38(8):3076–9.

28. Bessede E, Delcamp A, Sifre E, et al. New methods for detection of campylobacters in stool samples in comparison to culture. J Clin Microbiol 2011;49(3): 941–4.

29. Granato PA, Chen L, Holiday I, et al. Comparison of premier CAMPY enzyme immunoassay (EIA), ProSpecT Campylobacter EIA, and ImmunoCard STAT! CAMPY tests with culture for laboratory diagnosis of *Campylobacter* enteric infections. J Clin Microbiol 2010;48(11):4022–7.

30. Tribble DR, Baqar S, Pang LW, et al. Diagnostic approach to acute diarrheal illness in a military population on training exercises in Thailand, a region of *Campylobacter* hyperendemicity. J Clin Microbiol 2008;46(4):1418–25.

31. Floch P, Goret J, Bessede F, et al. Evaluation of the positive predictive value of a rapid immunochromatographic test to detect *Campylobacter* in stools. Gut Pathog 2012;4(1):17.

32. Giltner CL, Saeki S, Bobenchik AM, et al. Rapid detection of *Campylobacter* antigen by enzyme immunoassay leads to increased positivity rates. J Clin Microbiol 2013;51(2):618–20.

33. Myers AL, Jackson MA, Selvarangan R. False-positive results of *Campylobacter* rapid antigen testing. Pediatr Infect Dis J 2011;30(6):542.

34. Operario DJ, Moonah S, Houpt E. Hemolytic uremic syndrome following infection with O111 Shiga toxin-producing *Escherichia coli* revealed through molecular diagnostics. J Clin Microbiol 2014;52(3):1003–5.

35. de Boer RF, Ott A, Guren P, et al. Detection of *Campylobacter* species and *Arcobacter butzleri* in stool samples by use of real-time multiplex PCR. J Clin Microbiol 2013;51(1):253–9.

36. Kulkarni SP, Lever S, Logan JM, et al. Detection of *Campylobacter* species: a comparison of culture and polymerase chain reaction based methods. J Clin Pathol 2002;55(10):749–53.

37. Liu J, Gratz J, Amour C, et al. A laboratory-developed TaqMan array card for simultaneous detection of 19 enteropathogens. J Clin Microbiol 2013;51(2): 472–80.

38. Mengelle C, Mansuy JM, Prere MF, et al. Simultaneous detection of gastrointestinal pathogens with a multiplex Luminex-based molecular assay in stool samples from diarrhoeic patients. Clin Microbiol Infect 2013;19(10):E458–65.

39. Perry MD, Corden SA, Howe RA. Evaluation of the Luminex xTAG Gastrointestinal Pathogen Panel and the Savyon Diagnostics Gastrointestinal Infection Panel for the detection of enteric pathogens in clinical samples. J Med Microbiol 2014; 63(Pt 11):1419–26.

40. Buchan BW, Olson WJ, Pezewski M, et al. Clinical evaluation of a real-time PCR assay for identification of *Salmonella, Shigella, Campylobacter* (*Campylobacter jejuni* and *C coli*), and shiga toxin-producing *Escherichia coli* isolates in stool specimens. J Clin Microbiol 2013;51(12):4001–7.

41. Buss SN, Leber A, Chapin K, et al. Multicenter evaluation of the BioFire FilmArray gastrointestinal panel for etiologic diagnosis of infectious gastroenteritis. J Clin Microbiol 2015;53(3):915–25.

42. Anderson NW, Buchan BW, Ledeboer NA. Comparison of the BD MAX enteric bacterial panel to routine culture methods for detection of *Campylobacter*, enterohemorrhagic *Escherichia coli* (O157), *Salmonella*, and *Shigella* isolates in preserved stool specimens. J Clin Microbiol 2014;52(4):1222–4.

43. Siah SP, Merif J, Kaur K, et al. Improved detection of gastrointestinal pathogens using generalised sample processing and amplification panels. Pathology 2014; 46(1):53–9.

44. On SL, Jordan PJ. Evaluation of 11 PCR assays for species-level identification of *Campylobacter jejuni* and *Campylobacter coli*. J Clin Microbiol 2003;41(1):330–6.

45. Debruyne L, Samyn E, De Brandt E, et al. Comparative performance of different PCR assays for the identification of *Campylobacter jejuni* and *Campylobacter coli*. Res Microbiol 2008;159(2):88–93.

46. Korczak BM, Stieber R, Emler S, et al. Genetic relatedness within the genus *Campylobacter* inferred from rpoB sequences. Int J Syst Evol Microbiol 2006; 56(Pt 5):937–45.

47. Alispahic M, Hummel K, Jandreski-Cvetkovic D, et al. Species-specific identification and differentiation of *Arcobacter, Helicobacter* and *Campylobacter* by full-spectral matrix-associated laser desorption/ionization time of flight mass spectrometry analysis. J Med Microbiol 2010;59(Pt 3):295–301.

48. Bessede E, Solecki O, Sifre E, et al. Identification of *Campylobacter* species and related organisms by matrix assisted laser desorption ionization-time of flight (MALDI-TOF) mass spectrometry. Clin Microbiol Infect 2011;17(11):1735–9.

49. Martiny D, Dediste A, Debruyne L, et al. Accuracy of the API Campy system, the Vitek 2 Neisseria-Haemophilus card and matrix-assisted laser desorption ionization time-of-flight mass spectrometry for the identification of *Campylobacter* and related organisms. Clin Microbiol Infect 2011;17(7):1001–6.

# Optimizing the Laboratory Diagnosis of *Clostridium difficile* Infection

Peter H. Gilligan, PhD, D(ABMM)[a,b,*]

## KEYWORDS

- *Clostridium difficile* • Glutamate dehydrogenase • Algorithm • Diarrhea
- Nucleic acid amplification test (NAAT) • Toxin • Microbiome • Disease outcomes

## KEY POINTS

- *Clostridium difficile* is the most common cause of health care–associated infection in the United States; only toxigenic strains of *C difficile* cause disease.
- The optimal laboratory approach for diagnosing *C difficile* infection (CDI) remains controversial. A 2014 College of American Pathologists survey reported that nucleic acid amplification tests (NAAT) are the most widely used diagnostic test to establish this diagnosis in the United States.
- A large prospective multicenter outcome study of *C difficile* diagnostics showed that the detection of toxin was associated with more severe outcomes than detection of toxigenic organisms either by culture or NAAT.
- The United Kingdom's National Health Service requires only patients with positive toxin tests to be reported as having CDI.
- Laboratories that have switched from less sensitive solid-phase or immunochromatographic toxin assays to NAAT have higher CDI rates. Now that mandatory reporting of CDI rates is required in some states in the United States, there may be a disadvantage to institutions using a sensitive compared with less sensitive techniques.
- Laboratories that are using NAAT as stand-alone test for CDI should consider confirming NAAT-positive tests with a toxin-based assay.

## INTRODUCTION

In a recent multistate point prevalence survey, *Clostridium difficile* was the most common causal agent of health care–associated infections (HAIs).[1] During this century, the

---

Disclosures: None.
[a] Clinical Microbiology-Immunology Laboratories, Microbiology-Immunology, UNC Health Care, UNC School of Medicine, CB 7600, Chapel Hill, NC 27516, USA; [b] Pathology-Laboratory Medicine, UNC School of Medicine, CB 7600, Chapel Hill, NC 27516, USA
* Pathology-Laboratory Medicine, UNC School of Medicine, CB 7600, Chapel Hill, NC 27516.
*E-mail address:* gilliganncphd@gmail.com

Clin Lab Med 35 (2015) 299–312
http://dx.doi.org/10.1016/j.cll.2015.02.003
0272-2712/15/$ – see front matter © 2015 Elsevier Inc. All rights reserved.

labmed.theclinics.com

incidence, morbidity, and mortality of *C difficile* infection (CDI) have all increased.[2] The reasons for this increase are complex but include an aging population that is particularly susceptible to CDI with poor outcomes[3]; increased use of fluoroquinolones to which the organism is resistant[3]; emergence of at least 2 highly virulent ribotypes, 027 and 078, which produce increased toxin levels and perhaps more severe disease[3,4]; and improved diagnostic testing.[5]

Since the initial recognition of *C difficile* as causing a toxin-induced diarrheal disease,[6] prior or concurrent antimicrobial therapy was seen as an important risk factor for this infection.[7] Understanding of why antimicrobial treatment is central to the development of CDI is rapidly evolving as clinicians begin to understand the complexity of the gastrointestinal (GI) microbiome and its ability to protect against CDI. In a recent review, Taur and Palmer[8] suggested one way in which the microbiome might protect from CDI and how its disruption could provide an environment for the growth and toxin production essential for this infection. Primary bile salts stimulate the germination of *C difficile* spores in the intestinal tract, which can potentially result in *C difficile* growth and toxin production in colonized individuals. Individuals with an intact intestinal microbiome are able to metabolize bile salts from their primary form to secondary forms. Secondary bile salts inhibit the growth of toxin-producing *C difficile* vegetative cells, protecting the individual from this organism. When the protective microbiome is diminished or eliminated by antimicrobials, spore germination, organism growth, and toxin production may proceed, resulting in disease. Recent studies suggest that specific organisms within the intestinal microbiome may play a role in protecting from CDI, including species within the *Bacteroides*, Ruminococcaceae, Lachnospiraceae, and *Eubacterium*.[9,10] These organisms are often absent in the intestinal microbiome of patients with CDI. These data suggest that elimination of key components of the intestinal microbiome by antimicrobial therapy creates an environment in which toxigenic *C difficile* can proliferate and cause disease.[8–10] In studies of patients with recurrence of CDI, reintroducing these protective organisms by fecal microbiota transplant resulted in resolution of disease in 90% of patients, compared with a resolution of only 30% of patients receiving *C difficile*–specific antimicrobial therapy.[11–13] In another small study of only 2 patients with *C difficile* recurrence, organisms derived from the stool of a healthy donor were prepared in a chemostat. This mixture included species of organisms thought to protect from CDI. Both patients resolved their infections.[10] Taken together, these data provide important evidence of the value of reconstituting the protective microbiome in patients with CDI.

Although understanding of the microbiome has given clinicians new avenues for treatment and perhaps even prevention of disease, how best to diagnose CDI is a source of ongoing debate. Two recent clinical practice guidelines, one written in the United States,[7] the other in the United Kingdom,[14] take different approaches to defining CDI, with the US guideline advocating the use of the nucleic acid amplification test (NAAT) as the definite test for CDI either as a stand-alone test or part of a multistep algorithm. The UK guideline uses the detection of toxin in feces as the definite test for CDI and proposes NAAT as a screening test with toxin detection confirming CDI in NAAT-positive specimens. Further complicating this debate is the US requirement to report CDI rates as a measure of the quality of care at an institution. This requirement is part of a national effort to reduce HAIs, of which *C difficile* is the most common.[1] The definition of CDI is based on detection of *C difficile* toxin A and/or B, toxin genes by nucleic acid amplification, or toxigenic culture in unformed stools (stools taking the shape of the specimen container). More information can be found at http://www.cdc.gov/nhsn/PDFs/pscManual/12pscMDRO.CDADcurrent.pdf.

This article examines each stage in the CDI diagnostic process and how it may affect the infection rates at an institution. It focuses on *C difficile* carriage and how distinguishing carriage from infection can be difficult in selected populations. It reviews the new multiplex NAAT tests for enteric pathogens and comments on how they may need to be used in this new era of HAI accountability. It also discusses the problem of diagnosis of patients with recurrence of infection.

## PREANALYTICAL STAGE: WHO SHOULD BE TESTED?

Patients should be tested if they are currently receiving antimicrobials or have received antimicrobials in the past 8 weeks and have a minimum of 3 documented episodes of diarrhea per day.[5] The disease is most prevalent in individuals more than 65 years of age, especially those who have recently been in hospital or live in a long-term care facility.[3] The term antimicrobials needs to be defined broadly as any agent that has significant antimicrobial activity that can alter the intestinal microbiome and place an individual at risk for CDI. Agents such as azidothymidine and methotrexate (a cancer and rheumatologic chemotherapeutic agent) both have antimicrobial activity and have been associated with the induction of CDI.[15] Clinicians also are beginning to recognize patients with community-acquired CDI without evidence of prior or current antimicrobial therapy.[16] However, alternative medicines and nutritional supplements may contain substances with antimicrobial activity that may alter the GI microbiome.[15,17]

The more complicated problem is who has diarrhea and is it likely to be caused by *C difficile*? An important article by Dubberke and colleagues[18] showed that 19% of patients tested for CDI received laxatives in the 48 hours before having testing performed; another 17% did not meet the criteria for clinically significant diarrhea. Although the implementation of the electronic medical record in many institutions should make it possible for laboratory technologists to access patient history and to determine whether diarrhea has been documented in the patient being tested, laboratorians often do not have the time to review charts to determine the number of diarrhea episodes per day, which is central to both the definition and severity of CDI.[7] In addition, these data are often poorly documented. As a result, the most expedient approach to determining whether a patient has diarrhea is to have the technologist examine the stool to determine whether it represents a diarrheal specimen. One approach is to use a reference method called the Bristol Stool Form Scale.[19] The specimen's consistency is compared with the chart, with specimens giving a score of 5 to 7 deemed most likely to be associated with CDI.[19] Specimen that have a score of 6 or 7 are liquid or take the form of the cup, whereas specimens that score 1 to 4 are formed. Specimens with a score of 5 are soft and may conform to the shape of the specimen container. Most laboratories do not test specimens that have a score of 1 to 4.[19] A simpler approach, championed by Brecher and colleagues,[20] is the simple stick test. Its application is easily remembered. In the words of Brecher and colleagues[20]: "If the stick falls, test them all. If the stick stands, the test is banned."

Regardless of the approach used by the laboratory to characterize the stool, it is essential that only stools from patients with diarrhea be tested.

It is important to test only diarrheal specimens because the test most widely used in the United States, NAAT, detects toxigenic organisms rather than toxin in stool,[5] so there is a significant potential for false-positive test results. Asymptomatic carriage of *C difficile* is high in specific populations. The American Academy of Pediatrics actively discourages *C difficile* testing on children less than a year of age because asymptomatic carriage rates vary from 37% in the first month of life, to 30% between 1 and 6 months, to 14% in children 6 to 12 months old, making interpretation of test results difficult in this age group.[21] CDI seems to be rare in children between 12 and 24 months of age.[21] Only by the third birthday do carriage rates decrease to what is seen in adults.[21] *C difficile* testing is only recommended when children reach this age. When clinicians consider testing children between 1 and 3 years of age for CDI, it should be done in consultation with the laboratory. Only children in whom other, more common, causes of diarrheal disease, such as rotavirus and norovirus, are first ruled out and who have a typical clinical presentation of CDI, including more than 3 stools per day and concurrent or antimicrobial therapy in the prior 8 weeks, should be considered for testing.[21]

The carriage rates of *C difficile* in asymptomatic adults have been reported to vary from 3% to 15%.[22–25] In asymptomatic adults who are currently receiving or have recently received antimicrobials, the carriage rate can be as high as 25%.[22] In individuals cared for in long-term care facilities, carriage rates as high as 57% have been reported.[7] Many of these individuals have recently been hospitalized and/or were receiving antimicrobials, both of which are important risk factors for *C difficile* carriage. These high carriage rates may result in false-positive *C difficile* tests, especially if patients without diarrhea are tested using *C difficile* NAAT.[26]

Diarrhea is especially common in 2 patient populations: those with inflammatory bowel disease (IBD) and those with graft-versus-host disease (GVHD). CDI is reported to be a significant cause of flares in IBD.[7] Likewise, CDI may contribute to the diarrhea that is common in patients with GVHD.[27] It is recommended that diarrheal patients with these underlying conditions be tested and, if positive, treated for CDI.[7]

The frequency of testing is an issue that is frequently discussed, especially in patients who have an initial negative *C difficile* test and in whom diarrhea persists. Given the high sensitivity of algorithmic and NAAT testing for *C difficile* detection, multiple tests are generally not recommended.[7,28,29] Many laboratories test on a weekly basis in patients in whom diarrhea persists, although only 3% of repeat tests are positive and some of them may be falsely so.[28]

There are 2 other preanalytical issues that require consideration: test of cure, and the diagnosis of disease recurrence. Test of cure is not recommended by current guidelines, in part because the organism can persist for up to 30 days in as many as 20% of patients who have resolved their diarrhea.[7] The test of cure in CDI is the resolution of diarrhea because of organism persistence. However, laboratories may be asked to document the absence of *C difficile* for placement purposes in long-term care facilities. Our approach is to screen these patients for the presence of *C difficile* glutamate dehydrogenase (GDH) (discussed later) and to certify them as negative if they are GDH negative. Our rationale is that the organism must be actively growing in order to produce sufficient protein to give a positive result, whereas NAAT, because of the enhanced sensitivity, may be positive in the absence of active growth. However, this is strictly a working hypothesis that is not proved but is accepted by our infection prevention team that manages this issue.

The diagnosis of CDI recurrence can also be a difficult issue. CDI recurrences can be caused by relapse of a treated infection or reinfection with a different strain of *C difficile*. Evidence indicates that recurrences are increasing,[30] that they are seen most frequently in patients more than 75 years of age,[30] that patients who have recurrences are not able to mount a protective immune response against the toxin A and B produced by the organism,[31] and that patients who have one recurrence are more likely to have additional ones.[30] Our major recommendation to clinicians who are attempting to detect recurrence is to make sure that the patient has recurrence, and is not refractory to antimicrobial treatment or fecal microbiome transplant. Simply stated, patients must have resolved their diarrhea and had a period of normal bowel activity and then redevelop diarrhea of at least 3 stools a day. In that clinical setting, we would test for *C difficile*.

## ANALYTICAL STAGE: WHAT TESTING SCHEME IS BEST?

The initial clinical test used for the detection of CDI was the cytotoxin neutralization (CTN) test, which was developed in the 1970s.[32] In this test, stool filtrates were applied to tissue culture monolayers and examined for actinomorphic changes (the cells rounded up and had raylike projections). These actinomorphic changes could be neutralized by preincubating the stool filtrate with antitoxin specific for *C difficile* toxins.[32] *C difficile* toxins were found in 20% to 30% of patients with antimicrobial-associated diarrhea and in close to 100% of patients with pseudomembranous colitis, but were found in only 1% to 3% of patients without diarrhea.[6] Because animal studies showed that 2 toxins, called toxin A and toxin B,[33] were responsible for the disease associated with this organism in animal models and were present in stool of patients with diarrhea, this quickly became the standard diagnostic test for *C difficile*. However, this test was time consuming, required significant technical skill, had a slow turnaround time (TAT), and specimens often had to be transported to reference laboratories, lengthening already slow TATs.[5]

Shortly after the development of CTN, a selective medium, cycloserine cefoxitin fructose agar, was developed for the detection of *C difficile*.[34] Several modifications of this medium have been made that have improved the sensitivity of *C difficile* detection.[35] At the time, culture was considered the microbiologic gold standard. However, this gold standard was flawed because, although highly sensitive for CDI, it lacked specificity for primarily 2 reasons. As already reviewed, asymptomatic carriage rates were particularly high in certain patient populations, such as infants and individuals being treated or recently exposed to antimicrobials. Second some strains of *C difficile* did not produce toxins and therefore could not cause disease.[33] This observation resulted in the need for an additional step to prove whether cultured isolates produced toxins and thus could cause disease, which slowed down TAT.

CTN and toxigenic culture on a selective medium remain important reference methods for research into diagnostic tests for CDI but, given their complexity and slow TAT, neither is widely used currently for diagnostic purposes.[5]

An important innovation for the detection of CDI that occurred in the early 1990s was the commercial development and use of immunoassays for detection of *C difficile* toxins. The initial tests were solid-phase enzyme immunoassays (EIA) that detected toxin A, which was thought at the time to be the essential toxin in *C difficile* pathogenesis.[5] Subsequently, it was recognized that strains of *C difficile* that produced only toxin B could cause disease.[36,37] Commercial development of assays for both toxins A and B soon followed. These assays were reported to have a sensitivity of as high as 98% compared with CTN.[5] Solid-phase EIA tests for *C difficile* became the standard for CDI detection in most clinical laboratories until 2006, when the utility of this diagnostic approach was called into question by the seminal work of Dr Carroll's group.[38] Using CTN as a reference method, her group showed that a test that detected a *C difficile* cell wall–associated antigen, glutamate dehydrogenase (GDH), had a sensitivity of 100% compared with the toxin A/B EIA sensitivity of 38%. Although the negative predictive value was 100%, the positive predictive value of the GDH assay was only 59%, requiring confirmation of positive GDH results. Other studies confirmed this observation.[39,40] This work led our laboratory to implement a 2-stage algorithm using an immunochromatographic assay for GDH followed by CTN assay.[39] Because of the reported high sensitivity and negative predictive value of the GDH assay, negative GDH results were reported as negative, whereas GDH-positive specimens were subsequently assayed by CTN. Specimens positive in the CTN assay were reported as positive for *C difficile*; those that were negative were reported as negative for *C difficile*. The GDH assay, which took 15 minutes to perform, was done 3 times a day, resulting in a TAT of less than or equal to 8 hours for the approximately 80% to 85% of specimens that were GDH negative. However, the 15% to 20% of specimens that were GDH positive were assayed only once a day with the CTN, resulting in a TAT of as long as 56 hours for these specimens. Many CTN-positive specimens had a TAT closer to 30 hours. This slow TAT for potentially positive specimens was not well received by our clinicians. However, by early 2009, 2 innovations were available in *C difficile* diagnostics. First, the GDH immunoassay was coupled with a toxin A/B immunoassay. Although the toxin A/B EIA had a modest sensitivity of between 45% and 60%, its positive predictive value was between 90% and 100%, allowing specimens positive for both GDH and toxin A/B to be reported as positive for *C difficile*.[41,42] Second, NAATs for detection of toxigenic *C difficile* were becoming widely available commercially.[5]

As of this writing, there are 9 US Food and Drug Administration (FDA)–approved *C difficile* NAATs of varying complexity.[5] Six are polymerase chain reaction (PCR)-based assays and 3 are isothermal assays; 2 helicase-dependent amplification, and the other loop-mediated isothermal amplification (LAMP). The assays have similar performance characteristics, with sensitivities ranging from 80% to 100% and specificities ranging from 87% to 99% depending on the assay and the reference method used.[5] Meta-analysis data are not available for all of the NAATs but, for those for which there are data, the test performances are similar,[43,44] although individual studies might show modest differences in performance.[5]

These two innovations spawned different approaches to CDI diagnosis: a 2-step or 3-step testing algorithm or the use of a stand-alone NAAT.[15] The NAAT stand-alone approach has become the most common method used by laboratories who participated in the 2014 College of American Pathologists (CAP) proficiency testing program.[45] The most widely used NAATs were Cepheid Xpert PCR assay (Sunnyvale, CA), which is used by 25% of laboratories, and the Meridian illumigene LAMP assay (Cincinnati, OH) by 19%. Other PCR assays were used by 2% of the participants. The TECHLAB/Alere Quik/Chek Complete (Scarborough, ME), which detects GDH and toxin A/B, was used by 21% of participants. It is unclear what would be done if those laboratories had a GDH-positive/toxin-negative specimen. It is disappointing that 19% of laboratories used toxin A/B solid-phase immunoassay or immunochromatographic assays even though 2 recent clinical practice guidelines recommend against their use as stand-alone tests.[7,14] Other tests were used in 6% of laboratories.

Our laboratory has used a 3-stage algorithm since mid-2009. The initial step in this assay is to do the TECHLAB/Alere Quik/Chek Complete assay as a screening test on each laboratory shift. If the patient is negative for GDH and toxins A and B, the assay is reported as *C difficile* negative; if it is positive for both analytes it is reported as *C difficile* positive. If it is positive for GDH but negative for toxin A/B, it is reflexed to the Gene Xpert PCR assay, tested immediately, and the result of this assay is the final result. The major advantage of this approach compared with a NAAT-only approach is cost. We determined that the testing algorithm saved us approximately $90,000 in supply costs over a 1-year period compared with a NAAT-only approach.[46] In addition, we have a TAT of less than 8 hours for screen-positive and screen-negative specimens (87% of all specimens) and less than 12 hours for PCR specimens (13%), which are tested on demand in the Gene Xpert system.

A novel approach to *C difficile* testing is its detection as part of a multiplex NAAT panel for detection of GI pathogens. One panel detects 11 pathogens (7 bacterial,

2 viruses, and 2 parasites) (Luminex Corporation, Toronto, Canada), whereas a second panel detects 23 pathogens (14 bacteria, 5 viruses, and 4 parasites) (BioFire Diagnostics, Salt Lake City, UT). Both have gained FDA clearance. *C difficile* was the most common pathogen detected in a study comparing the 2 assays, and both assays were highly sensitive and specific compared with a laboratory-developed *C difficile* toxin A/B real-time PCR assay.[47] *C difficile* was the pathogen detected most frequently in mixed infections with the Luminex assay. The utility of detection of *C difficile* in a multiplex assay is currently difficult to assess, in part because there is little clinical detail in the current evaluation. Further, the patient population that is most likely to benefit from multiplex NAAT detection of GI pathogens is that with community-acquired diarrheal disease, and these patients are likely to be at comparatively low risk for *C difficile* disease. Given the high rate of asymptomatic carriage of *C difficile* in some populations, the finding of *C difficile* in the setting of mixed infections presents a conundrum for clinicians. Because of this, our laboratory does not report the *C difficile* analyte, although we do offer the Luminex multiplex GI panel. A further issue is that practice guidelines recommend that only *C difficile* testing be done on diarrheal patients who have been in hospital for longer than 3 days, making the multiplex approach of limited value in hospitalized patients.[7] In addition, the supply costs are considerably more for multiplex NAAT assays than for the *C difficile* specific NAAT. Because there is insufficient information on how to apply the multiplex NAAT assays to the detection of CDI, these tests currently cannot be recommended for CDI detection.

## POSTANALYTICAL PHASE
### What Do a Positive and Negative Test Result for Clostridium difficile Mean?

Two recent guidelines suggest different approaches to interpreting *C difficile* test results. The American College of Gastroenterology advocates that NAAT be the primary means of diagnosing CDI, preferably as a stand-alone test, because of superior sensitivity to an algorithmic approach.[7] The National Health System in the United Kingdom[14] proposes an algorithmic approach in which NAAT or GDH is used as a screening test, screening test negatives are reported as negative, and a sensitive toxin A/B assay be used as a confirmatory test with toxin-positive specimens being reported as positive, and a toxin-negative test indicating that the patient is a *C difficile* excretor. The most sensitive toxin A/B assay is the CTN but, for technical and TAT reasons already discussed, it is highly unlikely that this approach will find any support in the United States. The data on which the UK recommendations are based come from a prospective, multicenter study that examined the CDI outcome based on CTN and toxigenic culture as reference methods.[48] The investigators studied 6522 inpatients with diarrheal disease for whom outcomes were available. There were 3 groups in the study: patients who were CTN positive (group 1), patients who were toxigenic culture positive but CTN negative (group 2), and patients negative for both tests (group 3). Patients who were CTN positive (group 1) had a higher case mortality than patients in either group 2 or 3. Group 1 and 2 had longer hospital stays than group 3 patients in a univariate analysis but, when other predictors were added, multivariate analysis could not confirm this finding. Importantly, NAAT-positive, CTN-negative patients gave similar results to those who were toxigenic culture positive. At least 4 other, smaller studies have shown that stool toxin–positive patients, detected either by toxin EIA or CTN, seem to have more severe disease than those who are toxin negative but positive for toxigenic organisms by either NAAT or culture.[49–53] An important observation in 2 of these studies is that the crossing threshold (the number of cycles needed to get a positive NAAT) was higher in patients who were toxin negative.[49,51] This finding suggests that patients with specimens that are NAAT positive and toxin negative have lower numbers of organisms and, in at least some patients, likely represent asymptomatic carriage. A recent multicenter study of more than 600 specimens found that, when an NAAT (Lyra, Direct *C difficile* assay Quidel, San Diego, CA) was compared with CTN, the NAAT was highly sensitive, with poor positive predictive value but high negative predictive value; these are characteristics of a good screening test. The comparison of the NAAT with toxigenic culture showed that the sensitivity was lower but it had much better positive predictive value with still high negative predictive value, confirming that NAAT is more predictive of toxigenic culture results than CTN.[54] As discussed earlier, the UK National Health Service (NHS) guideline recommends that a positive NAAT test be confirmed by a "sensitive toxin EIA test."[14] Solid-phase toxin A/B EIA tests are more sensitive than immunochromatographic tests.[5] For example, when we evaluated a solid-phase EIA compared with an immunochromatographic test, we found the solid-phase assay to have a sensitivity of 60% compared with 43% for the immunochromatographic EIA.[39]

### Does Rapid Testing Affect Patient Care?

Because CTN is the most accurate toxin detection assay, the question is whether laboratories should return to using that assay to confirm either GDH or NAAT results. Based on CAP *C difficile* surveys, CTN is used in less than 1% of laboratories.[5] Therefore, laboratories would need to send their confirmatory testing to a reference laboratory. These data suggest that if laboratories choose to confirm GDH or NAAT results, they are likely to use more rapid but less sensitive EIA-based assays.

Reporting *C difficile* results rapidly does have a positive impact on patient care. A study that compared management of patients whose diagnosis of CDI was based either on CTN/toxigenic culture versus NAAT only or a GDH/NAAT algorithm found that patients who, by either NAAT or GDH/NAAT algorithm, had results reported sooner had fewer repeat tests, and were specifically treated sooner.[55] Furthermore, empiric CDI therapy was used less often in these patients. There also was a trend to fewer days on unneeded infection-control precautions. There was no difference in 30-day mortality, disease recurrence, or length of stay with any of the three approaches. The physicians surveyed preferred rapid result reporting, although there was no difference in satisfaction between NAAT stand-alone testing versus GDH/NAAT algorithm.[55] A second study comparing a CTN-based algorithm versus a NAAT-based algorithm showed that the NAAT-based algorithm reduced the use of unnecessary CDI therapy.[56]

### What Is the Impact of Molecular Testing on Health Care–associated Clostridium difficile Infection Rates?

At present, facilities in 30 states and the District of Columbia are required by law to report HAI rates, including CDI HAI rates, to the National Healthcare Safety Network (NHSN). The NHSN has established rules for reporting patients as having CDI. A positive laboratory test for CDI is defined as a positive result for toxin A and/or B (by molecular or toxin assays) or detection of toxin-producing *C difficile* by culture or other laboratory measures (http://www.cdc.gov/nhsn/PDFs/pscManual/12pscMDRO_CDADcurrent.pdf).

Laboratories that switched from toxin-based methods to NAAT methods have seen significant increases in their CDI infection rates.[15,57–59] In our laboratory, when we switched from a toxin-based method to an algorithm we saw a doubling in our CDI infection rate; a rate that has persisted for 3 years (**Fig. 1**). During a 1-year period in which 4321 specimens were tested using a 3-step algorithm, we found that

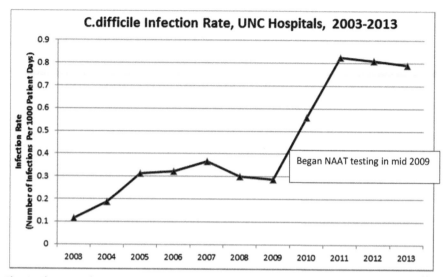

**Fig. 1.** The rate of CDI at the University of North Carolina (UNC) Hospitals. (*From* Gilligan P. Contemporary approaches for the laboratory diagnosis of *Clostridium difficile* infections. Semin Colon Rectal Surg 2014;25:141; with permission.)

approximately 12% of patients had CDI based on the NHSN definition, 4.4% positive by toxin A/B immunochromatographic assay, whereas 7.9% were positive by PCR.[46] **Fig. 2,** shows that our hospital has a significantly higher infection rate compared with all North Carolina hospitals but a similar infection rates compared with our peer

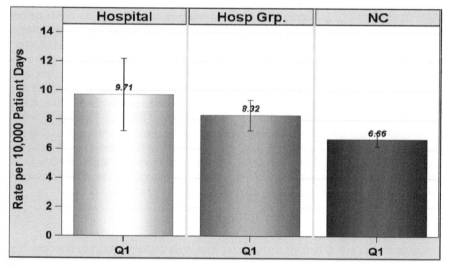

**Fig. 2.** CDI rates for UNC Health Care (Hospital) compared with North Carolina hospitals of similar size and care complexity (Hosp Grp) and all North Carolina hospitals (NC) from January 1 to March 31, 2014. (*From* North Carolina Department of Health and Human Services. Healthcare-Associated Infections in North Carolina. N.C. Healthcare-Associated Infections Prevention Program, N.C. Communicable Disease Branch; 2014. Available at: http://epi. publichealth.nc.gov/cd/hai/figures/hai_jul2014_consumers.pdf. Accessed October 30, 2014.)

institutions. Part of this increased infection rate is caused by the more complex patient populations that we care for, but part of it might be caused by our use of PCR as a confirmatory test. Based on CAP data,[45] it is likely that at least some North Carolina hospitals are using less sensitive assays and thus have lower reported infection rates.

### Should the Playing Field Be Leveled?

The NHS approach to C difficile test reporting is more proscriptive than that of the US NHSN. The NHS definition only considers patients as CDI positive if they have toxin present in stool, whereas the NHSN guidelines consider anyone with any positive test for toxigenic C difficile as having CDI. As a result, laboratories that use insensitive toxin immunochromatographic assays as stand-alone tests have much lower infection rates than those using NAAT.[57–59] Because of a growing body of evidence suggesting that at least some NAAT-positive, toxin-negative patients do not have disease,[49–53] testing approaches and interpretations in the United States should be reconsidered. At the least, laboratories that are using NAAT as a stand-alone test might consider confirming NAAT-positive specimens with a toxin assay, preferably by a solid-phase EIA because of its superior sensitivity.[5] The NHSN might then consider the NHS approach, in which only toxin-positive patients are reported as having CDI, whereas NAAT-positive, toxin-negative patients could be reviewed by an infection prevention-ist and using standardized definitions they would determine whether those patients were likely to have CDI or were C difficile excretors. In either case, the NAAT-positive patients would still require isolation, at least until their diarrhea resolved. This approach could also be applied to a 3-stage algorithm in which a less sensitive toxin immunochromatographic assay is used with the same infection preventionist re-view applying to the GDH-positive, toxin-negative, NAAT-positive individuals. Patients who are toxin positive in this scheme are considered as having CDI.

A hospital currently using an NAAT-only approach might be willing to add an addi-tional confirmatory step to the 10% to 15% of their specimens which are positive by NAAT. Starting in 2015, hospitals will have a financial incentive to do confirmatory testing since high CDI rates may result in Centers for Medicare and Medicaid Services penalties. This will depend on the willingness of the NHSN to modify their CDI definition to fit the emerging evidence that CDI outcomes are more closely linked to the presence of toxin in stool than the detection of organisms.[48–53] Importantly, the concept of C difficile excretors, defined as individuals without evidence of CDI based on the absence of toxin in stool and/or clinical review by infection preventionists, should be embraced. Given that these individuals may be a source of infection for other patients, they should remain on isolation until symptoms resolve. Studies are needed to deter-mine whether C difficile excretors should receive anti–C difficile therapy, although the emerging understanding of the interaction of the GI microbiome and C difficile likely argues against that approach.[9] These individuals may be candidates for microbiome replacement when stool substitutes currently in development are available.

### SELF-ASSESSMENT

1. A patient who is a C difficile excretor is most likely to have which of the following test results on a stool specimen?
   a. Toxin positive and NAAT positive
   b. Toxin positive and NAAT negative
   c. GDH positive, toxin positive, and NAAT positive
   d. GDH positive, toxin negative, and NAAT positive
   e. GDH positive, toxin negative, and NAAT negative

2. Which test results is or are most strongly indicative of CDI?
   a. GDH positive, toxin negative, and NAAT negative
   b. GDH or NAAT positive, toxin positive
   c. NAAT positive
   d. GDH negative, toxin negative
   e. GDH positive, toxin negative, and NAAT positive

3. Based on the NHSN guidelines for *C difficile* testing, the patient population with the highest rate of CDI will be:
   a. Patients tested with a stand-alone toxin EIA test
   b. Patients tested with an algorithm that uses GDH as a screening test and cyto-toxin neutralization as a confirmatory test for GDH-positive specimens
   c. Patients tested with an algorithm that uses GDH and toxin A/B EIA as a screening test and NAAT as a confirmatory test for GDH-positive or toxin-positive specimens
   d. Patients tested with a toxin A/B EIA test and positives confirmed by NAAT testing
   e. Patients tested with a stand-alone NAAT

ANSWERS

Answer 1: (d).

Because this is the definition of a *C difficile* excretor. Answers (a), (b), and (c) all meet the NHS guideline definition of CDI. The results in (e) do not indicate the presence of toxigenic *C difficile* and would be considered a false-positive for CDI.

Answer 2: (b).

The presence of *C difficile* toxin is most consistent with CDI. The other choices do not indicate the presence of *C difficile* toxin.

Answer 3: (e).

An NAAT is the most sensitive method for detection of *C difficile*. Hospitals that have adopted this approach have seen significant increases in CDI rates.

**REFERENCES**

1. Magill SS, Edwards JR, Bamberg W, et al. Multistate point-prevalence survey of health care-associated infections. N Engl J Med 2014;370:1198–208.
2. Peery AF, Dellon ES, Lund J, et al. Burden of gastrointestinal disease in the United States: 2012 update. Gastroenterology 2012;143:1179–87.e1–3.
3. Lessa FC, Gould CV, McDonald LC. Current status of *Clostridium difficile* infection epidemiology. Clin Infect Dis 2012;55(Suppl 2):S65–70.
4. Walker AS, Eyre DW, Wyllie DH, et al. Relationship between bacterial strain type, host biomarkers, and mortality in *Clostridium difficile* infection. Clin Infect Dis 2013;56:1589–600.
5. Burnham CA, Carroll KC. Diagnosis of *Clostridium difficile* infection: an ongoing conundrum for clinicians and for clinical laboratories. Clin Microbiol Rev 2013; 26:604–30.
6. Bartlett JG, Moon N, Chang TW, et al. Role of *Clostridium difficile* in antibiotic-associated pseudomembranous colitis. Gastroenterology 1978;75:778–82.

7. Surawicz CM, Brandt LJ, Binion DG, et al. Guidelines for diagnosis, treatment, and prevention of *Clostridium difficile* infections. Am J Gastroenterol 2013;108: 478–98 [quiz: 99].

8. Taur Y, Pamer EG. Harnessing microbiota to kill a pathogen: fixing the microbiota to treat *Clostridium difficile* infections. Nat Med 2014;20:246–7.

9. Schubert AM, Rogers MA, Ring C, et al. Microbiome data distinguish patients with *Clostridium difficile* infection and non-*C. difficile*-associated diarrhea from healthy controls. MBio 2014;5(3):e01021–14.

10. Petrof EO, Gloor GB, Vanner SJ, et al. Stool substitute transplant therapy for the eradication of *Clostridium difficile* infection: 'RePOOPulating' the gut. Microbiome 2013;1:3.

11. Youngster I, Russell GH, Pindar C, et al. Oral, capsulized, frozen fecal microbiota transplantation for relapsing *Clostridium difficile* infection. JAMA 2014;312:1772–8.

12. van Nood E, Vrieze A, Nieuwdorp M, et al. Duodenal infusion of donor feces for recurrent *Clostridium difficile*. N Engl J Med 2013;368:407–15.

13. Kassam Z, Lee CH, Yuan Y, et al. Fecal microbiota transplantation for *Clostridium difficile* infection: systematic review and meta-analysis. Am J Gastroenterol 2013; 108:500–8.

14. Advisory Committee on Antimicrobial Resistance and Healthcare Associated Infections. Updated guidance on the diagnosis and reporting of *Clostridium difficile*. United Kingdom: National Health Service; 2012.

15. Gilligan P. Contemporary approaches for the laboratory diagnosis of *Clostridium difficile* infections. Semin Colon Rectal Surg 2014;25:137–42.

16. Kutty PK, Woods CW, Sena AC, et al. Risk factors for and estimated incidence of community-associated *Clostridium difficile* infection, North Carolina, USA. Emerg Infect Dis 2010;16:197–204.

17. McCarthy K, Johnston S, Hepworth C. *Clostridium difficile*-associated colitis following the use of Chinese medicine. BMJ Case Rep 2009;2009. http://dx.doi.org/10.1136/bcr.08.2008.0716.

18. Dubberke ER, Han Z, Bobo L, et al. Impact of clinical symptoms on interpretation of diagnostic assays for *Clostridium difficile* infections. J Clin Microbiol 2011;49: 2887–93.

19. Caroff DA, Edelstein PH, Hamilton K, et al. The Bristol Stool Scale and its relationship to *Clostridium difficile* infection. J Clin Microbiol 2014;52:3437–9.

20. Brecher SM, Novak-Weekley SM, Nagy E. Laboratory diagnosis of *Clostridium difficile* infections: there is light at the end of the colon. Clin Infect Dis 2013;57: 1175–81.

21. Schutze GE, Willoughby RE. *Clostridium difficile* infection in infants and children. Pediatrics 2013;131:196–200.

22. Viscidi R, Willey S, Bartlett JG. Isolation rates and toxigenic potential of *Clostridium difficile* isolates from various patient populations. Gastroenterology 1981;81:5–9.

23. Galdys AL, Nelson JS, Shutt KA, et al. Prevalence and duration of asymptomatic *Clostridium difficile* carriage among healthy subjects in Pittsburgh, Pennsylvania. J Clin Microbiol 2014;52:2406–9.

24. Guerrero DM, Becker JC, Eckstein EC, et al. Asymptomatic carriage of toxigenic *Clostridium difficile* by hospitalized patients. J Hosp Infect 2013;85:155–8.

25. Alasmari F, Seiler SM, Hink T, et al. Prevalence and risk factors for asymptomatic *Clostridium difficile* carriage. Clin Infect Dis 2014;59:216–22.

26. Koo HL, Van JN, Zhao M, et al. Real-time polymerase chain reaction detection of asymptomatic *Clostridium difficile* colonization and rising *C. difficile*-associated disease rates. Infect Control Hosp Epidemiol 2014;35:667–73.

27. Willems L, Porcher R, Lafaurie M, et al. *Clostridium difficile* infection after alloge-neic hematopoietic stem cell transplantation: incidence, risk factors, and outcome. Biol Blood Marrow Transplantant 2012;18:1295–301.

28. Khanna S, Pardi DS, Rosenblatt JE, et al. An evaluation of repeat stool testing for *Clostridium difficile* infection by polymerase chain reaction. J Clin Gastroenterol 2012;46:846–9.

29. Nistico JA, Hage JE, Schoch PE, et al. Unnecessary repeat *Clostridium difficile* PCR testing in hospitalized adults with C. difficile-negative diarrhea. Eur J Clin Mi-crobiol Infect Dis 2012;32:97–9.

30. D'Agostino RB Sr, Collins SH, Pencina KM, et al. Risk estimation for recurrent *Clostridium difficile* infection based on clinical factors. Clin Infect Dis 2014;58:1386–93.

31. Leav BA, Blair B, Leney M, et al. Serum anti-toxin B antibody correlates with pro-tection from recurrent *Clostridium difficile* infection (CDI). Vaccine 2009;28:965–9.

32. Chang TW, Lin PS, Gorbach SL, et al. Ultrastructural changes of cultured human amnion cells by *Clostridium difficile* toxin. Infect Immun 1979;23:795–8.

33. Lyerly DM, Krivan HC, Wilkins TD. *Clostridium difficile*: its disease and toxins. Clin Microbiol Rev 1988;1:1–18.

34. George WL, Sutter VL, Citron D, et al. Selective and differential medium for isola-tion of *Clostridium difficile*. J Clin Microbiol 1979;9:214–9.

35. Lister M, Stevenson E, Heeg D, et al. Comparison of culture based methods for the isolation of *Clostridium difficile* from stool samples in a research setting. Anaerobe 2014;28:226–9.

36. Lyras D, O'Connor JR, Howarth PM, et al. Toxin B is essential for virulence of *Clos-tridium difficile*. Nature 2009;458:1176–9.

37. Kuehne SA, Cartman ST, Heap JT, et al. The role of toxin A and toxin B in *Clos-tridium difficile* infection. Nature 2010;467:711–3.

38. Ticehurst JR, Aird DZ, Dam LM, et al. Effective detection of toxigenic *Clostridium difficile* by a two-step algorithm including tests for antigen and cytotoxin. J Clin Microbiol 2006;44:1145–9.

39. Gilligan PH. Is a two-step glutamate dehyrogenase antigen-cytotoxicity neutraliza-tion assay algorithm superior to the premier toxin A and B enzyme immunoassay for laboratory detection of *Clostridium difficile*? J Clin Microbiol 2008;46:1523–5.

40. Fenner L, Widmer AF, Goy G, et al. Rapid and reliable diagnostic algorithm for detection of *Clostridium difficile*. J Clin Microbiol 2008;46:328–30.

41. Quinn CD, Sefers SE, Babiker W, et al. C. Diff Quik Chek complete enzyme immu-noassay provides a reliable first-line method for detection of *Clostridium difficile* in stool specimens. J Clin Microbiol 2009;48:603–5.

42. Sharp SE, Ruden LO, Pohl JC, et al. Evaluation of the C. Diff Quik Chek Complete Assay, a new glutamate dehydrogenase and A/B toxin combination lateral flow assay for use in rapid, simple diagnosis of *Clostridium difficile* disease. J Clin Microbiol 2010;48:2082–6.

43. O'Horo JC, Jones A, Sternke M, et al. Molecular techniques for diagnosis of *Clos-tridium difficile* infection: systematic review and meta-analysis. Mayo Clin Proc 2012;87:643–51.

44. Deshpande A, Pasupuleti V, Rolston DD, et al. Diagnostic accuracy of real-time polymerase chain reaction in detection of *Clostridium difficile* in the stool samples of patients with suspected *Clostridium difficile* infection: a meta-analysis. Clin Infect Dis 2011;53:e81–90.

45. College of American Pathologists. D-A Bacteriology participant survey. Northfield (IL): American College of Pathologists; 2014.

46. Culbreath K, Ager E, Nemeyer RJ, et al. Evolution of testing algorithms at a university hospital for detection of *Clostridium difficile* infections. J Clin Microbiol 2012;50:3073–6.

47. Khare R, Espy MJ, Cebelinski E, et al. Comparative evaluation of two commercial multiplex panels for detection of gastrointestinal pathogens by use of clinical stool specimens. J Clin Microbiol 2014;52:3667–73.

48. Planche TD, Davies KA, Coen PG, et al. Differences in outcome according to *Clostridium difficile* testing method: a prospective multicentre diagnostic validation study of *C difficile* infection. Lancet Infect Dis 2013;13:936–45.

49. Beaulieu C, Dionne LL, Julien AS, et al. Clinical characteristics and outcome of patients with *Clostridium difficile* infection diagnosed by PCR versus a three-step algorithm. Clin Microbiol Infect 2014;20:1067–73.

50. Landry ML, Ferguson D, Topal J. Comparison of Simplexa universal direct PCR with cytotoxicity assay for diagnosis of *Clostridium difficile* infection: performance, cost, and correlation with disease. J Clin Microbiol 2014;52:275–80.

51. Baker I, Leeming JP, Reynolds R, et al. Clinical relevance of a positive molecular test in the diagnosis of *Clostridium difficile* infection. J Hosp Infect 2013;84:311–5.

52. Leslie JL, Cohen SH, Solnick JV, et al. Role of fecal *Clostridium difficile* load in discrepancies between toxin tests and PCR: is quantitation the next step in *C. difficile* testing? Eur J Clin Microbiol Infect Dis 2012;31:3295–9.

53. Polage CR, Chin DL, Leslie JL, et al. Outcomes in patients tested for *Clostridium difficile* toxins. Diagn Microbiol Infect Dis 2012;74:369–73.

54. Beck ET, Buchan BW, Riebe KM, et al. Multicenter evaluation of the Quidel Lyra Direct *C. difficile* nucleic acid amplification assay. J Clin Microbiol 2014;52:1998–2002.

55. Barbut F, Surgers L, Eckert C, et al. Does a rapid diagnosis of *Clostridium difficile* infection impact on quality of patient management? Clin Microbiol Infect 2013;20:136–44.

56. Sydnor ER, Lenhart A, Trollinger B, et al. Antimicrobial prescribing practices in response to different *Clostridium difficile* diagnostic methodologies. Infect Control Hosp Epidemiol 2011;32:1133–6.

57. Gould CV, Edwards JR, Cohen J, et al. Effect of nucleic acid amplification testing on population-based incidence rates of *Clostridium difficile* infection. Clin Infect Dis 2013;57:1304–7.

58. Williamson DA, Basu I, Freeman J, et al. Improved detection of toxigenic *Clostridium difficile* using the Cepheid Xpert *C difficile* assay and impact on *C difficile* infection rates in a tertiary hospital: a double-edged sword. Am J Infect Control 2012;41:270–2.

59. Longtin Y, Trottier S, Brochu G, et al. Impact of the type of diagnostic assay on *Clostridium difficile* infection and complication rates in a mandatory reporting program. Clin Infect Dis 2013;56:67–73.

# Antimicrobial Susceptibility Testing of Bacteria That Cause Gastroenteritis

Romney M. Humphries, PhD, D(ABMM)[a],
Audrey N. Schuetz, MD, MPH, D(ABMM)[b],*

## KEYWORDS

- Susceptibility testing • *Campylobacter* • *Salmonella* • *Shigella* • *Vibrio* • *Aeromonas*
- *Clostridium difficile*

## KEY POINTS

- Infections due to most gastrointestinal pathogens are self-limiting in immunocompetent patients, and isolates from these patients generally do not require antimicrobial susceptibility testing (AST).
- The National Antimicrobial Resistance Monitoring System (NARMS) monitors antimicrobial resistance trends in enteric bacteria across the United States.
- New fluoroquinolone breakpoints should be used for all *Salmonella* spp.
- The Clinical and Laboratory Standards Institute (CLSI) has provided new azithromycin breakpoints for *Salmonella* Typhi.
- Although official breakpoints do not exist for azithromycin and *Campylobacter* or *Shigella*, epidemiologic cutoff values (ECOFFs) can be used for surveillance purposes.
- Antimicrobial resistance of various enteric pathogens isolated from animals and water is of concern due to transfer of resistance to humans.

Bacterial gastroenteritis is a self-limiting disease for which antimicrobial therapy is generally not indicated. In some cases, antimicrobial therapy can in fact be detrimental to the host. Such is the case when quinolones are used for the treatment of shiga-toxigenic *Escherichia coli* infection, resulting in a burst of toxin production by the organism that puts the patient at increased risk for hemolytic uremic syndrome (HUS).[1,2]

---

The authors have no disclosures to provide.
[a] Pathology & Laboratory Medicine, University of California Los Angeles, 10833 Le Conte Avenue, Brentwood Annex, Los Angeles, CA 90095, USA; [b] Department of Pathology and Laboratory Medicine, Weill Cornell Medical College/NewYork-Presbyterian Hospital, 525 East 68th Street, Starr 737C, New York, NY 10065, USA
* Corresponding author.
*E-mail address:* ans9112@med.cornell.edu

http://dx.doi.org/10.1016/j.cll.2015.02.005
0272-2712/15/$ – see front matter © 2015 Elsevier Inc. All rights reserved.
labmed.theclinics.com

Similarly, the use of antimicrobials for the treatment of uncomplicated, nontyphoidal *Salmonella* gastroenteritis has been shown to increase the rate of clinical relapse and prolong carriage of the organism by the host.[3] As a result, susceptibility testing of bacterial pathogens isolated from stool cultures should not be routinely performed by the laboratory for isolates from patients without underlying medical problems.[4,5] There are, however, some clinical circumstances in which antimicrobial therapy is indicated for bacterial gastroenteritis, including patients with severe or prolonged diarrhea (characterized by $\geq 6$ unformed stools per day, temperature $\geq 101°F$, tenesmus, or the presence of blood in stool or fecal leukocytes), the immunocompromised host, the elderly, and infants younger than 6 months.[6] In these cases, communication between the laboratory and the treating physician aids in determining the need for susceptibility testing and the antimicrobial agents to be tested. In addition, if the laboratory identifies *Salmonella enterica* ser. Typhi or *S enterica* ser. Paratyphi from stool, consideration should be given to susceptibility testing. Finally, isolation of any of the organisms described herein from an extraintestinal source (eg, blood, urine) warrants susceptibility testing.

In the United States, the NARMS monitors antimicrobial resistance in enteric bacteria isolated from humans, food-producing animals, and retail meat sources on an annual basis. This program, performed in collaboration between the Centers for Disease Control and Prevention (CDC), the US Food and Drug Administration (FDA), and the US Department of Agriculture, includes annual data on antimicrobial resistance in human isolates of *Salmonella, Shigella, Campylobacter, E coli* O157, and *Vibrio* species other than *Vibrio cholerae*. These data are publicly available on the CDC Web site and are an excellent reference for laboratories and physicians.

This article summarizes the current state of AST for the bacterial gastrointestinal pathogens.

## CAMPYLOBACTER

*Campylobacter* is one of the most common causes of bacterial food-borne illness in the United States, and 80% to 90% of reported infections are caused by *Campylobacter jejuni*.[7] Most cases of campylobacteriosis are characterized by acute, self-limiting diarrhea, for which antimicrobial therapy provides the limited benefit of 1.3 days of symptom relief and is therefore generally not indicated.[8] In contrast, severe, prolonged, or relapsing campylobacteriosis, which occurs predominantly in the very young, the elderly, and the immunocompromised, is treated. The macrolide azithromycin is now the preferred agent for treating campylobacteriosis because of recent concerns of the slight risk of cardiac arrest associated with erythromycin, in particular when given with medications that inhibit CYP3A4.[9] Resistance to both azithromycin and erythromycin remains low in the United States, with less than 2% of *C jejuni* and 9% of *Campylobacter coli* isolates reported as resistant to these agents in 2012 surveillance performed by CDC NARMS.[10] In contrast, *Campylobacter* resistance to the fluoroquinolones, which are second-line agents for campylobacteriosis, has been reported with increasing frequency in the United States. In 2012, 25% of *C jejuni* isolates and 34% of *C coli* were resistant to ciprofloxacin.[10] Worldwide, fluoroquinolone resistance in *Campylobacter* is increasing, with rates well more than 60% in Southeast Asia and some regions of Latin America, Africa, and India.[11] Doxycycline and tetracycline are alternative agents for antimicrobial therapy, but approximately half of *C jejuni* and *C coli* isolates in the United States are resistant to tetracycline.[10] Macrolide resistance in *Campylobacter* is usually due to ribosomal target mutations, whereas fluoroquinolone resistance is conferred by mutation of the DNA gyrase gene *gyrA*, typically by the point mutation C257 T.[12,13] The *tet*(O) gene, located on plasmids or chromosomes, confers high-level tetracycline resistance in *C jejuni* and *C coli*.

Mutations in efflux pumps can also lead to resistance to macrolides, fluoroquinolones, and/or tetracyclines.

Livestock are the primary reservoir for human *Campylobacter* infections. Resistance to both the macrolides and fluoroquinolones in animal isolates of *Campylobacter* has been associated with the practice of adding these agents to animal food or water as growth-promoting agents.[14] In 2005, the FDA withdrew its approval of the veterinary fluoroquinolone, enrofloxacin, for use in poultry water because of concern of increasing fluoroquinolone resistance in human *Campylobacter* isolates.[15] However, this action does not seem to have changed the trajectory of ciprofloxacin resistance among human isolates of *Campylobacter* in the United States. In 2005, 21.6% of *C jejuni* were resistant to ciprofloxacin, whereas in 2012, this number had increased to 25.3%.[10] Other countries have noted similar findings after withdrawal of veterinary fluoroquinolones.[16] Fluoroquinolone-resistant isolates have been shown to outcompete wild-type *Campylobacter* isolates in the chicken, suggesting that enhanced biological fitness is associated with fluoroquinolone resistance and explaining the persistence of resistance to this antimicrobial despite removal of selective pressure imposed by veterinary fluoroquinolones.[17] Human infections caused by fluoroquinolone-resistant *Campylobacter* do not seem to cause more severe disease than infections caused by fluoroquinolone-susceptible isolates[18]; nonetheless, fluoroquinolone-resistant *Campylobacter* is a significant clinical concern.

Because of increasing resistance, AST of isolates from individual patients with severe illness, with prolonged symptoms, or at risk for severe disease is warranted if antimicrobial treatment is under consideration. In addition, *Campylobacter* isolated from extraintestinal sites should be tested for antimicrobial susceptibility. Until recently, susceptibility testing for *Campylobacter* isolates was fraught with technical difficulties, making this task a challenge for clinical laboratories. However, starting with the standardization of agar dilution methods in 2004[19,20] and more recently broth microdilution (BMD) and disk diffusion (DD) by both the CLSI[4] and the European Committee on Antimicrobial Susceptibility Testing (EUCAST), the reliability of AST for this organism has greatly improved. The recent availability of standardized DD methods is of particular importance, as this technique is widely accessible to most laboratories that perform *Campylobacter* cultures.

The CLSI recommends BMD in cation-adjusted Mueller-Hinton broth supplemented with 2.5% to 5% (v/v) laked (lysed) horse blood, with incubation in a microaerobic atmosphere for *C jejuni* and *C coli*.[4] No standardized susceptibility test methods or breakpoints exist for *Campylobacter* spp other than *C jejuni* and *C coli*. Interpretive criteria for ciprofloxacin, erythromycin, doxycycline, and tetracycline are provided by the CLSI M45-A2 guideline for this method.[4] EUCAST suggests BMD be performed by International Standards Organization standards,[21] with the modification of adding 5% lysed horse blood and 20 mg/L β-nicotinamide adenine dinucleotide (NAD) to the test media. EUCAST provides breakpoints for ciprofloxacin, erythromycin, and tetracycline by this method. According to EUCAST, tetracycline can be used to determined susceptibility to doxycycline.

Both the CLSI and EUCAST have standardized the DD method for *Campylobacter*. Significant controversy exists in the literature regarding the performance of DD AST for *Campylobacter* spp.[22,23] The predominant technical challenge associated with DD for *Campylobacter* spp is measurement of zones of inhibition, as *Campylobacter* growth can be hazy or filmlike on DD plates (**Fig. 1**). DD by the CLSI method is performed on Mueller-Hinton agar with 5% sheep blood (BMHA) and incubated at 42°C for 24 to 48 hours. The EUCAST *Campylobacter* DD method is similar to that of the CLSI, with the exception that Mueller-Hinton agar (MHA) supplemented with 5%

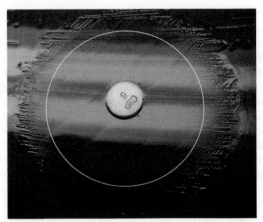

**Fig. 1.** *Campylobacter jejuni* ciprofloxacin disk diffusion test on Mueller-Hinton agar with 5% sheep blood. Testing should be performed following drying of media in an incubator before plating and by tilting the plate to read the innermost zone of inhibition (*white ring*). Note the filmlike growth surrounding the zone of inhibition.

defibrinated horse blood and 20 mg/L β-NAD is used in place of BMHA.[24] Key factors for improving the reproducibility of DD results include drying of the agar plates before inoculation to prevent swarming, and reading zone diameters by tilting the plate and reading the smallest zone of inhibition (see **Fig. 1**). Colonies within the zone are not ignored. Using these revised recommendations, the CLSI developed disk interpretive criteria for tetracycline and revised the criteria for ciprofloxacin and erythromycin, using data gathered through multicenter studies (**Table 1**). These criteria will be

**Table 1**
*Campylobacter* breakpoints and epidemiologic cutoff values

| Antimicrobial | Disk Diffusion (mm) | | | MIC (μg/mL) | | |
|---|---|---|---|---|---|---|
| | S | I | R | S | I | R |
| Azithromycin | | | | | | |
|   CDC ECOFF | — | — | — | ≤0.25 | | ≥0.5 |
| Erythromycin | | | | | | |
|   CLSI | ≥16 | 13–15 | ≤12 | ≤8 | 16 | ≥32 |
|   EUCAST *C jejuni*[a] | ≥20 | — | <20 | ≤4 | — | >4 |
|   EUCAST *C coli*[a] | ≥24 | — | <24 | ≤8 | — | >8 |
| Ciprofloxacin | | | | | | |
|   CLSI | ≥24 | 21–23 | ≤20 | ≤1 | 2 | ≥4 |
|   EUCAST | ≥26 | — | <26 | ≤0.5 | — | >0.5 |
| Tetracycline | | | | | | |
|   CLSI | ≥26 | 23–25 | ≤22 | ≤4 | 8 | ≥16 |
|   EUCAST[b] | ≥30 | — | <30 | ≤2 | — | >2 |
| Doxycycline | | | | | | |
|   CLSI | — | — | — | ≤2 | 4 | ≥8 |

*Abbreviations:* I, intermediate; MIC, minimal inhibitory concentration; R, resistant in legend; S, susceptible.
[a] Erythromycin can be used to determine susceptibility to azithromycin and clarithromycin.
[b] Tetracycline can be used to determine susceptibility to doxycycline.

published in the forthcoming CLSI M45-A3 document, and various documentation are provided on the CLSI Web site.[25] In these studies, no false susceptible interpretations were observed and only 1.0% minor errors were noted for ciprofloxacin (*C jejuni*) and 1.4% for tetracycline (*C coli*) by DD, as compared with CLSI BMD. These interpretations differ from the M45-A2 version, which included a resistance-only category for DD testing for erythromycin and ciprofloxacin and included no disk criteria for tetracycline.[4] EUCAST has also developed disk interpretive criteria for ciprofloxacin, erythromycin, and tetracycline, which differ from those of the CLSI (see **Table 1**).[24]

No commercial susceptibility test methods are presently cleared by the FDA for *Campylobacter* spp. However, Trek Sensititre (Thermo Fisher Scientific, Oakwood Village, OH, USA) has developed a *Campylobacter* minimal inhibitory concentration (MIC) plate, which is available as a research-use-only product. This lyophilized BMD panel includes 9 antimicrobials: azithromycin, erythromycin, telithromycin, ciprofloxacin, nalidixic acid, florfenicol, tetracycline, gentamicin, and clindamycin. In addition, Etest (bioMérieux, Marcy L'Etoile, France) has been evaluated in several studies for the determination of *Campylobacter* susceptibility testing, although many of these studies were performed before standardized reference methods existed for *Campylobacter* susceptibility testing, making the results difficult to interpret. Among the more recent studies, Valdivieso-Garcia and colleagues[26] compared the performance of Etest on MHA supplemented with 5% lysed horse blood to agar dilution for a collection of 103 chicken isolates of *Campylobacter*. In both methods, samples were incubated at 37°C under microaerobic conditions for 48 hours. In this study, Etest MICs were lower than agar dilution MICs for all antimicrobials tested and only 51.5% essential agreement (MIC agreement within 1 $\log_2$ dilution) was achieved for ciprofloxacin, 52.5% for erythromycin, and 82.6% for tetracycline.[26] No significant categorical errors were noted in this study.[26] van der Beek and colleagues[27] compared erythromycin Etest and BMD, which was performed on the Sensititre panels, for a collection of 36 *C jejuni* and 12 *C coli* human isolates. In this study, 100% essential and categorical agreement was achieved between the 2 methods.

No official breakpoints have been developed for azithromycin, which is the primary treatment choice for campylobacteriosis. However, the CDC has developed an ECOFF for azithromycin and *Campylobacter*, which is used for surveillance purposes (see **Table 1**).[10] In addition, both the CLSI and EUCAST indicate that azithromycin susceptibility can be inferred from an erythromycin-susceptible result.

Different breakpoint-setting organizations have used different methods to set interpretive criteria. It should be noted that the CLSI M45 breakpoints for *Campylobacter* are guidelines only and were predominantly established by evaluating MIC distributions of wild-type *C jejuni* and *C coli* isolates and those with known drug-resistance mechanisms. In contrast, breakpoints published in the M100 standard are established by the CLSI following evaluation of 4 data sets: (1) MIC distributions, (2) pharmacokinetics of the antimicrobial, (3) pharmacodynamics of the antimicrobial, and (4) evaluation of clinical outcome data for patients treated with the antimicrobial in the context of MIC of the infecting organism.[28] The CLSI ciprofloxacin and tetracycline MIC breakpoints for *Campylobacter* are based on Enterobacteriaceae breakpoints for these antimicrobials, which were confirmed for a collection of 417 *C jejuni* and *C coli* isolates, including both resistant and susceptible isolates.[4] CLSI doxycycline and erythromycin MIC breakpoints were determined by evaluating MIC population distributions for 150 isolates of wild-type *C jejuni* and *C coli* tested at 36°C to 37°C following CLSI recommendations. Similarly, because of the absence of pharmacokinetic/pharmacodynamic and clinical outcomes data, EUCAST breakpoints for *Campylobacter* are based on ECOFFs. ECOFFs are derived from analyses of MIC distribution data for a given organism and antimicrobial and are designed to differentiate isolates without resistance mechanisms (wild-type) from those with acquired resistance mechanisms. The CLSI breakpoints and EUCAST ECOFF values for *Campylobacter* are listed in **Table 1**. Several differences exist, but 1 key item to highlight is that EUCAST has developed a different ECOFF for *C jejuni* and *C coli* and erythromycin because of a different MIC distribution for erythromycin between these 2 species.

Although susceptibility testing for *Campylobacter* has vastly improved during the past decade, several factors remain lacking (**Table 2**). Carbapenems are often used for the treatment of extraintestinal campylobacteriosis, but little data are available regarding susceptibility testing and interpretation for this antimicrobial class. In addition, no testing methods have been validated or interpretive criteria developed by breakpoint-setting organizations for *Campylobacter* spp other than *C jejuni* or *C coli*, which may account for up to one-third of *Campylobacter* infections in some settings,[29] and for which susceptibility testing may be warranted if isolated from normally sterile body sites.

**Table 2**
**Outstanding issues regarding antimicrobial susceptibility testing of bacterial gastrointestinal pathogens**

| Dilemma | Interim Solution |
|---|---|
| *Campylobacter* spp | |
| Absence of azithromycin breakpoints | Azithromycin susceptibility can be predicted by susceptibility to erythromycin |
| No standardized susceptibility test methods or breakpoints exist for *Campylobacter* spp other than *C jejuni* and *C coli* (eg, *Campylobacter fetus, Campylobacter upsaliensis*) | No solution to date; consider modifying testing to 35°C |
| *Salmonella* spp | |
| Commercial test systems do not have ciprofloxacin or levofloxacin MIC concentrations low enough for current breakpoints | Use disk diffusion for ciprofloxacin, or Use Etest (following laboratory verification) for ciprofloxacin or levofloxacin, or Use pefloxacin disk (if available) as a surrogate agent |
| No levofloxacin disk diffusion breakpoints exist | Use Etest for levofloxacin MIC, or Use proposed disk breakpoints,[40,43] or Use pefloxacin disk (if available) as a surrogate agent |
| Pefloxacin disks are not available in all countries (including the United States); pefloxacin disk diffusion cannot detect *aac-6'-lb-cr* resistance | Test and report ciprofloxacin by disk diffusion or MIC method |
| No azithromycin breakpoints for non-Typhi *Salmonella* exist | Susceptibility testing is not generally required because of infrequent incidence of resistance Consider interpreting using *Salmonella* Typhi breakpoints, with caution |
| *Shigella* spp | |
| No azithromycin breakpoints or test method | Use EUCAST ECOFF as a guideline (≤16 μg/mL, susceptible), or Use Etest in several studies |

## SALMONELLA

As with *Campylobacter*, gastroenteritis due to *Salmonella* spp is generally a self-limiting disease, for which antimicrobial treatment is not required and may in fact prolong the carrier state.[30] However, antimicrobial therapy may be of benefit for patients with severe infection, characterized by severe diarrhea and high fever, or those who require hospitalization.[30] Certain patient populations, including the immunocompromised, children younger than 3 months,[31] and adults with atherosclerotic disease,[32] may also be considered for preemptive antimicrobial therapy for mild salmonellosis, in an attempt to prevent complications. Antimicrobial treatment is crucial for the roughly 5% of patients with nontyphoidal *Salmonella* gastroenteritis who develop bacteremia,[33,34] which can lead to endocarditis, mycotic aneurysm, and osteomyelitis. Susceptibility testing is indicated for typhoidal *Salmonella* (*S enterica* serovars Typhi and Paratyphi A-C) isolated from intestinal and nonintestinal sources because of the concern for enteric fever. Enteric fever is a severe systemic illness characterized by fever and abdominal pain caused by typhoidal strains of *Salmonella*.

According to NARMS, resistance to the primary antimicrobials used for the treatment of nontyphoidal *Salmonella*, that is, fluoroquinolones, azithromycin, or the third-generation cephalosporins if intravenous therapy is required,[3] remains infrequent in the United States. In 2012, less than 1% of nontyphoidal *Salmonella* were resistant to ciprofloxacin and 2.5% were resistant to ceftriaxone.[10] Less than 1% of isolates demonstrated azithromycin MICs of 32 μg/mL or more. Antimicrobial susceptibility varies by serotype, and in 2012, only 0.8% of *S enterica* ser. Enteritidis were resistant to ceftriaxone, whereas 5.4% and 6.6% of *S enterica* ser. Typhimurium and Newport, respectively, were resistant to ceftriaxone.[10] Of concern, 15.7% of *Salmonella* isolated from retail meat and 10.6% of isolates from food animals were resistant to cephalosporins in a recent study; these sources are thought to be the main reservoirs for human infection.[35] Ampicillin and trimethoprim-sulfamethoxazole (TMP-SMX) resistance of nontyphoidal *Salmonella* in 2011 were approximately 10% and less than 2%, respectively.[10] However, antimicrobial resistance among the serovars of *Salmonella* that cause enteric fever, predominantly *Salmonella* ser. Typhi and *Salmonella* ser. Paratyphi A, differs significantly for some antimicrobials as compared with nontyphoidal isolates. Multidrug resistant isolates of these serovars, which are defined as resistant to ampicillin, TMP-SMX, and chloramphenicol, have rapidly disseminated across the Indian subcontinent, Southeast Asia, Mexico, the Arabian Gulf, and Africa.[36] For these isolates, a fluoroquinolone is the preferred therapy for adults,[9] with the exception of patients returning from South Asia, where high rates of fluoroquinolone resistance preclude use of this antimicrobial class.[37] In the United States, fluoroquinolone nonsusceptibility (intermediate or resistant MIC) among typhoidal *Salmonella* isolated from returning travelers was 68.4% among *Salmonella* ser. Typhi and 95.5% among *Salmonella* ser. Paratyphi A, as compared with approximately 3% for nontyphoidal isolates.[10] Therapy options for fluoroquinolone nonsusceptible isolates include ceftriaxone or azithromycin.[38,39]

Current standards for susceptibility testing conditions and interpretive criteria for *Salmonella* are provided along with other members of Enterobacteriaceae in the CLSI M100 standard.[5] Two recent changes are important to highlight for susceptibility testing of *Salmonella* spp. The first is the change of the CLSI and FDA interpretive criteria for the fluoroquinolones, and the second is the recent addition of azithromycin breakpoints for *Salmonella* ser. Typhi.

The CLSI fluoroquinolone breakpoints for *Salmonella* have been subject to much scrutiny and revision, in part because of the emerging resistance mechanisms, reevaluation of fluoroquinolone pharmacokinetics and pharmacodynamics, and documented unfavorable treatment outcomes for patients with enteric fever who were treated with a fluoroquinolone when the infecting isolate harbored low-level fluoroquinolone resistance.[37] The most common mechanism of fluoroquinolone resistance is mutation to the quinolone resistance determining regions (QRDRs) of the *gyrA* gene, which results in MICs that are greater than the wild-type MICs of 0.06 µg/mL to ciprofloxacin or 0.12 µg/mL to levofloxacin and frank resistance to nalidixic acid (MIC $\geq$32 µg/mL). Less frequently, fluoroquinolone resistance can occur following mutation to the QRDRs of *gyrB* or the topoisomerase genes, *parC* and *parE*, or by acquisition of plasmid-mediated quinolone resistance determinant, such as *qnr* or *aac-6'-Ib-cr* genes.[37] Resistance via these pathways does not necessarily confer resistance to nalidixic acid, which was historically used as an indicator of fluoroquinolone resistance for *Salmonella* spp. As such, in 2012 and 2013, the CLSI lowered the ciprofloxacin, levofloxacin, and ofloxacin MIC breakpoints for *Salmonella* (**Table 3**) to better reflect the wild-type distribution of *Salmonella* MICs to these antimicrobials.[5] The FDA subsequently revised the ciprofloxacin MIC breakpoint to match those of the CLSI but for *Salmonella* ser. Typhi alone. EUCAST has similarly published *Salmonella*-specific MIC breakpoints for ciprofloxacin (see **Table 3**). In 2012, the CLSI established *Salmonella* DD breakpoints for ciprofloxacin,[5] but levofloxacin and ofloxacin disk breakpoints have not yet been established, although these have been proposed by Sjolund-Karlsson and colleagues.[40]

Laboratories in resource-limited countries, where enteric fever is endemic and fluoroquinolone resistance is prevalent, often must rely on DD rather than MIC testing because of cost restraints. These laboratories have noted difficulties in interpreting ciprofloxacin DD results.[37] To address this concern, the CLSI has added recommendations to the M100 S25 document for the use of a 5-µg pefloxacin DD test as a surrogate marker by which to detect fluoroquinolone resistance in *Salmonella*.[41] Pefloxacin screening is also recommended by EUCAST in place of ciprofloxacin DD

**Table 3**
*Salmonella* MIC and disk diffusion breakpoints for fluoroquinolones and nalidixic acid

| Antimicrobial | Disk Diffusion (mm) | | | MIC (µg/mL) | | |
|---|---|---|---|---|---|---|
| | S | I | R | S | I | R |
| Ciprofloxacin | | | | | | |
| CLSI | $\geq$31 | 21–30 | $\leq$20 | $\leq$0.06 | 0.12–0.5 | $\geq$1.0 |
| EUCAST | (Use 5 µg pefloxacin disk) | | | $\leq$0.06 | — | >0.06 |
| FDA (*Salmonella* Typhi only) | $\geq$31 | 21–30 | $\leq$20 | $\leq$0.06 | 0.12–0.5 | $\geq$1.0 |
| Levofloxacin | | | | | | |
| CLSI | — | — | — | $\leq$0.12 | 0.25–1.0 | $\geq$2.0 |
| Ofloxacin | | | | | | |
| CLSI | — | — | — | $\leq$0.12 | 0.25–1.0 | $\geq$2.0 |
| Surrogate/Screening Agents For Detection of Fluoroquinolone Resistance | | | | | | |
| Nalidixic acid | | | | | | |
| CLSI | $\geq$19 | 15–18 | $\leq$13 | $\leq$16 | — | $\geq$32 |
| Pefloxacin | | | | | | |
| CLSI | $\geq$24 | — | $\leq$23 | — | — | — |
| EUCAST | $\geq$24 | — | <24 | — | — | — |

(see **Table 3**). In studies performed in both Europe and the United States, and presented to the CLSI Microbiology Subcommittee on Antimicrobial Susceptibility Testing in July 2014, pefloxacin zone diameters of 24 mm or more were found to be an excellent indicator of wild-type isolates (ie, those without fluoroquinolone resistance mechanisms) and in 1 laboratory were found to agree with ciprofloxacin-susceptible MICs in 96.5% of cases (R. M. H, unpublished observation, 2014[26]). The caveat to the use of pefloxacin as a surrogate for fluoroquinolone susceptibility is that isolates with *aac-6'-lb-cr* do not necessarily test resistant to pefloxacin, as this enzyme has no effect on the activity of the quinolones.[42] Furthermore, with some lots of MHA, several discrete colonies within the zone of inhibition were noted for *Salmonella* with ciprofloxacin-intermediate MICs (**Fig. 2**), making interpretation of pefloxacin disk results difficult to read. In such instances, the zone of inhibition should be read inside these colonies (see **Fig. 2**A). Such difficult-to-read isolates also display difficult-to-read nalidixic acid zones of inhibition; again, colonies within the zone should not be ignored for nalidixic acid (see **Fig. 2**B).

Despite recent advances, several outstanding challenges exist for fluoroquinolone susceptibility testing of *Salmonella* isolates, and these are summarized in **Table 2**. First, pefloxacin disks are not available in the United States and because of regulatory issues are unlikely to become available in the near future. Second, no commercial MIC susceptibility test panels manufactured in the United States contain ciprofloxacin or levofloxacin concentrations low enough to allow use of the current CLSI susceptible breakpoints ($\leq$0.06 µg/mL for ciprofloxacin or $\leq$0.12 µg/mL for levofloxacin). Laboratories in the United States have the option of performing a ciprofloxacin DD or Etest to determine if an isolate is susceptible to this drug. However, levofloxacin DD breakpoints have not yet been established by the CLSI. Ciprofloxacin DD results cannot be used necessarily to extrapolate levofloxacin susceptibility, leaving laboratories no immediate option for levofloxacin testing. One potential solution is the use of Etest, although laboratories would have to verify the CLSI *Salmonella* breakpoints for Etest

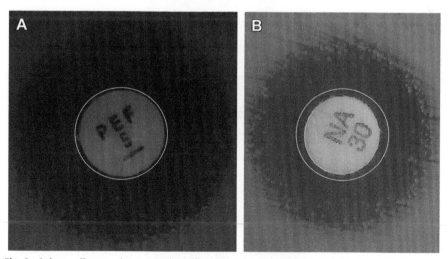

**Fig. 2.** *Salmonella enterica* ser. Typhi pefloxacin (*A*) and nalidixic acid (*B*) disk diffusion tests, demonstrating discrete colonies within the zone of inhibition. These colonies should not be ignored; the white rings indicate the appropriate zone to be read. This isolate had a ciprofloxacin MIC of 0.5 µg/mL.

before use for clinical testing, as such testing would be considered a laboratory modification of an FDA-cleared product. The performance of both ciprofloxacin and levofloxacin Etest was evaluated for a collection of 135 *Salmonella* isolates with a wide range of ciprofloxacin and levofloxacin MICs.[43] In this study, categorical agreement was 89.6% for ciprofloxacin and 83.7% for levofloxacin, as compared with BMD. In both cases, only minor errors were observed, in which the Etest MIC was interpreted as resistant and BMD MIC was intermediate. Because no data exist to suggest that higher doses of fluoroquinolone are effective for the treatment of isolates with MICs in the intermediate rage, these errors are unlikely to affect treatment decisions, and Etest may be an option for laboratories that need to perform a fluoroquinolone susceptibility test.

Several studies have demonstrated azithromycin to be an excellent treatment option for enteric fever.[38,39] The CLSI published azithromycin MIC and DD breakpoints for *S enterica* ser. Typhi in the M100 S25 document, but these have not yet been developed for *Salmonella* ser. Paratyphi A, which displays a statistically significant higher azithromycin MIC distribution.[44] The *S enterica* ser. Typhi breakpoints are the following: susceptible less than or equal to 16 µg/mL; resistant more than or equal to 32 µg/mL, resistant. An ECOFF of greater than or equal to 32 µg/mL has been used to indicate resistance for *Salmonella* ser. Typhi by EUCAST.[24] No commercial test systems are cleared by the FDA at present for azithromycin testing of *Salmonella* isolates. Some laboratories have noted double zones of inhibition for azithromycin (**Fig. 3**), making interpretation of these results difficult on some media. When interpreting azithromycin, the innermost zone or ellipse should be read and reflective light should be used.

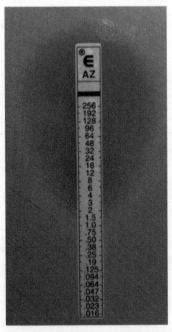

**Fig. 3.** *Salmonella enterica* ser. Typhi azithromycin Etest on Mueller-Hinton agar, demonstrating a double ellipse and an unclear zone. The MIC was interpreted in this case as 8 µg/mL.

Finally, although infrequent, ceftriaxone resistance has been noted in the United States for isolates of nontyphoidal *Salmonella*. The main resistance mechanisms include Ambler class C cephamycinases, encoded by $bla_{CMY}$ genes, and occasionally $bla_{CTX-M-15}$ or $bla_{TEM}$ extended-spectrum β-lactamases (ESBLs).[35] The old CLSI ESBL confirmatory test is not validated for *Salmonella* isolates; rather, laboratories should attempt to use the current CLSI breakpoints for the cephems (ie, MIC $\leq$1 µg/mL to ceftriaxone to indicate susceptibility). Rare *Salmonella* expressing acquired carbapenemases ((New Delhi metallo-β-lactamase [NDM], Klebsiella pneumoniae beta-lactamase [KPC], Verona integron-encoded metallo-β-lactamase [VIM], or oxacillinase-48 [OXA-48]) have also been isolated from humans and animals, raising concerns about zoonotic transmission.[45]

## SHIGELLA

In the United States, the burden of shigellosis is predominantly on children younger than 5 years. Children are treated with antimicrobials for shigellosis, as these can shorten the duration and severity of illness, as well as eradicate the organism and prevent transmission to others in settings such as day care centers.[46,47] Resistance among isolates in the United States to ampicillin and TMP-SMX, which are historical treatment options for shigellosis, is 25.5% and 43.3%, respectively, precluding their routine use. Ciprofloxacin is a treatment option for patients 18 years or older. In the United States, ciprofloxacin resistance rates are low at 2.0%.[10] Ceftriaxone is also frequently used for immunocompromised patients with severe infection, and resistance was 1.1% in 2012.[10]

Azithromycin is currently recommended by the American Academy of Pediatrics and the Infectious Diseases Society of America as one of the alternative treatment options for shigellosis.[3,31] In children, azithromycin has been shown to be clinically superior to cefixime.[48] Like the non-Typhi serovars of *Salmonella*, no susceptibility testing guidelines or breakpoints have been developed for azithromycin and *Shigella*, although EUCAST recommends an ECOFF of 16 µg/mL or less (see **Table 2**).[24] Jain and colleagues[49] reported difficulty in interpreting azithromycin susceptibilities for *Shigella sonnei* using Etest and DD methods because of double zones of growth, similar to that reported for *Salmonella*. The susceptible wild-type distribution of *Shigella* azithromycin MICs ranges from 4 to 16 µg/mL,[50] and the CDC uses the susceptible breakpoint of 16 µg/mL or less for surveillance purposes in the NARMS program. In 2012, 4.2% azithromycin resistance was documented in *Shigella* spp.[10] However, resistance to azithromycin was species dependent, with 15.3% of *Shigella flexneri* (n = 59) testing resistant in 2012.[10] In 2012, an outbreak of azithromycin-resistant *S sonnei* was reported in Los Angeles County and was associated with a plasmid-borne *mphA* resistance determinant.[51] Outbreaks of azithromycin-resistant shigellosis have subsequently been reported in Canada[52] and the United States[53] among men who have sex with men, underscoring the need for standardized test methodologies and interpretive criteria for azithromycin and *Shigella*.

## VIBRIO

Antimicrobial therapy is not required to manage cholera, but such therapy may shorten the duration and severity of disease and reduce shedding of bacilli in the stool by at least 3 days.[54] Similarly, otherwise healthy individuals with diarrhea due to *Vibrio* spp other than V *cholerae* usually recover spontaneously without treatment. AST is warranted when *Vibrio* spp are isolated from sources associated with serious infections. CLSI suggests use of BMD or DD using methodology similar to that for testing

Enterobacteriaceae. For testing of the halophilic *Vibrio* spp, CLSI recommends preparation of the inoculum suspension in 0.85% NaCl solution and preparation for BMD or DD testing in media without NaCl supplementation.[41]

*Vibrio cholerae* possesses efflux pumps that act on multiple antimicrobial classes; it also possesses enzymes that hydrolyze various antimicrobials.[54] Both *V cholerae* and the *Vibrio* spp other than V *cholerae* are often susceptible to most antimicrobial agents, including cephalosporins, aminoglycosides, fluoroquinolones, and tetracyclines.[55] However, a *V cholerae* El Tor Ogawa strain harboring an inducible, plasmid-mediated *bla*$_{DHA}$ gene and the *bla*$_{NDM-1}$ gene was described.[54] According to NARMS data, ampicillin resistance rates in 2012 of *Vibrio alginolyticus* approximated 98%, whereas ampicillin rates of *Vibrio parahemolyticus*, the most common *Vibrio* spp other than V *cholerae* isolated in the United States, were only 14%.[10] In the same year, no *Vibrio* isolates were resistant to quinolones or TMP-SMX, and only 0.2% of isolates were resistant to tetracycline.

Some studies have demonstrated poor clinical outcomes in patients with *V cholerae* serogroup O1 isolates with susceptible but elevated MICs to ciprofloxacin, highlighting the possibility that the ciprofloxacin breakpoint of less than or equal to 1 μg/mL is too high.[56] Resistance surveys of isolates from the 2010 Haitian *V cholerae* O1 outbreak showed reduced susceptibility to ciprofloxacin in the 0.25-1.0-μg/mL range, which was associated with mutation of the QRDR region of *gyrA* and *parC*.[57]

## AEROMONAS

Most published susceptibility studies on *Aeromonas* have been performed using the 3 most common species that infect humans: *Aeromonas hydrophila, Aeromonas caviae*, and *Aeromonas veronii* var. *sobria*. The M45 CLSI document covering infrequently isolated bacteria such as *Aeromonas* is currently being updated and will cover BMD and DD for a wider range of *Aeromonas* species.[4,58]

*Aeromonas* can produce several β-lactamases spanning all Ambler molecular classes A–D.[59] Expression of various β-lactamases is species specific (**Table 4**).[59] The most common metallo-β-lactamase (MBL) in *Aeromonas* is CphA, which hydrolyzes carbapenems but not penicillins or cephalosporins. CphA is found in *A hydrophila, A veronii*, and *A jandaei* but not in *A caviae*. A chromosomal NDM-1 was detected in *A caviae* from seepage water in New Delhi.[59] The meropenem and imipenem MICs of this isolate were 8 to 16 μg/mL. CphA MBL production is not easily detected with the ethylenediaminetetraacetic acid (EDTA) test usually used for MBL confirmation in Enterobacteriaceae unless a large inoculum is used.[60,61] This inoculum effect was demonstrated in a study of 34 *cphA*-positive *Aeromonas* spp, in which 33 of 34 (97%) were susceptible to imipenem using the standard inoculum (10⁴ colony-forming units [CFU]), whereas the same number was resistant by the agar dilution method using a larger inoculum of 10⁷ CFU.[61] The modified Hodge test detects 97% of *cphA*-

**Table 4**
**Species-specific distribution of β-lactamases by Ambler class in *Aeromonas* spp**

|  | Class A ESBL | Class B MBL | Class C AmpC | Class D Penicillinase |
|---|---|---|---|---|
| A hydrophila | + | + | + | + |
| A caviae | + | − | + | + |
| A veronii var. sobria | + | ± | + | + |

*Abbreviations:* AmpC, AmpC β-lactamase; MBL, metallo-β-lactamase.

positive organisms.[61] The MBL Etest also does not perform well for MBL detection in *Aeromonas* and is likely influenced by the inoculum effect.[61]

The most common AmpC in *Aeromonas* spp is the CepS cephalosporinase. ESBLs also have been detected in *Aeromonas*. Nonsusceptibility to third-generation cephalosporins may be a clue to the presence of an ESBL. However, ESBL confirmatory testing for *Aeromonas* is generally not helpful because of the common presence of the AmpC β-lactamase, which can mask the clavulanate effect. In the CLSI M45-A3 document, interpretive criteria for ampicillin, ampicillin-sulbactam, and cefazolin are no longer included for *Aeromonas* to reflect inherent resistance.[58]

*Aeromonas* spp are generally resistant to ampicillin but show variable susceptibility to cephalosporins.[28] In an antimicrobial surveillance study of 260 *Aeromonas* spp from the Asia-Pacific region, the most active antibiotics included amikacin, cefepime, and levofloxacin.[62] Susceptibility rates of less than 80% existed for ceftazidime, piperacillin-tazobactam, and imipenem. Susceptibility rates were stable for most antimicrobials over time, except for ciprofloxacin (92.2% susceptible [S] in 2003 to 2006 to 83.4% S in 2007 to 2010).

A variety of other antibiotic resistance determinants have been found in *Aeromonas* isolates from wastewater plants, fish, and various food isolates, and there is concern for transfer of resistance genes from environmental isolates to humans.[63]

## MISCELLANEOUS

Antimicrobial therapy options for *Clostridium difficile* include vancomycin, metronidazole, and fidaxomicin. Metronidazole-resistant strains are rare but have been documented.[64,65] Fidaxomicin shows excellent activity against *C difficile*, but high MICs have been documented in vitro and have been associated with mutations leading to target modifications.[66] *Clostridium difficile* is resistant to many β-lactam agents, including cephalosporins, fluoroquinolones, and clindamycin, and outbreaks of fluoroquinolone-resistant *C difficile* strains have been associated with increased mortality.[67] Thus, although resistance to the antimicrobials that are commonly used to treat *C difficile* infections is rare, the bacteria can spread rapidly because of resistance to antimicrobials used to treat other infections.

There is generally no need to test *C difficile* isolates for antimicrobial susceptibility because resistance to the commonly used antimicrobials is rare in the United States. In addition, the significance of breakpoints for vancomycin and fidaxomicin is questionable because fecal concentrations of these antimicrobials are extremely high and are hypothesized to be much higher than the organism MICs. However, fecal concentrations of metronidazole are believed to be close to the MIC of the organism.

The suggested AST method for *C difficile* is agar dilution, but it is difficult to perform because of the time, labor, and expertise required. The BMD method using brucella broth supplemented with hemin, vitamin K1, and 5% (v/v) laked horse blood is easier to perform. DD tests should not be performed for anaerobic bacteria, as the testing results are generally inaccurate.[68]

*Plesiomonas shigelloides* are generally susceptible to most antibiotics, excluding ampicillin and other penicillins such as piperacillin, and the organism has been moved from the CLSI M45-A2 document to M100 to be included with the interpretive breakpoint table for Enterobacteriaceae.[69] Antimicrobial therapy for *Yersinia enterocolitica* commonly includes ciprofloxacin, TMP-SMX, or a third-generation cephalosporin. The organism shows more than 90% susceptibility to these antimicrobials.[70] It is intrinsically resistant to ampicillin, amoxicillin, ticarcillin, cefazolin, and cephalothin. Enterobacteriaceae susceptibility testing criteria should also be followed for *Y enterocolitica*.

## SELF-ASSESSMENT

1. For which of the following organisms should AST be performed and reported when the isolate is recovered from the stool of an otherwise healthy adult with gastroenteritis?
   a. *Clostridium difficile*
   b. *Escherichia coli* O157:H7
   c. *Campylobacter jejuni*
   d. *Vibrio parahemolyticus*
   e. *Salmonella enterica* ser. Paratyphi A
2. Which of the following statements regarding azithromycin is true?
   a. *Salmonella* Typhi displays a statistically significant higher azithromycin MIC distribution than *Salmonella* Paratyphi A.
   b. Azithromycin DD testing for *Salmonella* typically demonstrates discrete colonies within the zone of inhibition.
   c. Nontyphoidal *Salmonella* demonstrates almost complete (99%) resistance to azithromycin.
   d. Azithromycin is currently recommended as a treatment option for shigellosis.
   e. The CLSI has recently set breakpoints for azithromycin and *Campylobacter*.
3. Which of the following statements is true regarding fluoroquinolone susceptibility testing and *Salmonella*?
   a. Susceptibility to the pefloxacin disk may be used as a surrogate test for ciprofloxacin susceptibility.
   b. The nalidixic acid DD test is the most sensitive indicator of fluoroquinolone resistance.
   c. Commercial test systems do not have levofloxacin concentrations high enough for current CLSI breakpoints.
   d. Mutation in the QRDR of the *gyrA* gene often is associated with nalidixic acid susceptibility.
   e. Levofloxacin DD CLSI breakpoints have recently been established.

ANSWERS
   Answer 1: E.
   A. Routine susceptibility for C difficile from stool is not necessary because resistance to the commonly used antimicrobials is rare and significance of susceptibility testing is questionable.
   B. Antimicrobial therapy for E coli O157:H7 can be detrimental to the host by putting the patient at increased risk of HUS. Therefore, AST is not performed.
   C. Routine susceptibility testing for C jejuni stool is not necessary because intestinal disease is usually acute and self-limiting.
   D. Routine susceptibility testing for V parahemolyticus from stool is only necessary when associated with serious infections.
   E. Routine susceptibility testing for S enterica ser. Paratyphi A from stool is indicated (as is S enterica serovars Typhi and Paratyphi B and C) because of the concern for enteric fever.
   Answer 2: D.
   A. S enterica ser. Paratyphi A displays a higher azithromycin MIC distribution than *Salmonella* Typhi.
   B. Azithromycin DD testing typically demonstrates a double ellipse and an unclear zone. Pefloxacin and nalidixic acid disk tests can demonstrate discrete colonies within the zone of inhibition when testing *Salmonella* spp.

C. Resistance of nontyphoidal *Salmonella* to azithromycin is rare; in 2012, less than 1% of US isolates were resistant.

D. Azithromycin is currently recommended by the American Academy of Pediatrics and the Infectious Diseases Society of America as one of the alternative treatment options for shigellosis.

E. The CLSI has not set breakpoints for azithromycin and *Campylobacter*. The CLSI has set azithromycin breakpoints for *Salmonella*.

Answer 3: A.

A. Susceptibility to the pefloxacin disk may be used as a surrogate test for ciprofloxacin susceptibility and is a good indicator of wild-type isolates.

B. Resistance via the non-QRDR gyrA pathways does not often confer resistance to nalidixic acid; thus, nalidixic acid may be falsely susceptible.

C. No commercial MIC susceptibility test panels manufactured in the United States contain ciprofloxacin or levofloxacin concentrations low enough to allow use of the current CLSI susceptible breakpoints.

D. The most common mechanism of fluoroquinolone resistance is mutation to the QRDRs of the *gyrA* gene, which results in frank resistance to nalidixic acid (MIC $\geq$32 $\mu$g/mL).

E. Levofloxacin DD CLSI breakpoints do not exist.

## REFERENCES

1. Zhang X, McDaniel AD, Wolf LE, et al. Quinolone antibiotics induce shiga toxin-encoding bacteriophages, toxin production, and death in mice. J Infect Dis 2000;181:664–70.

2. Wong CS, Mooney JC, Brandt JR, et al. Risk factors for the hemolytic uremic syndrome in children infected with *Escherichia coli* O157:H7: a multivariable analysis. Clin Infect Dis 2012;55:33–41.

3. Guerrant RL, Van Gilder T, Steiner TS, et al. Infectious Diseases Society of America. Practice guidelines for the management of infectious diarrhea. Clin Infect Dis 2001;32:331–51.

4. Clinical and Laboratory Standards Institute. Methods for antimicrobial dilution and disk susceptibility testing of infrequently isolated or fastidious bacteria; Approved guideline - second edition. CLSI document M45-A2. Wayne (PA): Clinical and Laboratory Standards Institute; 2010.

5. Clinical and Laboratory Standards Institute. Performance standards for antimicrobial susceptibility testing; Twenty-fourth informational supplement. M100 S24. Wayne (PA): Clinical and Laboratory Standards Institute; 2014.

6. DuPont HL. Clinical practice. Bacterial diarrhea. N Engl J Med 2009;361:1560–9.

7. Centers for Disease Control and Prevention. Incidence and trends of infection with pathogens transmitted commonly through food – foodborne diseases active surveillance network, 10 U.S. sites, 1996-2012. MMWR 2013;62:283–7.

8. Ternhag A, Asikainen T, Giesecke J, et al. A meta-analysis on the effects of antibiotic treatment on duration of symptoms caused by infection with *Campylobacter* species. Clin Infect Dis 2007;44:696–700.

9. Gilbert DN, Chambers HF, Eliopoulos GM, et al. The Sanford guide to antimicrobial therapy. 44th edition. Sperryville (VA): Antimicrobial Therapy, Inc; 2014.

10. National Antimicrobial Resistance Monitoring System for Enteric Bacteria (NARMS): Human Isolates Final Report. Atlanta (GA): U.S. Department of Health and Human Services, CDC; 2012. Available at: http://www.cdc.gov/narms/disease.html. Accessed March 17, 2015.

11. Vlieghe ER, Jacobs JA, Van Esbroeck M, et al. Trends of norfloxacin and erythromycin resistance of *Campylobacter jejuni/Campylobacter coli* isolates recovered from international travelers, 1994 to 2006. J Travel Med 2008;15:419–25.

12. Aarestrup FM, McDermott PF, Wegener HC. Transmission of antibiotic resistance from food animals to humans. In: Nachamkin I, Szymanski CM, Blaser MJ, editors. Campylobacter. Washington, DC: ASM Press; 2008. p. 645–65.

13. Bakeli G, Sato K, Kumita W, et al. Antimicrobial susceptibility and mechanism of quinolone resistance in *Campylobacter jejuni* strains isolated from diarrheal patients in a hospital in Tokyo. J Infect Chemother 2008;14:342–8.

14. Engberg J, Aarestrup FM, Taylor DE, et al. Quinolone and macrolide resistance in *Campylobacter jejuni* and *C. coli*: resistance mechanisms and trends in human isolates. Emerg Infect Dis 2001;7:24–34.

15. Nelson JM, Chiller TM, Powers JH, et al. Fluoroquinolone-resistant *Campylobacter* species and the withdrawal of fluoroquinolones from use in poultry: a public health success story. Clin Infect Dis 2007;44:977–80.

16. Griggs DJ, Johnson MM, Frost JA, et al. Incidence and mechanism of ciprofloxacin resistance in *Campylobacter* spp. isolated from commercial poultry flocks in the United Kingdom before, during, and after fluoroquinolone treatment. Antimicrob Agents Chemother 2005;49:699–707.

17. Luo N, Pereira S, Sahin O, et al. Enhanced in vivo fitness of fluoroquinolone-resistant *Campylobacter jejuni* in the absence of antibiotic selection pressure. Proc Natl Acad Sci U S A 2005;102:541–6.

18. Wassenaar TM, Kist M, de Jong A. Re-analysis of the risks attributed to ciprofloxacin-resistant *Campylobacter jejuni* infections. Int J Antimicrob Agents 2007;30:195–201.

19. McDermott PF, Bodeis SM, Aarestrup FM, et al. Development of a standardized susceptibility test for *Campylobacter* with quality-control ranges for ciprofloxacin, doxycycline, erythromycin, gentamicin, and meropenem. Microb Drug Resist 2004;10:124–31.

20. Clinical and Laboratory Standards Institute. Performance standards for antimicrobial disk and dilution susceptibility tests for bacteria isolated from animals; Approved standard - third edition. CLSI document M31-A3. Wayne (PA): Clinical and Laboratory Standards Institute; 2008.

21. International Organization for Standardization (ISO) Standards. Clinical laboratory testing and in vitro diagnostic test systems - Susceptibility testing of infectious agents and evaluation of performance of antimicrobial susceptibility test devices - Part 1: Reference method for testing the in vitro activity of antimicrobial agents against rapidly growing aerobic bacteria involved in infectious diseases (ISO 20776–1). Switzerland: ISO; 2006.

22. Gaudreau C. Disk diffusion method for erythromycin and ciprofloxacin susceptibility testing of *Campylobacter jejuni* and *Campylobacter coli*. J Clin Microbiol 2013;51:380.

23. Lehtopolku M, Kotilainen P, Puukka P, et al. Inaccuracy of the disk diffusion method compared with the agar dilution method for susceptibility testing of *Campylobacter* spp. J Clin Microbiol 2012;50:52–6.

24. European Committee on Antimicrobial Susceptibility Testing - EUCAST. Breakpoint tables for interpretation of MICs and zone diameters, Version 4.0. 2014. Available at: http://www.eucast.org/clinical_breakpoints/. Accessed March 17, 2015.

25. CLSI. Subcommittee of the Antimicrobial Susceptibility Testing, June 2014 meeting minutes. Available at: http://clsi.org/standards/micro/microbiology-files/. Accessed March 16, 2015.

26. Valdivieso-Garcia A, Imgrund R, Deckert A, et al. Cost analysis and antimicrobial susceptibility testing comparing the E test and the agar dilution method in *Campylobacter jejuni* and *Campylobacter coli*. Diagn Microbiol Infect Dis 2009; 65:168–74.

27. van der Beek MT, Claas EC, Mevius DJ, et al. Inaccuracy of routine susceptibility tests for detection of erythromycin resistance of *Campylobacter jejuni* and *Campylobacter coli*. Clin Microbiol Infect 2010;16:51–6.

28. Jorgensen JH, Hindler JF. New consensus guidelines from the Clinical and Laboratory Standards Institute for antimicrobial susceptibility testing of infrequently isolated or fastidious bacteria. Clin Infect Dis 2007;44:280–6.

29. Platts-Mills JA, Liu J, Gratz J, et al. Detection of *Campylobacter* in stool and determination of significance by culture, enzyme immunoassay, and PCR in developing countries. J Clin Microbiol 2014;52:1074–80.

30. Wistrom J, Jertborn M, Ekwall E, et al. Empiric treatment of acute diarrheal disease with norfloxacin. A randomized, placebo-controlled study. Swedish Study Group. Ann Intern Med 1992;117:202–8.

31. American Academy of Pediatrics. Shigella infections. In: Pickering LK, Baker CJ, Kimberlin DW, et al, editors. Red book: 2012 report of the Committee on Infectious Diseases. 29th edition. Elk Grove Village (IL): American Academy of Pediatrics; 2012. p. 645–7.

32. Benenson S, Raveh D, Schlesinger Y, et al. The risk of vascular infection in adult patients with nontyphi *Salmonella* bacteremia. Am J Med 2001;110:60–3.

33. Helms M, Simonsen J, Molbak K. Quinolone resistance is associated with increased risk of invasive illness or death during infection with *Salmonella* serotype Typhimurium. J Infect Dis 2004;190:1652–4.

34. Saphra I, Winter JW. Clinical manifestations of salmonellosis in man; an evaluation of 7779 human infections identified at the New York Salmonella Center. N Engl J Med 1957;256:1128–34.

35. Sjolund-Karlsson M, Howie R, Krueger A, et al. CTX-M-producing non-Typhi *Salmonella* spp. isolated from humans, United States. Emerg Infect Dis 2011;17:97–9.

36. Rowe B, Ward LR, Threlfall EJ. Multidrug-resistant *Salmonella typhi*: a worldwide epidemic. Clin Infect Dis 1997;24(Suppl 1):S106–9.

37. Humphries RM, Fang FC, Aarestrup FM, et al. In vitro susceptibility testing of fluoroquinolone activity against *Salmonella*: recent changes to CLSI standards. Clin Infect Dis 2012;55:1107–13.

38. Girgis NI, Butler T, Frenck RW, et al. Azithromycin versus ciprofloxacin for treatment of uncomplicated typhoid fever in a randomized trial in Egypt that included patients with multidrug resistance. Antimicrob Agents Chemother 1999;43:1441–4.

39. Frenck RW Jr, Mansour A, Nakhla I, et al. Short-course azithromycin for the treatment of uncomplicated typhoid fever in children and adolescents. Clin Infect Dis 2004;38:951–7.

40. Sjolund-Karlsson M, Howie RL, Crump JA, et al. Fluoroquinolone susceptibility testing of *Salmonella enterica*: detection of acquired resistance and selection of zone diameter breakpoints for levofloxacin and ofloxacin. J Clin Microbiol 2014;52:877–84.

41. Clinical and Laboratory Standards Institute. Performance standards for antimicrobial susceptibility testing; Twenty-fourth informational supplement. M100 S25. Wayne (PA): Clinical and Laboratory Standards Institute; 2015.

42. Robicsek A, Strahilevitz J, Jacoby GA, et al. Fluoroquinolone-modifying enzyme: a new adaptation of a common aminoglycoside acetyltransferase. Nat Med 2006; 12:83–8.

43. Deak E, Hindler JA, Skov R, et al. Performance of Etest and disk diffusion for the detection of ciprofloxacin and levofloxacin resistance in *Salmonella*. J Clin Microbiol 2015;53:298–301.

44. Butler T, Sridhar CB, Daga MK, et al. Treatment of typhoid fever with azithromycin versus chloramphenicol in a randomized multicentre trial in India. J Antimicrob Chemother 1999;44:243–50.

45. Woodford N, Wareham DW, Guerra B, et al. Carbapenemase-producing Entero-bacteriaceae and non-Enterobacteriaceae from animals and the environment: an emerging public health risk of our own making? J Antimicrob Chemother 2014;69:287–91.

46. Christopher PR, David KV, John SM, et al. Antibiotic therapy for *Shigella* dysen-tery. Cochrane Database Syst Rev 2010;(4):CD006784.

47. Haltalin KC, Nelson JD, Ring R, et al. Double-blind treatment study of shigellosis comparing ampicillin, sulfadiazine, and placebo. J Pediatr 1967;70:970–81.

48. Basualdo W, Arbo A. Randomized comparison of azithromycin versus cefixime for treatment of shigellosis in children. Pediatr Infect Dis J 2003;22:374–7.

49. Jain SK, Gupta A, Glanz B, et al. Antimicrobial-resistant *Shigella sonnei*: limited antimicrobial treatment options for children and challenges of interpreting in vitro azithromycin susceptibility. Pediatr Infect Dis J 2005;24:494–7.

50. Howie RL, Folster JP, Bowen A, et al. Reduced azithromycin susceptibility in *Shigella sonnei*, United States. Microb Drug Resist 2010;16:245–8.

51. Sjolund-Karlsson M, Bowen A, Reporter R, et al. Outbreak of infections caused by *Shigella sonnei* with reduced susceptibility to azithromycin in the United States. Antimicrob Agents Chemother 2013;57:1559–60.

52. Gaudreau C, Barkati S, Leduc JM, et al. *Shigella* spp. with reduced azithromy-cin susceptibility, Quebec, Canada, 2012-2013. Emerg Infect Dis 2014;20:854–6.

53. Heiman KE, Karlsson M, Grass J, et al. Notes from the field: *Shigella* with decreased susceptibility to azithromycin among men who have sex with men - United States, 2002-2013. MMWR 2014;63:132–3.

54. Mandal J, Sangeetha V, Ganesan V, et al. Third-generation cephalosporin-resistant *Vibrio cholerae*, India. Emerg Infect Dis 2012;18:1326–8.

55. Ismail H, Smith AM, Tau NP, et al. Group for Enteric, Respiratory and Meningeal Disease Surveillance in South Africa. Cholera outbreak in South Africa, 2008-2009: laboratory analysis of *Vibrio cholerae* O1 strains. J Infect Dis 2013;208(Suppl 1):S39–45.

56. Saha D, Karim MM, Khan WA, et al. Single-dose azithromycin for the treatment of cholera in adults. N Engl J Med 2006;354:2452–62.

57. Sjolund-Karlsson M, Reimer A, Folster JP, et al. Drug-resistance mechanisms in *Vibrio cholerae* O1 outbreak strain, Haiti, 2010. Emerg Infect Dis 2011;17:2151–4.

58. Clinical and Laboratory Standards Institute. Methods for antimicrobial dilution and disk susceptibility testing of infrequently isolated or fastidious bacteria; approved guideline - third edition. CLSI document M45–A3. Wayne (PA): Clinical and Laboratory Standards Institute, in press.

59. Walsh TR, Weeks J, Livermore DM, et al. Dissemination of NDM-1 positive bacte-ria in the New Delhi environment and its implications for human health: an envi-ronmental point prevalence study. Lancet Infect Dis 2011;11:355–62.

60. Rossolini GM, Walsh T, Amicosante G. The *Aeromonas* metallo-beta-lactamases: genetics, enzymology, and contribution to drug resistance. Microb Drug Resist 1996;2:245–52.

61. Wu CJ, Chen PL, Wu JJ, et al. Distribution and phenotypic and genotypic detection of a metallo-β-lactamase, CphA, among bacteraemic *Aeromonas* isolates. J Med Microbiol 2012;61(Pt 5):712–9.
62. Liu YM, Chen YS, Toh HS, et al. In vitro susceptibilities of non-Enterobacteriaceae isolates from patients with intra-abdominal infections in the Asia-Pacific region from 2003 to 2010: results from the Study for Monitoring Antimicrobial Resistance Trends (SMART). Int J Antimicrob Agents 2012;40(Suppl):S11–7.
63. Igbinosa IH, Okoh AI. Antibiotic susceptibility profile of *Aeromonas* species isolated from wastewater treatment plant. ScientificWorldJournal 2012;2012:764563.
64. Kunishima H, Chiba J, Saito M, et al. Antimicrobial susceptibilities of *Clostridium difficile* isolated in Japan. J Infect Chemother 2013;19:360–2.
65. Peláez T, Cercenado E, Alcalá L, et al. Metronidazole resistance in *Clostridium difficile* is heterogeneous. J Clin Microbiol 2008;46:3028–32.
66. Leeds JA, Sachdeva M, Mullin S, et al. In vitro selection, via serial passage, of *Clostridium difficile* mutants with reduced susceptibility to fidaxomicin or vancomycin. J Antimicrob Chemother 2013;69:41–4.
67. Labbé AC, Poirier L, Maccannell D, et al. *Clostridium difficile* infections in a Canadian tertiary care hospital before and during a regional epidemic associated with the BI/NAP1/027 strain. Antimicrob Agents Chemother 2008;52:3180–7.
68. Clinical and Laboratory Standards Institute. Performance standards for antimicrobial susceptibility testing; twenty-third informational supplement. CLSI document M100–S23. Wayne (PA): Clinical and Laboratory Standards Institute; 2013.
69. Chen X, Chen Y, Yang Q, et al. *Plesiomonas shigelloides* infection in Southeast China. PLoS One 2013;8:e77877.
70. Zhong H, Sun Y, Lin S, et al. *Yersinia enterocolitica* infection in diarrheal patients. Eur J Clin Microbiol Infect Dis 2008;27:741–52.

# Markers of Intestinal Inflammation for the Diagnosis of Infectious Gastroenteritis

Mark D. Gonzalez, PhD[a,1], Craig B. Wilen, MD, PhD[b,1], Carey-Ann D. Burnham, PhD[b,*]

## KEYWORDS

- Biomarker • C-reactive protein • Erythrocyte sedimentation reaction • IL-6 • IL-8
- IFN-$\gamma$ • TNF-$\alpha$ • Fecal leukocyte

## KEY POINTS

- It can be difficult to differentiate infectious versus noninfectious causes of diarrhea using clinical information.
- One approach to include or exclude an infectious cause of diarrhea is to measure a serum or fecal biomarker that is designed to detect the host's response to infection.
- An ideal biomarker would be inexpensive, rapid, and easy to perform, with high sensitivity and specificity.
- Systemic biomarkers, such as C-reactive protein, erythrocyte sedimentation rate, and serum cytokines, cannot be reliably used to include or exclude an infectious cause of diarrhea.
- Fecal biomarkers, such as fecal lactoferrin, fecal calprotectin, and fecal occult blood, cannot be reliably used to include or exclude an infectious cause of diarrhea.
- At this time, biomarker analysis cannot supplant diagnostic methods that specifically detect pathogens associated with infectious gastroenteritis, such as culture, nucleic acid detection, or antigen detection methods.

Disclosures: M.D. Gonzalez and C.B. Wilen have no relevant financial relationships to disclose. C.A. Burnham has received research support from Cepheid, bioMerieux, and Accelerate Diagnostics.
[a] Division of Laboratory and Genomic Medicine, Department of Pathology and Immunology, Washington University School of Medicine, Washington University in St. Louis, 660 South Euclid Avenue, St Louis, MO 63110, USA; [b] Department of Pathology and Immunology, Washington University School of Medicine, Washington University in St. Louis, 660 South Euclid Avenue, St. Louis, MO 63110, USA
[1] These authors contributed equally to this work.
* Corresponding author. Washington University School of Medicine, Washington University in St. Louis, 660 South Euclid Avenue, Campus Box 8118, St. Louis, MO 63110.
E-mail address: cburnham@path.wustl.edu

## INTRODUCTION

Infectious diarrhea is a major cause of morbidity; globally, gastrointestinal infections result in an estimated 2200 pediatric deaths each day, predominantly in the developing world.[1] In the United States, it is estimated that there are 178.8 million gastrointestinal infections per year, resulting in at least 474,000 hospitalizations and more than 5000 deaths annually.[2] Numerous types of microorganisms can cause gastrointestinal infections, including parasites, viruses, and bacteria. These organisms can be acquired through contaminated food and/or water sources and person-person or environmental transmission or may cause disease as a consequence of dysbiosis secondary to antibiotic therapy.

The identification of an etiologic agent causing infectious gastroenteritis can be labor intensive and expensive, and many commonly used methodologies have suboptimal analytical sensitivity. Traditionally, bacterial pathogens have been routinely identified using culture-based techniques, nucleic acid detection, or antigen detection. Viral pathogens are typically identified by nucleic acid detection or antigen detection methods, while parasites are identified by antigen detection methods combined with microscopic examination and special staining methods. Although some of these testing methods can be completed within a few hours, others require days, can be costly, and can require considerable laboratory resources and expertise. Newer US Food and Drug Administration–approved multiplexed nucleic acid detection assays are now available and allow for the simultaneous identification of a panel of bacterial, viral, and parasitic pathogens.[3-7]

The most appropriate course of therapy for a patient with diarrhea can be a significant clinical conundrum. Numerous noninfectious diseases, such as inflammatory bowel disease (IBD; eg, ulcerative colitis and Crohn disease), gastrointestinal malignancy, irritable bowel syndrome (IBS), and food allergies/intolerances, may present very similarly to infectious gastroenteritis. A biomarker that could rapidly differentiate between infectious and noninfectious causes of gastroenteritis with a very high negative predictive value for infection would be clinically useful in the triage of these patients. In addition, the ideal biomarker could rapidly differentiate between bacterial, viral, and parasitic causes. Based on these results, and before the identification of the etiologic agent, clinicians could identify which patients might require hospitalization, order the appropriate testing for pathogen identification, initiate the optimal therapy or supportive measures, and/or invoke appropriate infection prevention precautions. Such biomarkers would facilitate appropriate testing of patients with active infections (and thereby reduce potential false positives due to asymptomatic colonization), would reduce hospital costs by eliminating unnecessary testing, and could prevent patient morbidity and mortality related to more invasive procedures.

This article summarizes the data regarding the analytical performance characteristics of many of the common biomarkers that have been examined for the identification of gastrointestinal infections. An overview of the methods discussed can be found in **Table 1**.

## SYSTEMIC MARKERS
### C-Reactive Protein

C-reactive protein (CRP) and erythrocyte sedimentation rate (ESR) were 2 of the first markers of systemic inflammation to be described. Although both inflammatory markers are widely available, easy to perform, and well-described, they lack specificity, limiting their use as markers for infectious gastroenteritis.

**Table 1**
**Summary of biomarkers for gastrointestinal infections**

| Biomarker | Method(s) for Measurement | Reported Sensitivity Range (%) | Reported Specificity Range (%) | Charge[a] | References |
|---|---|---|---|---|---|
| **Systemic biomarkers** | | | | | |
| CRP | Immunoassay | 54–92 | 52–89 | $10 $24 HS | [10–19] |
| ESR | Gravity/centrifugation | NA | NA | $5 | [10,14,15,19] |
| Serum cytokines | Immunoassay | 50–79 | 63–91 | $24 | [11–13,16,18,21] |
| **Fecal biomarkers** | | | | | |
| Direct leukocyte detection | Methylene blue staining with microscopic analysis | 10–57 | 87–89 | $7 | [27–30] |
| Fecal lactoferrin | Immunoassay | 95 | 29 | $36 | [36] |
| Fecal occult blood | Peroxidase reaction Immunochemical | ND | ND | $29 | [36] |
| Fecal calprotectin | Immunoassay | 83–93 | 65–88 | $36 | [15,16,47–49] |

*Abbreviations:* HS, high sensitivity; NA, not available.
[a] 2014 CMS mid-point price rounded to the nearest US dollar (http://www.cms.gov/Medicare/Medicare-Fee-for-Service-Payment/ClinicalLabFeeSched/clinlab.html). Accessed November 11, 2014.
*Data from* Refs.[10–19,21,27–30,36,47–49]

CRP is synthesized by the liver in response to interleukin (IL)-6 as part of the host inflammatory response. It is an acute phase reactant that functions in part by activating the complement cascade.[8] It was first detected in the 1930s when serum from humans acutely infected with a variety of pathogens precipitated with the C polysaccharide of *Streptococcus pneumoniae*.[9] CRP can be measured with several immunologic methods. Immunoturbidimetry is the most commonly used method today, according to the 2014 College of American Pathologists Cardiac Risk Proficiency Testing Survey. High-sensitivity CRP assays have been developed relatively recently; these are performed by mixing patient serum with latex particles coated with CRP antibodies. The presence of CRP in serum causes the latex particles to agglutinate, resulting in turbidity that is measured by nephelometry and is proportional to the CRP concentration. CRP assays are accurate and inexpensive and can be performed in less than an hour. The role of CRP as a marker for gastroenteritis has been studied primarily in pediatric populations.

Many studies in children have assessed the utility of serum CRP in distinguishing bacterial from viral gastroenteritis, particularly that due to rotavirus. In these studies, the area under the receiver operating characteristic (ROC) curve for CRP ranged between 0.75 and 0.91[10–16] with a sensitivity of 54% to 92% and specificity of 52% to 89%.[10,12–18]

In comparison, 3 studies of adults with gastroenteritis demonstrated that CRP had an area under the ROC curve between 0.75 and 0.91, a sensitivity of 82% to 85%, and specificity of 55% to 85% for the diagnosis of bacterial gastroenteritis.[11,16,19] Thus, the data in adults and children for CRP are similar and suggest that CRP may have modest utility in certain clinical settings to distinguish bacterial from viral gastroenteritis. However, although CRP is a relatively sensitive marker for inflammation, it lacks specificity because it cannot distinguish the tissue source of the inflammation nor whether the inciting factor is autoimmune or infectious, much less bacterial or viral.

## Erythrocyte Sedimentation Rate

Like CRP, the ESR, first described in 1897 by Edmund Biernacki,[20] is a nonspecific inflammatory marker. ESR refers to the rate at which red blood cells settle in a glass cylinder in 1 hour; however, more recent methods use centrifugation to generate analogous results in 5 minutes. The main plasma factor promoting sedimentation is fibrinogen, an acute phase reactant, whereas the electrostatic charge, or zeta potential, of erythrocytes is the predominant antisedimentation force. The ESR can be prolonged in a variety of proinflammatory conditions, including autoimmune disease and infection, whereas a decreased ESR can be seen with certain hereditary red blood cell defects and congestive heart failure, among others. Because of the ease of use, rapid turn-around time, and correlation with systemic inflammation, ESR has been evaluated as a marker for gastroenteritis.

At least 4 studies, 3 of which were of children, have compared the diagnostic value of ESR in differentiating bacterial from viral gastroenteritis.[10,14,15,19] In these studies, ESR tended to be higher in cases of bacterial infection with the area under the ROC curves ranging from 0.57 to 0.84. However, in all 4 studies, CRP had a superior area under the ROC curve, suggesting ESR is relatively inferior in discriminating bacterial from viral gastroenteritis.

Despite the historical utilization of ESR, it has significant limitations. First, ESR can vary with gender, age, pregnancy, serum immunoglobulin concentration, red blood cell shape and concentration, and interfering substances such as drugs.[8] Second, the lag between onset of inflammation and change in ESR, as well as the slow rate of normalization of the ESR after resolution of inflammation, is inferior to that of CRP.[8] Such factors limit the reproducibility and predictive value of the ESR, making it less clinically useful than CRP in most settings.

## Serum Cytokines

Measurements of cytokines have been postulated to be useful as biomarkers to indicate whether the causative agent of gastroenteritis is a bacterial or viral cause. In addition, it has been proposed that cytokine concentrations may serve as broad markers to identify patients infected with gastrointestinal pathogens. Several cytokines have been evaluated from serum specimens, including interleukins (IL-6, IL-8), interferon (IFN-$\alpha$, IFN-$\gamma$), and tumor necrosis factor-$\alpha$ (TNF-$\alpha$). These cytokines play a variety of important roles in induction and regulation of the immune system response to infections, both bacterial and viral. Commercially available ELISA testing is available for the measurement of these cytokines from serum specimens.

Several studies have focused on the use of cytokines for the diagnosis of bacterial versus viral gastrointestinal infections in children.[12,13,18,21] Yeung and colleagues[18] evaluated a total of 115 patients; the study cohort included 75 bacterial and 43 viral infections and specimens were tested for the concentrations of IL-6, IL-8, INF-$\alpha$, and TNF-$\alpha$. The serum concentrations of IL-6 and IL-8 were significantly higher in patients with bacterial infections compared with viral infections. The sensitivity and specificity of IL-6 were 75% and 91%, whereas lower values were found with IL-8 of 46% and 71%, respectively. However, evaluation of INF-$\alpha$ and TNF-$\alpha$ in serum was much less sensitive and specific for differentiation of bacterial from viral gastrointestinal infections. These findings regarding IL-6 are similar to other reports with smaller cohorts, which reported sensitivity of 79% and specificity of 86%.[13,21] The use of serum IL-8 was also found to be less sensitive (50%) and specific (67%) for pathogen type discrimination.[13] Analysis of serum IL-10 concentrations in 2 separate studies suggests that it was significantly elevated in patients with either bacterial or viral infections relative to healthy controls, but did not reliably discriminate between viral and bacterial infections.[12,21] In contrast with the larger study by Yeung and colleagues,[18] another group (analyzing 17 patients positive for viral gastroenteritis and 14 patients with bacterial gastroenteritis) illustrated that serum TNF-α concentrations were 78% sensitive and 88% specific for distinguishing between pathogens.[12]

Studies evaluating serum cytokines for pathogen discrimination have failed to recapitulate the data demonstrating the utility of serum IL-6 in adults.[11,16] However, Weh and colleagues[16] found that in adult patients the serum levels of IFN-γ were significantly elevated in viral infections compared with bacterial infections, but with a sensitivity of 67% and specificity of 63%, the use of IFN-γ for pathogen discrimination would be suboptimal for routine clinical use.

The quantitative analysis of serum cytokine levels to differentiate between bacterial and viral gastrointestinal infections has yet to identify markers that yield similar results through several studies. In part, many of the studies were underpowered; this is compounded by the fact that serum cytokines are elevated in systemic infections or inflammatory conditions, which would likely decrease specificity in the context of diagnosis of gastrointestinal infections.[22–24]

## FECAL MARKERS
### Fecal Leukocyte Detection

Given the lack of specificity of systemic markers of infectious gastroenteritis, fecal biomarkers may increase specificity by differentiating gastrointestinal from extraintestinal inflammatory conditions. Direct or indirect detection of fecal leukocytes may overcome some of the challenges of inadequate specificity with systemic inflammatory markers such as CRP and ESR. The presence of fecal leukocytes can be detected either directly or indirectly.

### Direct Fecal Leukocyte Detection

One method to directly localize leukocytes is using scintigraphy to visualize autologous radiolabeled leukocytes. This method requires patients have their blood collected, and then the leukocytes are purified and labeled with either [111]Indium or [99]Technetium. The radiolabeled cells are reinfused; then the patient undergoes imaging to localize the labeled leukocytes. This method can identify the anatomic location of inflammation but is costly and invasive, requires highly specialized personnel, and has limited availability. Radiolabeled leukocyte scans have been primarily studied in the setting of IBD in which they correlate fairly well with histologic findings from endoscopy.[25]

A more practical and semiquantitative method to assess gastrointestinal leukocytes involves the direct enumeration of methylene blue–stained leukocytes from stool samples. Stool from healthy patients lack detectable fecal leukocytes, while they can be elevated in enteroinvasive gastrointestinal infections. Specifically, *Shigella*, *Salmonella*, enteroinvasive *Escherichia coli*, and amebic infections typically result in increased fecal polymorphonuclear leukocytes,[26] in contrast with fecal mononuclear leukocytes, which are more commonly elevated in typhoid fever. However, noninfectious causes, such as IBD, also cause elevated fecal leukocytes.[26] Notably, fecal leukocytes are rare in those with idiopathic and viral diarrhea as well as that due to *Vibrio cholera* or enterotoxigenic *E coli*. In one study of experimentally induced infection of healthy adults with *Shigella*, *Salmonella*, *V cholera*, invasive *E coli*, or viral causes of diarrhea, fecal leukocyte detection by microscopy was 89% specific in differentiating bacterial versus nonbacterial causes of diarrhea.[26]

Arguably the most common cause of infectious diarrhea in hospital settings is *Clostridium difficile*, although it can be difficult to distinguish between true disease and asymptomatic colonization with this bacterium.[27–29] Fecal leukocyte detection is of limited value in differentiating *C difficile* infection from other causes, with a reported sensitivity of only 10% compared with *C difficile* toxin assays, and thus direct fecal leukocyte detection should not play a significant role in evaluation for *C difficile* colitis.[30] In addition, Savola and colleagues[30] demonstrated that the sensitivity of direct fecal leukocyte detection (at a cutoff of 1 cell per high power field) varies significantly between inpatients (25%) and outpatients (57%) with similar specificities of 87% and 89%, respectively. Such poor sensitivity suggests a more limited role for fecal leukocyte detection in hospitalized patients.

### Indirect Fecal Leukocyte Detection

Although direct detection of fecal leukocytes by methylene blue staining and microscopy is relatively rapid and inexpensive, it requires skilled personnel and special specimen collection and handling, and interpretation is subjective. It is also poorly suited to automation, which is common in modern laboratories. Fecal lactoferrin and calprotectin assays were developed in part to overcome these limitations.

### Fecal Lactoferrin

Lactoferrin is an iron-binding glycoprotein found in neutrophil granules and in a variety of secretory fluids including breast milk. Its name is derived from its presence in breast milk and its structural homology to transferrin. Lactoferrin plays a broad role in innate immune defense.[31] Intestinal inflammation characterized by the recruitment of neutrophils results in elevated fecal lactoferrin levels. In contrast, monocytic and lymphocytic infiltration does not result in elevated fecal lactoferrin levels, because these cell types do not express lactoferrin.[32,33]

The major advantage of lactoferrin is that it has increased stability relative to other fecal biomarkers of intestinal inflammation, including fecal leukocytes, myeloperoxidase, and leukocyte esterase.[34] Fecal lactoferrin is relatively resistant to both freeze-thaw cycles and proteolysis with in vitro stability of up to 2 weeks when kept at 4°C, although the purported benefit of this property in the setting of diagnosis of acute gastrointestinal infection is unclear.

Several commercial assays for lactoferrin are available, including a qualitative immunochromatographic lateral flow assay called Leuko EZ Vue (Alere) and IBD-SCAN, a quantitative ELISA (Alere). In the differentiation of IBD from IBS in a single study from Switzerland, IBD-SCAN has an area under the ROC curve of 0.84.[35] In a meta-analysis of the use of lactoferrin to differentiate inflammatory from noninflammatory causes of diarrhea in resource-poor settings, lactoferrin had an area under the ROC curve of 0.79 with 95% sensitivity and 29% specificity at a cutoff of +1 at 1:50.[36]

### Fecal Occult Blood Test

Fecal occult blood testing (FOBT) has also been evaluated for the differentiation of viral from bacterial gastroenteritis. Occult blood in stool can be detected either biochemically or immunologically. Biochemical detection depends on the reaction of exogenous hydrogen peroxide with heme in the stool. Heme has peroxidase activity, which in the presence of hydrogen peroxide oxidizes guaiac acid, resulting in a blue color. False positives can be due to consumption of foods with peroxidase activity, such as red meat and radishes. More recently, fecal immunochemical tests (FIT) have been developed. These tests use antibodies against human hemoglobin to overcome the dietary limitations of peroxidase-based methods; however, FIT testing is substantially more expensive.[37]

In a meta-analysis assessing the utility of FOBT diagnosing inflammatory bacterial gastroenteritis, the area under the ROC curve was 0.63 for studies in resource-poor countries compared with 0.81 in developing countries.[36] In this study, FOBT had modestly inferior performance to fecal leukocyte microscopy and similar performance to fecal lactoferrin.[36] Thus, FOBT cannot be used reliably to include or exclude a diagnosis of infectious gastroenteritis.

### Fecal Calprotectin

Calprotectin is a heterodimeric protein complex composed of S100A8 and S100A9 that is present in neutrophils, monocytes, and macrophages. It binds to and sequesters calcium and zinc from bacterial inhabitants of the gastrointestinal tract. It is estimated that calprotectin composes 60% of the cytoplasmic protein content of neutrophils, which accounts for its large influx at sites of neutrophil activation. The levels of fecal calprotectin were found to correlate well with [111]Indium-labeled neutrophilic granulocyte infiltration in stool specimens of patients with IBD.[38] Calprotectin is stable at room temperature in feces for up to 7 days and is resistant to degradation by microbes; thus, no special specimen transport or preservative is required.[39]

In healthy patients, the levels of fecal calprotectin are inversely proportional to patient age, with higher levels found in young, healthy infants.[40–42] Although these studies evaluated this phenomenon in children from developed countries, similar trends were also observed in Ugandan children.[43] Intraindividual variability of fecal calprotectin levels has been noted in past studies when the levels when monitored over several days.[44,45] Of note, fecal calprotectin levels are elevated in patients with IBD and are used to monitor IBD treatment.[35] The measurement of fecal calprotectin levels can also be used to differentiate between IBD and IBS.[46] Numerous other conditions are also noted to lead to increased fecal calprotectin levels, including cystic fibrosis, Crohn disease, ulcerative colitis, gastrointestinal malignancy, and rheumatoid arthritis.[35]

Quantitative levels of fecal calprotectin levels can be determined with commercially available ELISA kits, with results usually reported as micrograms of calprotectin per gram of feces, or milligrams of calprotectin per kilogram of feces. Point-of-care chromatographic immunoassays are also available for quantitative measurement of fecal calprotectin levels.

One large, multicenter, prospective study in Germany enrolled nearly 2200 adults presenting with acute gastroenteritis to evaluate the use of fecal calprotectin levels to screen patients for bacterial causes of gastrointestinal symptoms.[47] Patients were excluded from the study if they had conditions known to result in elevated fecal calprotectin levels (eg, IBD, gastrointestinal malignancy). From this study group, 195 specimens had culture-confirmed infections, which were used to analyze the fecal calprotectin levels against 196 pathogen-negative specimens as controls. The authors found that when using greater than 15 mg/L of fecal calprotectin as the cutoff, calprotectin results had a sensitivity of 83% and specificity of 87% in patients with acute bacterial gastroenteritis.

The fecal calprotectin levels do not always appear to be elevated in patients with bacterial gastroenteritis. In one study from Denmark, the fecal calprotectin levels were evaluated in patients with *Campylobacter jejuni/coli* or *Campylobacter concisus* gastroenteritis.[48] Patients with underlying pathologic conditions were excluded from the study (ie, IBD, gastrointestinal malignancies, and cirrhosis). The authors identified 99 patients with *C concisus*–positive cultures, and 140 patients with *C jejuni/coli*–positive cultures. Patients infected with *C concisus* tended to have milder symptoms relative to patients infected with *C jejuni/coli*. The mean fecal calprotectin levels were lower in the *C concisus*–positive patients relative to the *C jejuni/coli* patients, and 41 of the *C concisus* culture–positive patients had normal levels of fecal calprotectin (<50 mg/kg).

Other studies evaluated fecal calprotectin levels with both viral and bacterial causes of gastrointestinal infections in children[15,49] and in adults.[16] In the article by Chen and colleagues, 153 children were identified with pathogen-positive testing, 91 for viral pathogens and 62 for bacterial pathogens. Fecal calprotectin levels were significantly higher (*P*<.05) in patients with bacterial infections (median value of 754 µg/g) when compared with viral infections (median value of 89 µg/g). Similar findings were observed in another study by Sýkora and colleagues,[15] with 66 children with pathogen-positive testing: 32 for viral pathogens and 34 for bacterial pathogens. Fecal calprotectin levels were significantly elevated in patients with bacterial infections when compared with either control, healthy patients or patients with viral infections (*P*<.001). No statistical difference in fecal calprotectin levels were observed in patients with viral infections when compared with the control, healthy patients. The ROC for fecal calprotectin in patients with bacterial infections was 0.95, with a sensitivity of 93% and specificity of 88%. Finally, in adults, Weh and colleagues[16] also found that fecal calprotectin levels were significantly elevated in patients with bacterial versus viral gastrointestinal infections (*P* = .0032). The ROC was 0.746, whereas the sensitivity and specificity were 87% and 65%, respectively.

Although a comprehensive evaluation of calprotectin in the context of a wide variety of bacterial causes of bacterial gastroenteritis is lacking, the above studies suggest that fecal calprotectin might be an adequate marker for bacterial gastrointestinal infections, excluding at least *C concisus*. However, fecal calprotectin is not a good marker for viral infections nor would be useful in patients with underlying gastrointestinal disorders that are known to result in elevated calprotectin levels.

## SUMMARY

A rapid and inexpensive assay that is sensitive and specific for the diagnosis of infectious gastroenteritis would be of significant clinical value. Such a test would enable clinicians to quickly triage patients, expedite appropriate treatment and avoid unnecessary invasive diagnostic testing. When laboratory confirmation of the cause of gastroenteritis is sought, diagnostic methods include culture, microscopy, immunoassay, or nucleic acid amplification testing. However, many of these methods are labor-intensive, slow, or expensive and may have limited sensitivity for rare or fastidious organisms. A diagnostic assay with the ability to rule in or out infectious gastroenteritis based on the host response, rather than relying exclusively on pathogen detection, may be synergistic with current diagnostic methods. For example, if a rapid marker of host response was to test negative for infectious gastroenteritis, this could prevent a costly and unnecessary infectious workup; although if the host marker suggested an infectious cause, it would expedite the use of appropriate antimicrobials when indicated and reduce unnecessary invasive testing such as colonoscopies and imaging studies.

However, the identification of a host marker with adequate analytical performance characteristics remains elusive. An ideal host marker for intestinal inflammation would be sensitive and specific, have rapid turn-around time and high reproducibility, and would work in all host backgrounds regardless of the immune status of the patient, which is important in developed countries, where many patients with suspected gastrointestinal infection are immunocompromised or have IBD. In addition, it is possible that recent advances in pathogen diagnostics, such as rapid multiplexed nucleic amplification tests,[3–7] may obviate the need for improved host biomarkers.

## SELF ASSESSMENT

Question 1

In which of the following patient populations or conditions would elevated fecal calprotectin levels be expected?
A. Irritable bowel syndrome
B. Healthy infants
C. Norovirus infection
D. Rotavirus infection
E. Healthy teenagers in the developing world

Question 2

Which of the following conditions is *not* associated with an elevated erythrocyte sedimentation rate?
A. Pregnancy
B. Systemic lupus erythematosus (SLE)
C. *Salmonella* gastroenteritis
D. *C difficile* colonization
E. *Campylobacter* gastroenteritis

Question 3

Which of the following inflammatory markers are typically measured in feces (not from blood)?
A. CRP
B. ESR
C. IL-6
D. Lactoferrin
E. TNF-α

ANSWERS

Answer 1: B. Healthy infants.

The levels of fecal calprotectin are notably higher in healthy infants without gastrointestinal symptoms, with levels being inversely proportional to age. Similar elevations in fecal calprotectin levels were noted in infants from Uganda, but the levels also decreased with age. Viral gastrointestinal infections, such as norovirus or rotavirus, tend not to result in elevated fecal calprotectin levels, whereas the levels are elevated in several bacterial infections. Finally, fecal calprotectin levels tend to be elevated in patients with inflammatory bowel disease but not in irritable bowel syndrome.

Answer 2: D. *C difficile* colonization.

ESR is a nonspecific marker of inflammation. *C difficile* colonization generally does not result in a significant systemic inflammatory response and thus is not typically associated with an elevated ESR. However, ESR may be increased in *C difficile* colitis. *Salmonella* and *Campylobacter* infection and autoimmune diseases including SLE typically cause elevated ESRs. Pregnancy has been associated with an increased ESR.

Answer 3: D. Lactoferrin.

Lactoferrin is measured from feces. Lactoferrin is an iron-binding protein found in neutrophil granules. IL-6 is a cytokine that increases CRP, an acute phase reactant. IL-6, TNF-α, and CRP are typically measured in serum. ESR is measured in whole blood anticoagulated with EDTA.

## REFERENCES

1. Liu L, Johnson HL, Cousens S, et al. Global, regional, and national causes of child mortality: an updated systematic analysis for 2010 with time trends since 2000. Lancet 2012;379(9832):2151–61.
2. Scallan E, Griffin PM, Angulo FJ, et al. Foodborne illness acquired in the United States–unspecified agents. Emerg Infect Dis 2011;17(1):16–22.
3. Perry MD, Corden SA, Howe RA. Evaluation of the Luminex xTAG Gastrointestinal Pathogen Panel and the Savyon Diagnostics Gastrointestinal Infection Panel for the detection of enteric pathogens in clinical samples. J Med Microbiol 2014; 63(Pt 11):1419–26.
4. Khare R, Espy MJ, Cebelinski E, et al. Comparative evaluation of two commercial multiplex panels for detection of gastrointestinal pathogens by use of clinical stool specimens. J Clin Microbiol 2014;52(10):3667–73.
5. Halligan E, Edgeworth J, Bisnauthsing K, et al. Multiplex molecular testing for management of infectious gastroenteritis in a hospital setting: a comparative diagnostic and clinical utility study. Clin Microbiol Infect 2014;20(8):O460–7.
6. Wessels E, Rusman LG, van Bussel MJ, et al. Added value of multiplex Luminex Gastrointestinal Pathogen Panel (xTAG® GPP) testing in the diagnosis of infectious gastroenteritis. Clin Microbiol Infect 2014;20(3):O182–7.
7. Claas EC, Burnham CA, Mazzulli T, et al. Performance of the xTAG® gastrointestinal pathogen panel, a multiplex molecular assay for simultaneous detection of bacterial, viral, and parasitic causes of infectious gastroenteritis. J Microbiol Biotechnol 2013;23(7):1041–5.
8. Gabay C, Kushner I. Acute-phase proteins and other systemic responses to inflammation. N Engl J Med 1999;340(6):448–54.
9. Abernethy TJ, Avery OT. The occurrence during acute infections of a protein not normally present in the blood: I. Distribution of the reactive protein in patients' sera and the effect of calcium on the flocculation reaction with C polysaccharide of pneumococcus. J Exp Med 1941;73(2):173–82.
10. Borgnolo G, Barbone F, Guidobaldi G, et al. C-reactive protein in viral and bacterial gastroenteritis in childhood. Acta Paediatr 1996;85(6):670–4.
11. Elsing C, Ernst S, Kayali N, et al. Lipopolysaccharide binding protein, interleukin-6 and C-reactive protein in acute gastrointestinal infections: value as biomarkers to reduce unnecessary antibiotic therapy. Infection 2011;39(4):327–31.
12. Hsu TR, Chen SJ, Wu TC, et al. Tumor necrosis factor-alpha and interleukin-10 in viral and bacterial gastroenteritis in children. J Chin Med Assoc 2005;68(6):250–3.
13. Lin CH, Hsieh CC, Chen SJ, et al. The diagnostic value of serum interleukins 6 and 8 in children with acute gastroenteritis. J Pediatr Gastroenterol Nutr 2006; 43(1):25–9.
14. Meloni GF, Tomasi PA, Spanu P, et al. C-reactive protein levels for diagnosis of Salmonella gastroenteritis. Pediatr Infect Dis J 1999;18(5):471–3.
15. Sýkora J, Siala K, Huml M, et al. Evaluation of faecal calprotectin as a valuable non-invasive marker in distinguishing gut pathogens in young children with acute gastroenteritis. Acta Paediatr 2010;99(9):1389–95.
16. Weh J, Antoni C, Weiß C, et al. Discriminatory potential of C-reactive protein, cytokines, and fecal markers in infectious gastroenteritis in adults. Diagn Microbiol Infect Dis 2013;77(1):79–84.
17. Mangiarotti P, Moulin F, Palmer P, et al. Interferon-alpha in viral and bacterial gastroenteritis: a comparison with C-reactive protein and interleukin-6. Acta Paediatr 1999;88(6):592–4.

18. Yeung CY, Lee HC, Lin SP, et al. Serum cytokines in differentiating between viral and bacterial enterocolitis. Ann Trop Paediatr 2004;24(4):337–43.
19. Kim DH, Kang SH, Jeong WS, et al. Serum C-reactive protein (CRP) levels in young adults can be used to discriminate between inflammatory and non-inflammatory diarrhea. Dig Dis Sci 2013;58(2):504–8.
20. Grzybowski A, Sak J. Edmund Biernacki (1866–1911): discoverer of the erythrocyte sedimentation rate. On the 100th anniversary of his death. Clin Dermatol 2011;29(6):697–703.
21. Chen SM, Ku MS, Lee MY, et al. Diagnostic performance of serum interleukin-6 and interleukin-10 levels and clinical predictors in children with rotavirus and norovirus gastroenteritis. Cytokine 2012;59(2):299–304.
22. Riedel S, Carroll KC. Laboratory detection of sepsis: biomarkers and molecular approaches. Clin Lab Med 2013;33(3):413–37.
23. Tanaka T, Narazaki M, Kishimoto T. IL-6 in inflammation, immunity, and disease. Cold Spring Harb Perspect Biol 2014;6(10):a016295.
24. Popa C, Netea MG, van Riel PL, et al. The role of TNF-alpha in chronic inflammatory conditions, intermediary metabolism, and cardiovascular risk. J Lipid Res 2007;48(4):751–62.
25. Stathaki MI, Koukouraki SI, Karkavitsas NS, et al. Role of scintigraphy in inflammatory bowel disease. World J Gastroenterol 2009;15(22):2693–700.
26. Harris JC, Dupont HL, Hornick RB. Fecal leukocytes in diarrheal illness. Ann Intern Med 1972;76(5):697–703.
27. Alasmari F, Seiler SM, Hink T, et al. Prevalence and risk factors for asymptomatic Clostridium difficile carriage. Clin Infect Dis 2014;59(2):216–22.
28. Burnham CA, Carroll KC. Diagnosis of Clostridium difficile infection: an ongoing conundrum for clinicians and for clinical laboratories. Clin Microbiol Rev 2013; 26(3):604–30.
29. Dubberke ER, Han Z, Bobo L, et al. Impact of clinical symptoms on interpretation of diagnostic assays for Clostridium difficile infections. J Clin Microbiol 2011; 49(8):2887–93.
30. Savola KL, Baron EJ, Tompkins LS, et al. Fecal leukocyte stain has diagnostic value for outpatients but not inpatients. J Clin Microbiol 2001;39(1): 266–9.
31. Däbritz J, Musci J, Foell D. Diagnostic utility of faecal biomarkers in patients with irritable bowel syndrome. World J Gastroenterol 2014;20(2):363–75.
32. Guerrant RL, Araujo V, Soares E, et al. Measurement of fecal lactoferrin as a marker of fecal leukocytes. J Clin Microbiol 1992;30(5):1238–42.
33. Naidu AS, Arnold RR. Influence of lactoferrin on host-microbe interactions. In: Hutchens TW, Lonnerdal B, editors. Lactoferrin—interactions and biological functions, vol. 28. Totowa (NJ): Humana Press; 1997. p. 259–75.
34. Uchida K, Matsuse R, Tomita S, et al. Immunochemical detection of human lactoferrin in feces as a new marker for inflammatory gastrointestinal disorders and colon cancer. Clin Biochem 1994;27(4):259–64.
35. Burri E, Beglinger C. The use of fecal calprotectin as a biomarker in gastrointestinal disease. Expert Rev Gastroenterol Hepatol 2014;8(2):197–210.
36. Gill CJ, Lau J, Gorbach SL, et al. Diagnostic accuracy of stool assays for inflammatory bacterial gastroenteritis in developed and resource-poor countries. Clin Infect Dis 2003;37(3):365–75.
37. Greenwald B. From guaiac to immune fecal occult blood tests: the emergence of technology in colorectal cancer screening. Gastroenterol Nurs 2005;28(2): 90–6.

38. Røseth AG, Schmidt PN, Fagerhol MK. Correlation between faecal excretion of indium-111-labelled granulocytes and calprotectin, a granulocyte marker protein, in patients with inflammatory bowel disease. Scand J Gastroenterol 1999;34(1): 50–4.

39. Dolwani S, Metzner M, Wassell JJ, et al. Diagnostic accuracy of faecal calprotectin estimation in prediction of abnormal small bowel radiology. Aliment Pharmacol Ther 2004;20(6):615–21.

40. Savino F, Castagno E, Calabrese R, et al. High faecal calprotectin levels in healthy, exclusively breast-fed infants. Neonatology 2010;97(4):299–304.

41. Campeotto F, Butel MJ, Kalach N, et al. High faecal calprotectin concentrations in newborn infants. Arch Dis Child Fetal Neonatal Ed 2004;89(4):F353–5.

42. Olafsdottir E, Aksnes L, Fluge G, et al. Faecal calprotectin levels in infants with infantile colic, healthy infants, children with inflammatory bowel disease, children with recurrent abdominal pain and healthy children. Acta Paediatr 2002;91(1): 45–50.

43. Hestvik E, Tumwine JK, Tylleskar T, et al. Faecal calprotectin concentrations in apparently healthy children aged 0–12 years in urban Kampala, Uganda: a community-based survey. BMC Pediatr 2011;11:9.

44. Husebye E, Tøn H, Johne B. Biological variability of fecal calprotectin in patients referred for colonoscopy without colonic inflammation or neoplasm. Am J Gastroenterol 2001;96(9):2683–7.

45. Naismith GD, Smith LA, Barry SJ, et al. A prospective single-centre evaluation of the intra-individual variability of faecal calprotectin in quiescent Crohn's disease. Aliment Pharmacol Ther 2013;37(6):613–21.

46. Sherwood RA. Faecal markers of gastrointestinal inflammation. J Clin Pathol 2012;65(11):981–5.

47. Shastri YM, Bergis D, Povse N, et al. Prospective multicenter study evaluating fecal calprotectin in adult acute bacterial diarrhea. Am J Med 2008;121(12): 1099–106.

48. Nielsen HL, Engberg J, Ejlertsen T, et al. Evaluation of fecal calprotectin in Campylobacter concisus and Campylobacter jejuni/coli gastroenteritis. Scand J Gastroenterol 2013;48(5):633–5.

49. Chen CC, Huang JL, Chang CJ, et al. Fecal calprotectin as a correlative marker in clinical severity of infectious diarrhea and usefulness in evaluating bacterial or viral pathogens in children. J Pediatr Gastroenterol Nutr 2012;55(5):541–7.

# Laboratory Diagnosis of Noroviruses: Present and Future

Xiaoli Pang, PhD[a,b,*], Bonita E. Lee, MD, MSc[c]

## KEYWORDS

- Norovirus • Genotypes • Sporadic and outbreak gastroenteritis • Laboratory test
- Diagnosis

## KEY POINTS

- There is no test for infectious norovirus (NoV) because of the absence of *in vitro* culture system.
- Electron microscopy is no longer an adequate detection method for NoV.
- The highly diversified genome and antigens of NoV present challenges for the development of antigen-based immunoassays.
- Real-time reverse transcription polymerase chain reaction (RT-PCR) is currently considered as the gold standard test for NoV.
- Rectal and oral swabs, which are convenient to collect, may be good alternatives to stool samples for testing of NoV.
- Genotyping is an important tool for NoV molecular epidemiologic surveillance and vaccine development.
- Further development of nanotechnology-based platforms might provide point-of-care testing.
- Each laboratory needs to select a testing platform that is best fitted for its needs and feasibilities.

## INTRODUCTION

With the development and application of advanced diagnostic assays to detect norovirus (NoV) in public health and clinical laboratories, NoV is well known as one of the top 5 causative agents of global epidemics of gastroenteritis outbreaks and is increasingly being recognized as one of the most important pathogens of sporadic gastroenteritis.[1,2]

Disclosures: Both authors declare no conflicts of interest with the preparation of this article.
[a] Provincial Laboratory for Public Health, Walter Mackenzie Health Sciences Centre, University of Alberta Hospital, 8440 - 112 Street, Edmonton, Alberta T6G 2J2, Canada; [b] Department of Laboratory Medicine and Pathology, University of Alberta, 8440-112 Street, Edmonton, Alberta T6G 2B7, Canada; [c] Department of Pediatrics, University of Alberta, 11405, 87 Avenue, Edmonton, Alberta T6G 1C9, Canada
* Corresponding author. Provincial Laboratory for Public Health, Walter Mackenzie Health Sciences Centre, University of Alberta Hospital, 8440 - 112 Street, Edmonton, Alberta T6G 2J2, Canada.
*E-mail address:* xiao-li.pang@albertahealthservices.ca

Clin Lab Med 35 (2015) 345–362
http://dx.doi.org/10.1016/j.cll.2015.02.008
labmed.theclinics.com

Based on a systematic review of 31 studies in both developed and developing countries, it was estimated that NoV accounted for 10% to 15% of severe gastroenteritis cases in children younger than 5 years and 9% to 15% of mild and moderate diarrheal disorders in populations of various ages, leading to 1.7 million to 1.9 million outpatient visits and 19 million to 21 million total illnesses per year in the United States.[3] NoV is becoming the predominant cause of sporadic gastroenteritis in young children, especially in regions where rotavirus vaccine programs have been implemented.[4,5]

Laboratory testing for NoV has undergone development during the last 4 decades since the virus was discovered by Dr Kapikian using immunoelectron microscopy (EM).[6] There are still knowledge and technical gaps, with no method to detect infectious NoV particles because of the absence of *in vitro* viral culture system and small animal model. Although research laboratories can produce recombinant p particles and viruslike particles (VLPs) that have NoV characteristics and can be used as a vehicle for vaccine development,[7,8] the inability to produce large volume of naturally occurring viral particles hampers the development of diagnostic assays. At present, real-time RT-PCR is considered the best assay to detect NoV in both research and clinical settings. However, there are still limitations with this approach, including the need for multistep procedure, high cost, need for special instruments, and being too sensitive to provide results relevant to clinical situations. Simple, more affordable, and rapid testing methods such as enzyme immune assay (EIA) or enzyme-linked immunosorbent assay (ELISA) to detect NoV have been developed but generally have low sensitivity and thus limited utility. Novel nanotechnology array-based assays to detect NoV are in development and under validation. A major breakthrough with nanotechnology array-based assays will be the development of point-of-care tests, featuring rapidity and potential utility in many settings including resource-poor countries depending on affordability. It will take time to validate some of these prototypes before their application in clinical diagnostics. The future directions of technology development for NoV detection likely focus on method simplification, cost-effectiveness, analytical precision, and accuracy. This review summarizes technologies used in the detection of NoV and highlights some of their features.

## NOROVIRUS AND ITS CLINICAL RELEVANCE
### Structures and Taxonomy

NoV is a small (30–38 nm), round, nonenveloped virus with a single-stranded, positive-sense RNA genome. NoV was initially called small round-structured virus, deriving from the smooth surface of its morphologic structure.[9] Using cryoelectron microscopy and x-ray crystallography analysis of VLPs, the 3-icosahedral capsid of NoV was shown to be composed of 90 dimeric capsomers made up of 180 capsid proteins. Each capsid protein possesses 2 major domains, the shell and the protrusion domains. The RNA genome of NoV is ~7.5 kb in length with a poly A tail.[10] Three open reading frames (ORFs) have been characterized, with ORF1 encoding the nonstructural proteins, ORF2 the VP1 capsid protein, and ORF3 a minor structural protein.

NoV family is classified into 5 genogroups (GI-V) with GI, GII, and GIV found mainly in human infections, GII and GIII in pigs and cattle, and GV in mice.[11] Zoonotic transmission of NoV has been postulated only based on seroprevalence studies.[12] At least 14 genotypes of GI, 29 genotypes of GII, and 2 genotypes of GIV have been identified.[13–15] Most human infections are caused by NoV GI or GII. Up to 85% of global epidemics of NoV infections have been caused by different GII.4 (GII genotype 4) variants that emerge every 2 to 3 years. NoV GII.4 was found to have a higher mutation rate and a faster pace of evolution than other NoV strains, enhancing its epidemiologic fitness.[16] In addition to causing global epidemics of outbreaks, GII.4 variants play an important role in sporadic gastroenteritis.[14,17]

### Epidemiology

NoV is highly contagious and is becoming the most common cause of nonbacterial acute gastroenteritis globally.[18] People of all ages can be infected likely because of the diversity of NoV strains, incomplete protective immunity following childhood infection, and reinfection in their lifetime. The susceptibility to NoV infections has been found to be associated with the human histo-blood group antigen (HBGA) genotype; nonsecretors, who do not express HBGA in tissue and body fluids, are more resistant to NoV infection.[19] NoV gastroenteritis and its common association with outbreaks in closed communities is an important public health issue. NoV outbreaks occur in a variety of settings, including hospitals, day care centers, schools, nursing homes, cruise ships, and military camps. NoV has also been identified as the leading cause of acute gastroenteritis in children in the United States and in regions with routine rotavirus vaccination programs.[4,5] Sporadic NoV disease and outbreaks impose a significant burden on health and economic resources.

NoV is transmitted by the fecal-oral route through person-to-person contact or indirectly through contaminated fomites (eg, shared eating utensils, environmental surfaces, toys in playrooms). Transmission is highly efficient because of the physical hardiness of the viruses, the high amounts of viral particles shed in stool, and low infectious dose. NoV is also readily transmitted by eating or drinking contaminated foods or beverages, which usually results in outbreaks in social gatherings. Another well-known cause of NoV outbreaks is from eating raw or undercooked contaminated shellfish or drinking contaminated water. In temperate climate, NoV gastroenteritis is more prevalent in cold seasons, typically with a winter peak.

### Clinical Aspects

Infection with NoV usually has a sudden onset following a short incubation period of 1 to 2 days. The symptoms are variable and can include diarrhea, nausea, vomiting (in >50% of cases), abdominal cramps, and malaise. The duration of symptoms is usually less than 7 days. In most cases, virus shedding in stool lasts about 1 to 2 weeks but can be longer depending on the virus and the host.[20,21] The diarrheal stool is usually watery or loose with no mucus or blood, and leukocytes are typically absent. The illness is self-limited in well-nourished individuals with normal immune system. Asymptomatic infections or mild disease are common, but severe illnesses can occur in infants, the elderly, and immunocompromised individuals, resulting in significant morbidity. Chronic diarrhea, prolonged viral shedding up to months, and increased mortality are seen in immunocompromised hosts. NoV has been reported to be associated with necrotizing enterocolitis in neonates.[22,23]

Because NoV is associated with epidemics and outbreaks and contributes to a high burden of gastroenteritis, the development of vaccines and antivirals is urgently needed. Randomized, double-blinded, and placebo-controlled trial of an NoV genotype GI.1 VLP vaccine has found that immunization with the vaccine reduced the frequencies of vomiting and/or diarrhea and shedding of NoV in a challenge study.[24,25] However, a better understanding of immunity after NoV infection and vaccination is still needed. At present, preventive and control strategies for NoV infections are focused on identifying and eliminating the infectious source, promoting good personal hygienic practices, performing proper disinfection of environmental surfaces, identifying and avoiding sick contacts, and stopping other mechanisms of transmission.

## SAMPLE COLLECTIONS AND REQUIREMENTS FOR NOROVIRUS TESTING
### Clinical Sample Types

#### Stool sample

Stool is the classic specimen of choice for laboratory testing of NoV. A few grams of stool sample (pea size) are sufficient for NoV detection by EM, antigen testing, or nucleic acid testing (NAT) methods. It is best to urinate before collection of stool samples to avoid mixing of the 2 specimen types. For patients in a health care setting, a bed pan, catching device, or portable commode is often used to collect the stool, from which a small amount can be transferred to nonleak plastic containers usually equipped with a screwcap and small scoop. However, often stool samples need to be collected from outpatients at home, which is inconvenient and can be messy. For adults or toilet-trained children, a catching device that is provided by clinics or emergency departments or a piece of plastic (eg, Saran wrap) can be placed over the toilet seat with a dip in the center. After defecation, a small amount of the stool sample can be collected into the nonleak container prelabeled with patient identifiers. For babies and infants, stool samples can be obtained from a diaper using either a wooden tongue depressor or the scoop of the nonleak container for transportation to the laboratory. It is important to wash hands after collection of the stool sample. It is preferable to collect stool sample within the first 48 hours of illness when viral shedding is at its maximum, which increases the likelihood of virus detection.

#### Rectal swab

Obtaining bulk stool specimens is challenging especially in the home setting. There is some recent evidence supporting the use of rectal swab, which gave equivalent results of detecting NoV using real-time RT-PCR.[26,27] However, rectal swabs are not recommended for testing by EM and antigen detection test (EIA/ELISA) because of insufficient quantity of feces. It is easier and more convenient to collect a rectal swab, but more data and validation are needed to support its use as a routine diagnostic sample.

#### Serum

Serum samples can be tested to detect NoV viremia in patients with severe illness or complications, for example, extraintestinal manifestations such as seizures and encephalopathy.[23,28–31] Another use of serum is the detection of antibodies to NoV, but serologic testing for NoV only has limited application in research and epidemiologic seroprevalance studies. Acute-phase serum sample should be collected as soon as possible after illness onset; the acute and convalescent samples should be tested simultaneously.

#### Oral swab

The oral swab has also been used as an alternate specimen type for the detection of NoV infections, especially in patients presenting only with vomiting, as it is difficult to collect and test vomitus. However, like rectal swab, oral swab is not routinely accepted for diagnostic testing and needs further studies to understand its test characteristics such as sensitivity and specificity.

#### Beyond clinical samples

Drinking water, food, beverages, and other environmental specimens are sometimes collected for the investigation of outbreaks associated with NoV. If a food item or water is suspected to be the source of an outbreak, specimens should be obtained as early as possible and stored under appropriate conditions. Because testing of these types of specimen is not routinely performed in most diagnostic laboratories and they often require special handling and processing, reference laboratory with the capability to perform these specialized tests should be contacted to obtain appropriate instructions before specimen collection.

### Storage and Transportation

In general, the best test results are obtained by testing fresh stool samples, especially for those methods that depend on the morphologic appearance of virus, that is, EM. For EM, stool samples should be stored at 4°C immediately after collection and promptly transported to the laboratory for processing. If repeat testing is expected for the same sample, single-use aliquots of the sample should be prepared and stored for future testing. Processing and storing samples in this manner can minimize the degradation of viral particles, proteins, and/or nucleic acids (NAs) and cross-contamination. The ideal storage temperature for aliquots, especially in terms of preserving NAs, is −70°C. On the other hand, local experience has shown that NoV can be detected in stool samples using molecular tests after storage at −20°C for 3 years. Stool samples can be shipped on wet or dry ice, depending on their storage conditions (eg, short- or long-term storage). Repeat freezing and thawing should be avoided. Processed serum specimens can be stored at 2°C to 8°C up to several days then stored at −20°C or colder for prolonged storage.

### Testing Frequency

For investigation of NoV outbreaks, testing up to 6 samples per outbreak is considered sufficient for identification of NoV and ruling out of NoV as the causative agent.[32] Once 2 stool samples from the same outbreak are tested as positive, NoV can be confirmed as a causative agent. If all 6 samples are tested as negative, an outbreak can be defined as non-NoV associated, and further investigation for other pathogens may be required.[33] Repeat testing of NoV for the same patient using molecular testing should not be performed except for special clinical reasons, as NoV can be shed for weeks to months especially in immunosuppressed patients.[20,21]

## LABORATORY TESTING OF NOROVIRUSES FOR DIAGNOSTICS
### Direct Detection

### Electron microscopy
Viruses can be identified using EM by visualizing the shape and size of intact viral particles during examination of a very small amount of stool sample. This traditional method offers the advantages of short processing time and the ability to detect multiple viruses with different morphologic types if present. However, EM has low sensitivity for small round-structured viruses and cannot differentiate NoV, sapovirus, and astrovirus, as their morphology is similar.[6] In a 1-year prospective study, of 2486 stool samples, EM missed all 403 NoV-positive samples as detected by real-time RT-PCR.[34] There is also high cost associated with the maintenance of the EM instrument and the requirement for specialized technical expertise; thus, EM is usually only performed in public health or large clinical laboratories. Electron microscopy with its low sensitivity and specificity has largely been replaced by molecular methods for the detection of NoV.

### Immunoassays for norovirus antigen detection
Antigenic detection assays have the advantages of being rapid, inexpensive, simple to perform, and highly adoptable for use in many laboratories; therefore, these assays, usually EIA, have been developed for direct detection of NoV since 2003.[35–48] Common formats of antigen detection assays include the conventional 96-well microplate

EIA, rapid membrane-based immunochromatographic assays, and most recently bioluminescent EIA.[48] However, the number of antigen detection assays remains limited for NoV because of the absence of specific antibodies that can capture and detect conserved viral antigens in this highly diversified virus. The performance of existing antigen detection assays needs to be vastly improved to achieve better sensitivity and specificity. Because of the high degree of genetic and antigenic diversity of NoV, the sensitivity of many antigen detection assays is still low, even though their test performance is better than EM.

Although several antigen detection assays for NoV have been commercialized, most of these assays are only CE mark in Europe for *in vitro* diagnostic use and are not yet available in North America. Only 1 NoV assay (RIDASCREEN Norovirus 3rd Generation EIA) from R-Biopharm AG (Darmstadt, Germany) has been licensed by the US Food and Drug Administration for preliminary identification of NoV during outbreak screening. Because of the limited sensitivity and specificity, NoV antigen detection assays have been used mainly in research settings and are not recommended for routine clinical diagnosis.[49] Several evaluation studies on commercial EIA and immunochromatographic kits for NoV showed much lower sensitivity compared with RT-PCR for detection of NoV GI and GII.[32]

## Nucleic Acid–Based Detection

NAT methods based on reverse transcription and polymerase chain reaction (RT-PCR), available since the 1990s with the cloning of NoV, are currently considered as the gold standard for NoV diagnostics.[10] These molecular amplification methods are sensitive and have become increasingly important for accurate detection of NoV.[49] On the other hand, the clinical interpretation of a positive NoV NAT test result in patients who might have prolonged shedding, for example, patients with solid organ or bone marrow transplant, is complicated. Moreover, the inability to assess infectious human NoV also presents unanswered questions for infection control and isolation practice for these patients.

### Extraction and preparation of norovirus RNA for amplification testing

One of the major challenges of viral detection in stool specimens by NAT is the presence of inhibitors, which can lead to false-negative results. Different approaches have been developed and undertaken to reduce inhibitory substances and their effects, for example, dilution of stool samples and/or extracted NAs; addition of chelating agents, detergents, or denaturing chemicals during RNA extraction; and inclusion of amplification facilitators such as bovine serum albumin and betaine during PCR.[50,51] An inhibitory effect on PCR can be monitored by adding known NA to the sample as an internal control during NA extraction. Most commercial NA extraction protocols now use silica- or magnetic bead–based extraction technologies that are simple and efficient and provide adequate amounts of high-quality NA. Having an efficient NA extraction method is essential for the removal of contaminants from cellular proteins, carbohydrates, and lipids and to eliminate inhibitors or interference in the downstream amplification step.

NA extracts from stool specimens usually contain large amounts of nonviral RNA from different microorganisms and host cells that can be nonspecifically amplified by primers specifically designed for NoV. These nonspecific PCR products cannot be eliminated even under the high-stringency conditions of the reactions. Thus, hybridization with NoV-specific probes is usually required as part of the PCR process to confirm the results.

### Conventional reverse transcription polymerase chain reaction

Conventional RT-PCR (cRT-PCR) refers to the traditional amplification process whereby the amplified product is allowed to accumulate as the thermal cycling continues to an end point and the reaction reaches a plateau before detection or analysis steps are conducted. Amplified PCR products are usually detected by size fractionation using agarose or polyacrylamide gel electrophoresis. Jiang and colleagues[52] first used cRT-PCR to detect human NoV using specific primers targeting Norwalk virus. As a detection method, cRT-PCR has issues of a complex multistep procedure that is associated with high variability, low throughput, being labor intensive and time consuming, and posing significant risk of contamination because of the need to manipulate postamplified products in an open system. Although cRT-PCR is still commonly used to detect NoV in epidemiologic studies of gastroenteritis, it is not widely adopted by diagnostic laboratories.

A different application of cRT-PCR in NoV diagnostics is the development of primer sets to target various genetic regions to study the evolution and molecular epidemiology of NoV. Combining cRT-PCR with genetic sequencing of the amplicons is being used to study the genetic variations among NoV strains.[11,53]

### Real-time reverse transcription polymerase chain reaction

At present, real-time RT-PCR is commonly used by clinical laboratories to detect NoV using a variety of primers, probes, and amplification conditions (**Table 1**). Real-time RT-PCR detects NoV RNA in a real-time manner (at each PCR cycle) using either nonspecific intercalating dyes or fluorescent dyes bound to target-specific probes. Advantages of this technology include preoptimized universal reagents and conditions for amplification, simplified assay platforms and software for designing primers and probes, multiple detection chemistries, high-throughput capabilities, enhanced reproducibility, flexibility to develop multiplex assays for different NoV genogroups in a single reaction, low risk of contamination, increased sensitivity and specificity in comparison with cRT-PCR, and automation with software-driven operation.

The ORF1-ORF2 junction region is a conserved region of the NoV genome. This region is a common target for designing primers for real-time RT-PCR assays to achieve high analytical sensitivity as well as broad detection of many NoV genotypes.[54] With primers specific to individual genogroups (GI and GII), a multiplex real-time PCR was developed to detect and differentiate NoV by genogroups.[55] The multiplex assay increases testing efficiency by decreasing test time by 50% and reduces reagent costs significantly. A real-time RT-PCR assay with additional primers and probe targeting GIV NoV was also developed using the LightCycler instrument (Roche Diagnostics, GmbH, Germany).[56] The multiplex assay platforms are widely used in clinical laboratories worldwide, especially in North America.[57–61] There are a few commercial kits available, such as the NoV Type I and Type II kits (Generon, Castelnuovo Rangone, Italy) and the AnDiaTec NoV real-time RT-PCR kit (AnDiaTec GmbH & Co KG, Kornwestheim, Germany). However, these 2 commercial kits failed to detect the most common NoV GI strains in a validation study.[62] Another commercial assay, Xpert NoV kit (Cepheid, Sunnyvale, CA, USA), obtained clearance in Europe and is commercially available for NoV detection from April 2014 (www.cepheidinternational.com/). There is no information yet in terms of its clinical applicability and analytical precision.

### Isothermal amplification assays

Nucleic acid sequence–based amplification (NASBA) and loop-mediated isothermal amplification (LAMP) have been used to detect NoV from stool specimens. In contrast to thermal cycle–based amplification, these assays use a simple isotemperature for NA amplification. Similar to real-time RT-PCR, the assays have high sensitivity. In a study, specificity was reported as a critical concern using NASBA because of

**Table 1**
**Overview of real-time RT-PCR for the detection of norovirus**

| Genogroup | Primer/Probe | Sequence (5′ → 3′)[a] | Probe/Dye | Length (bp) | Type/Platform | Reference |
|---|---|---|---|---|---|---|
| GI | COG1-F | CGYTGGATGCGNTTYCATGA | TaqMan | 85 | Multiplex PCR ABI 7700/7000/7300/7500 | 54,55 |
|  | COG1-R | CTTAGACGCCATCATCATTYAC |  |  |  |  |
|  | Probe (a)-R | AGATYGCGATCYCCTGTCCA | VIC/TAMRA |  |  |  |
|  | Probe (b)-R | AGATCGCGGTCTCCTGTCCA | FAM/TAMRA |  |  |  |
| GII | COG2-F | CARGARBCNATGTTYAGRTGGATGAG | TaqMan | 98 |  |  |
|  | COG2-R | TCGACGCCATCTTCATTCACA |  |  |  |  |
|  | Probe-F | TGGGAGGGCGATCGCAATCT | FAM/TAMRA |  |  |  |
| GI | NV192-F | GCYATGTTCCGCTGGATGC | MGB | 98 | Multiplex PCR ABI 7700 | 57 |
|  | NV193-R | CGTCCTTAGACGCCATCATCA |  |  |  |  |
|  | Probe-F | TGGGAGGGCGATCGCAATCTGGC | VIC/NFQ |  |  |  |
| GII | NV107(a)-F | AGCCAATGTTCAGATGGATG | TaqMan | 94 |  |  |
|  | NV107(b)-F | AICCIATGTTYAGITGGATG |  |  |  |  |
|  | NV119-R | TCGACGCCATCTTCATTCAC |  |  |  |  |
|  | Probe-F | TGGGAGGGCGATCGCAATCTGGC | FAM/NFQ |  |  |  |
| GI | JJV1-F | GCCATGTTCCGITGGATG | TaqMan | 96 | Multiplex PCR Bio-Rad iCycler, Cepheid SmartCycler and ABI 5700 | 58 |
|  | JJV1-R | TCCTTAGACGCCATCATCAT |  |  |  |  |
|  | Probe-F | TGTGGACAGGAGATCGCA ATCTC | FAM/BHQ |  |  |  |
| GII | JJV2-F | CAAGAGTCA ATGTTAGGTGGATGAG | TaqMan | 98 |  |  |
|  | COG2-R | TCGACGCCATCTTCATTCACA |  |  |  |  |
|  | Probe-F | TGGGAGGGCGATCGCAATCT | JOE/BHQ |  |  |  |
| GI | COG1-F | CGYTGGATGCGNTTYCATGA | TaqMan | 85 | Monoplex PCR for GI, GII, and GIV Roche LightCycler | 56 |
|  | COG1-R | CTTAGACGCCATCATCATTYAC |  |  |  |  |
|  | Probe (a)-R | AGATYGCGATCYCCTGTCCA | FAM/BHQ |  |  |  |
|  | Probe (b)-R | AGATCGCGGTCTCCTGTCCA | FAM/BHQ |  |  |  |
| GII | COG2-F | CARGARBCNATGTTYAGRTGGATGAG | TaqMan | 98 |  |  |
|  | COG2-R | TCGACGCCATCTTCATTCACA |  |  |  |  |
|  | Probe-F | TGGGAGGGCGATCGCAATCT | FAM/BHQ |  |  |  |
| GIV | Mon 4-F | TTTGAGTCYATGTACAAGTGGATGC |  | 98 |  |  |
|  | Mon 4-R | TCGACGCCATCTTCATTCACA |  |  |  |  |
|  | Probe-F | TGGGAGGGGGATCGCGATCT | FAM/BHQ |  |  |  |

| Target | Primer/Probe | Sequence | Reporter | Position | Method | Ref |
|---|---|---|---|---|---|---|
| GI | COG1-F | CGYTGGATGCGNTTYCATGA | MGB | 87 | Monoplex PCR for GI; Multiplex PCR for GII and GIV; ABI 7000 | 59 |
|  | GI-R | TCCTTAGACGCCATCATCATTYAC |  |  |  |  |
|  | Probe (a)-R | AGATYGCGATCYCCTGTCCA | VIC/NFQ |  |  |  |
|  | Probe (b)-R | AGATCGCGGTCTCCTGTCCA | VIC/NFQ |  |  |  |
| GII | GII-F | CARGARBCNATGTTYAGRTGGATGAG | MGB | 97 |  |  |
|  | Probe-R | ATTGCGATGCCCTC | FAM/NFQ |  |  |  |
| GIV | GIV-F | CCAAAGTTTGAGTCYATGTACAAGTG | MGB | 103 |  |  |
|  | Probe-F | CGATCTCGCTCCCG | VIC/NFQ |  |  |  |
| GII/GIV[b] | GII/GIV-R | CGACGCCATCTTCATTCACA |  |  |  |  |
| GI | QNIF4-F | CGCTGGATGCGNTTCCAT | TaqMan | 86 | Multiplex PCR; Roche LightCycler 480 | 60 |
|  | NV1LC-R | CCTTAGACGCCATCATCATTTAC |  |  |  |  |
|  | Probe-F | TGGACAGGAGAYCGCRATCT | FAM/BHQ |  |  |  |
| GII | QNIF2-F | ATGTTCAGRTGGATGAGRTTCTCWGA | TaqMan | 89 |  |  |
|  | COG2-R | TCGACGCCATCTCATTCACA |  |  |  |  |
|  | Probe-F | AGCACGTGGGAGGGCGATCG | Texas Red/BHQ |  |  |  |
| GI | GI1-F | ATGTTCCGYTGGATGCGIT | TaqMan | Variable | Multiplex PCR; ABI 7900 | 61 |
|  | GI2-F | TTGGATGCGITTYCATGA |  |  |  |  |
|  | GI1-R | GGTCAGAAGCATTAACCTCCG |  |  |  |  |
|  | GI2-R | GGTCAGCTGTATTAACCTCCG |  |  |  |  |
|  | GI3-R | AGCTGRCCGGCACCACT |  |  |  |  |
|  | GI4-R | CACTRGTGCCATCCATGTTT |  |  |  |  |
|  | Probe-R | GCGTCCTTAGACGCCATCTTCATTTAC | VIC? |  |  |  |
| GII | GII-F | BCIATGTTYAGRTGGATGAG | TaqMan | 91 |  |  |
|  | GII-R | CGACGCCATCTTCATTCAC |  |  |  |  |
|  | Probe-R | AGATTGCGATGCCCTCCCA | FAM? |  |  |  |

*Abbreviations:* BHQ, Black Hole quencher; F, forward (virus sense); FAM, 6-carboxyfluorescein reporter; MGB, minor groove binder; NFQ, nonfluorescent quencher; R, reverse (anti–virus sense); TAMRA, 6-carboxy-tetramethylrhodamine quencher; VIC, proprietary fluorescent reporter.
a Mixed bases in degenerate primers and probes are indicated as follows: Y, C, or T; R, A, or G; I, inosin; B, not A; N, any.
b GII and GIV sharing same reverse primer.
*Data from* Refs.[54–61]

decreased stringency when amplifying NoV RNA at low temperatures (~40°C).[63] The LAMP technology has the added advantages of speed and simplicity, with the reaction being performed in a single tube and requiring no more than 1 hour to complete.[64] Reactions normally show high tolerance to biological products so that extensive NA preparation is not needed. LAMP does not require sophisticated equipment, and a simple heat block or water bath can be used because amplification occurs at low and constant temperature, ranging from 60°C to 65°C. When there is a positive reaction using LAMP, magnesium pyrophosphate precipitates out of the solution causing turbidity, which can easily be detected using a turbidity meter. A fluorescent indicator can also be added to enhance the readability. The simplicity of the LAMP platform makes it a superior choice for laboratories with limited resources and experience in performing NAT. Laboratory-developed LAMP assays have been used to detect NoV GI and GII and have demonstrated compatible results with real-time RT-PCR.[65–67] A commercial LAMP kit for the detection of NoV GI and GII was developed by Eiken Chemical Co (Tokyo, Japan), showing assay sensitivity that was as good as laboratory-developed LAMP assay.[66] However, LAMP is still not broadly used because of specific requirements for primer design. In the near future, LAMP might provide an alternate method for fast and reliable detection of NoV in diagnostic laboratories.

### Nanotechnology for norovirus detection

Nanotechnology has been developed to create commercial medical devices. Advances in microelectronics, microfluidics, and microfabrication have paved the way for novel and miniature technologies to reach an ultimate goal of creating simple, affordable, and point-of-care molecular diagnostic device. Nanotechnology is being used to develop sample-in/answer-out testing for laboratories regardless of size, resources, or capacity, with the use of the smallest quantities of reagents and samples. It also supports multiplex diagnostic testing for comprehensive syndrome-specific assessment of various diseases.

The liquid array–based technology has been used to develop the first commercial multiplex, syndrome-specific molecular testing assay for the detection of enteric pathogens, the xTAG gastrointestinal pathogen panel (GPP). The xTAG GPP was developed by Luminex (Austin, TX, USA) and approved by the US Food and Drug Administration. This advanced platform provides simultaneous detection of 11 pathogens associated with gastroenteritis, including 7 enteric bacteria, 2 parasites, and 2 viruses (rotavirus and NoV GI/GII).[49,68] The in vitro diagnostic product licensed in Canada and Europe includes the detection of adenovirus types 40/41 and 2 additional bacteria and 1 parasitic pathogen. The platform couples PCR with suspension microarray to screen for multiple enteric pathogens in a simple run. A preliminary assessment has been reported to have better sensitivity than the rapid immunochromatographic test for NoV detection and comparable performance as laboratory-developed molecular methods.[69,70]

Another multiplex assay, the FilmArray Gastrointestinal Panel, is under development by BioFire Diagnostics (Salt Lake City, UT, USA). This assay platform is designed to provide rapid sample-in/answer-out testing by simultaneous detection of 23 gastrointestinal pathogens in stool samples, including NoV GI, GII, and 4 common gastroenteritis viruses (rotavirus, EAdV types 40/41, human astrovirus serotypes 1–8, and sapovirus serotypes I, II, IV, and V). The FilmArray platform is a fully closed and automated system for sample preparation, multiplex nested PCR, and result analysis using integrated electropneumatics and chemical circuits in a reaction pouch with an approximate turnaround time of 1 hour and total hands-on time of 2 to 5 minutes.

The xTAG GPP and FilmArray Gastrointestinal Panel A showed comparable results in the detection of multiple gastroenteritis pathogens in a comparison study by Khare and colleagues.[71] This fully automated system shows great potential for use as point-of-care test to identify enteric pathogens associated with sporadic gastroenteritis and outbreaks while saving significant time in terms of clinical intervention and disease control. Similar devices being developed include Verigene Enteric Pathogens Nucleic Acid Test (Nanosphere, Northbrook, IL, USA). A summary of those commercial robotic assay platforms is showed in **Table 2**.

### Genetic Typing of Norovirus

Genetic typing provides essential information to further the understanding of NoV genetic evolution, classification, and molecular epidemiology. Information on genetic traits of NoV causing regional gastroenteritis outbreaks in a spatiotemporal manner can be exchanged nationally and internationally to map the trend of NoV strains causing endemic, epidemic, or pandemic events. Genetic information of NoV is also critical for the development of preventive strategies against NoV infections such as vaccines.

NoV genotyping is largely performed in research and public health laboratories because genotyping usually has no direct impact on clinical decision making and patient management except in special outbreak investigations or clinical settings. Human NoV is classified into genogroups, subgenogroups, genotypes, and variants based on genotyping. With the highly diversified genome of NoV, genotyping requires further testing, that is, sequencing, of postamplified RT-PCR products. Primers targeting the highly conserved RNA-dependent RNA polymerase genes have traditionally been used to perform RT-PCR–based NoV genotyping. In recent years, primers targeting NoV viral capsid proteins are preferred for genotyping because viral capsid is directly involved in host-receptor interaction and immune response and contain relevant genetic variations. Hasing and colleagues[72] reported that the primers in ORF1/2 junction region worked better for identifying NoV antigenic drift than recombination events. Sequence alignment followed by phylogenetic analysis is being used to classify NoV. More than 40 genotypes associated with NoV gastroenteritis have been categorized into the 2 major NoV genogroups (GI and GII).

More recently, Next-Generation Sequencing (NGS), a fundamentally different approach to genetic sequencing, has triggered numerous groundbreaking discoveries and ignited a revolution in genomic science. The principle of NGS is similar to that of capillary electrophoresis (CE)-based Sanger sequencing—the bases of a small DNA fragment are sequentially identified from signals emitted as each fragment is resynthesized from a DNA template strand. NGS extends this process across millions of reactions in a massively parallel manner. This technological advancement enables rapid sequencing of large stretches of DNA spanning entire genomes, with the latest instruments capable of producing hundreds of gigabases of data in a single sequencing run.[73,74] NGS has good features including high throughput, powerful scalability, tunable resolution, ever-fast speed, and unlimited dynamic range and sensitivity. Because NoV has a small viral genome and is noncultivable, characterization using direct genetic sequencing can become a new approach to study NoV. The latest NGS amplicon library preparation kits allow researchers to perform rapid amplification of custom-targeted regions from NoV genome. Using this approach, thousands of amplicons spanning multiple samples can be simultaneously prepared and indexed. With the ability to process numerous amplicons and samples on a single run, NGS enables researchers to simultaneously analyze all genomic content of interest in a single experiment in a cost-effective manner.[75] With sufficient depth of coverage, NGS

**Table 2**
Overview of commercial molecular assays for the detection of norovirus

| Assay | License/Approval Information | Principle of the Test | Instrument | Vendor | Reference with Validation/Evaluation Data |
|---|---|---|---|---|---|
| AndiaTee Norovirus real RT-PCR kit | CE mark-IVD | Real-time RT-PCR TaqMan | ABI system and a comparable instrument (eg, Roche 480, Stratagene, Qiagen/Corbett) | AndiaTee GmbH Komvesthein, Germany | 62 |
| RealStar Norovirus RT-PCR kit | CE mark-IVD | Real-time RT-PCR TaqMan | m2000rt, Mx 3005P VERSANT kPCR ABI 7500/7500 Fast LightCycler 480 Rotor-Gene 3000/6000, Rotor-Gene Q 5/6 plex | Altona Diagnostics GmbH Hamburg, Germany | www.altona-diagnostics.com |
| Xpert Norovirus kit | CE mark-IVD | Real-time RT-PCR | Xpert system | Cepheid, CA, USA | www.cepheid.com |
| Luminex xTAG GPP | FDA cleared/Health Canada approved; IVD | Multiplex RT-PCR and liquid array | Luminex system | Luminex, TX, USA | 68–70 |
| FilmArray GI panel | FDA cleared; IVD | Nested RT-PCR and film array | FilmArray platform | BioFire Diagnostics, UT, USA | 70 |
| Verigene Enteric Pathogens Nucleic Acid Test (EP) | FDA cleared; IVD | Multiplex RT-PCR and array hybridization | Verigene platform | Nanosphere, Inc, IL, USA | http://www.nanosphere.us |

Abbreviations: FDA, US Food and Drug Administration; IVD, in vitro diagnostic use.
Data from Refs. 62,68–70

sequencing can identify common and rare sequence variations of NoV in clinical samples. This application is particularly useful for tracking genetic evolution of NoV and the discovery of emerging variants, which may potentially cause pandemic outbreaks of NoV gastroenteritis. NGS is increasingly used by research laboratories and anticipated to be included into clinical diagnostic laboratory work flows with further development of standard reagents and kits in the near future.[76–79]

## SUMMARY

With the advantages and disadvantages of each method, none of the current assays used to detect NoV is prefect. Each laboratory needs to select an adequate detection platform that meets its needs and objectives (diagnostic vs research), laboratory setting (reference vs regional diagnostic laboratories), test volume and throughput, instrument availability, and technical expertise. Immunoassays for NoV can be used as preliminary tests for suspected NoV gastroenteritis outbreaks but are not recommended for routine diagnostic use because of their low sensitivity. Real-time RT-PCR is considered to be a superb method for NoV detection in stool, food, and environmental samples. However, genetically diverse NoV with 3 major genogroups can still result in false-negative test results, especially when a single pair of specific primers is being used. Multiple primer sets targeting different fragments of the NoV genome or degenerated primers based on sequence variations of known NoV references are being used to improve the sensitivity and accuracy of NoV detection. Some other technologies, such as LAMP, nanotechnology array-based multiplex panel, and NGS, have been developed and used to detect NoV, mostly in research settings. It is anticipated that these new technologies will be used in the routine diagnosis of NoV infections in clinical laboratories in the future.

## SELF-ASSESSMENT

1. What is the preferred method for detecting NoV in clinical samples?
   a. Viral culture
   b. Electron microscopy
   c. Real-time RT-PCR
   d. Antigen detection, for example, EIA

2. What is a characteristic of NoV that makes it difficult to develop diagnostics assay?
   a. NoV is shed at high amounts in stool sample.
   b. NoV is stable in the environment.
   c. NoV has highly diversified genome and viral antigens.
   d. There is variation in host susceptibility to NoV based on HBGA genotype.

3. What are the factors that laboratories need to consider when they are choosing a test for NoV?
   a. Test performance: sensitivity, specificity, and precision
   b. Test volume and throughput
   c. Availability of testing instruments or platforms
   d. All of the above

## ANSWERS

Answer 1: C.

Real-time RT-PCR is the most sensitive and specific test for NoV.

Answer 2: C.

The diverse genome and viral antigens make detection by molecular methods and immunologic methods challenging.

Answer 3: D.

Each of these factors must be considered in the selection of the most appropriate test for each laboratory.

## REFERENCES

1. Siebenga JJ, Vennema H, Zheng DP, et al. Norovirus illness is a global problem: emergence and spread of norovirus GII.4 variants, 2001–2007. J Infect Dis 2009; 200:802–12.
2. Ahmed SM, Hall AJ, Robinson AE, et al. Global prevalence of norovirus in cases of gastroenteritis: a systematic review and meta-analysis. Lancet Infect Dis 2014; 14:725–30.
3. Patel MM, Widdowson MA, Glass RI, et al. Systematic literature review of role of noroviruses in sporadic gastroenteritis. Emerg Infect Dis 2008;4:1224–31.
4. Payne DC, Vinjé J, Szilagyi PG, et al. Norovirus and medically attended gastro-enteritis in U.S. children. N Engl J Med 2013;368:1121–30.
5. Bucardo F, Reyes Y, Svensson L, et al. Predominance of norovirus and sapovirus in Nicaragua after implementation of universal rotavirus vaccination. PLoS One 2014;9:e98201.
6. Kapikian AZ, Wyatt RG, Dolin R, et al. Visualization by immune electron micro-scopy of a 27-nm particle associated with acute infectious nonbacterial gastroen-teritis. J Virol 1972;10:1075–81.
7. Tan M, Jiang X. Norovirus P particle: a subviral nanoparticle for vaccine develop-ment against norovirus, rotavirus and influenza virus. Nanomedicine 2012;7: 889–97.
8. Debbink K, Costantini V, Swanstrom J, et al. Human norovirus detection and pro-duction, quantification, and storage of virus-like particles. Curr Protoc Microbiol 2013;31:15.
9. Green YK. Caliciviridae: the noroviruses. In: Knipe DM, Howley PM, Griffin DE, et al, editors. Fields virology. 5th edition. Philadelphia: Lippincott Williams & Wilkins; 2007. p. 949–79.
10. Jiang X, Wang M, Wang K, et al. Sequence and genomic organization of Norwalk virus. Virology 1993;195:51–61.
11. Zheng DP, Ando T, Fankhauser RL, et al. Norovirus classification and proposed strain nomenclature. Virology 2006;346:312–23.
12. Menon VK, George S, Shanti AA, et al. Exposure to human and bovine norovi-ruses in a birth cohort in southern India from 2002 to 2006. J Clin Microbiol 2013;51:2391–5.
13. Bruggink LD, Oluwatoyin O, Sameer R, et al. Molecular and epidemiological fea-tures of gastroenteritis outbreaks involving genogroup I norovirus in Victoria, Australia, 2002-2010. J Med Virol 2012;84:1437–48.
14. Hoa Tran TN, Trainor E, Nakagomi T, et al. Molecular epidemiology of noroviruses associated with acute sporadic gastroenteritis in children: global distribution of genogroups, genotypes and GII.4 variants. J Clin Virol 2013;56:185–93.
15. Vinjé J. Advances in laboratory methods for detection and typing of norovirus. J Clin Microbiol 2015;53:373–81.

16. Bull RA, Eden JS, Rawlinson WD, et al. Rapid evolution of pandemic noroviruses of the GII.4 lineage. PLoS Pathog 2010;6:e1000831.
17. Lee BE, Preiksaitis JK, Chui N, et al. Genetic relatedness of noroviruses identified in sporadic gastroenteritis in children and gastroenteritis outbreaks in northern Alberta. J Med Virol 2008;80:330–7.
18. Glass RI, Parashar UD, Estes MK. Norovirus gastroenteritis. N Engl J Med 2009; 361:1776–85.
19. Huang P, Farkas T, Zhong W, et al. Norovirus and histo-blood group antigens: demonstration of a wide spectrum of strain specificities and classification of two major binding groups among multiple binding patterns. J Virol 2005;79:6714–22.
20. Krones E, Högenauer C. Diarrhea in the immunocompromised patient. Gastroenterol Clin North Am 2012;41:677–701.
21. Bok K, Green KY. Norovirus gastroenteritis in immunocompromised patients. N Engl J Med 2012;367:2126–32.
22. Long SS. Evidence of norovirus causing necrotizing enterocolitis (NEC) in a NICU. J Pediatr 2008;153:A2.
23. Turcios-Ruiz RM, Axelrod P, St. John K, et al. Outbreak of necrotizing enterocolitis caused by norovirus in a neonatal intensive care unit. J Pediatr 2008;153:339–44.
24. Atmar RL, Bernstein DI, Harro CD, et al. Norovirus vaccine against experimental human Norwalk virus illness. N Engl J Med 2011;365:2178–87.
25. Atmar RL, Opekun AR, Gilger MA, et al. Determination of the 50% human infectious dose for Norwalk virus. J Infect Dis 2014;209:1016–22.
26. Arvelo W, Hall AJ, Estevez A, et al. Diagnostic performance of rectal swab versus bulk stool specimens for the detection of rotavirus and norovirus: implications for outbreak investigations. J Clin Virol 2013;58:678–82.
27. Sidler JA, Käch R, Noppen C, et al. Rectal swab for detection of norovirus by real-time PCR: similar sensitivity compared to faecal specimens. Clin Microbiol Infect 2014;20:O1017–9.
28. Ito S, Takeshita S, Nezu A, et al. Norovirus-associated encephalopathy. Pediatr Infect Dis J 2006;25:651–2.
29. Takanashi S, Hashira S, Matsunaga T, et al. Detection, genetic characterization, and quantification of norovirus RNA from sera of children with gastroenteritis. J Clin Virol 2009;44:161–3.
30. Fumian TM, Justino MC, D'Arc Pereira Mascarenhas J, et al. Quantitative and molecular analysis of noroviruses RNA in blood from children hospitalized for acute gastroenteritis in Belém, Brazil. J Clin Virol 2013;58:31–5.
31. Medici MC, Abelli LA, Dodi I, et al. Norovirus RNA in the blood of a child with gastroenteritis and convulsions – a case report. J Clin Virol 2010;48:147–9.
32. Duizer E, Pielaat A, Vennema H, et al. Probabilities in norovirus outbreak diagnosis. J Clin Virol 2007;40:38–42.
33. Pang XL, Preiksaitis JK, Wong S, et al. Influence of novel norovirus GII.4 variants on gastroenteritis outbreak dynamics in Alberta and the Northern Territories, Canada between 2000 and 2008. PLoS One 2010;5:e11599.
34. Pang XL, Preiksaitis JK, Lee BE. Enhanced enteric virus detection in sporadic gastroenteritis using a multi-target real-time PCR panel – a one-year study. J Med Virol 2014;86:1594–601.
35. Richards AF, Lopman B, Gunn A, et al. Evaluation of a commercial ELISA for detecting Norwalk-like virus antigen in faeces. J Clin Virol 2003;26:109–15.
36. Burton-MacLeod JA, Kane EM, Beard RS, et al. Evaluation and comparison of two commercial enzyme-linked immunosorbent assay kits for detection of antigenically diverse human noroviruses in stool samples. J Clin Microbiol 2004;42:2587–95.

37. Gray JJ, Kohli E, Ruggeri FM, et al. European multicenter evaluation of commercial enzyme immunoassays for detecting norovirus antigen in fecal samples. Clin Vaccine Immunol 2007;14:1349–55.
38. Takanashi S, Okame M, Shiota T, et al. Development of a rapid immunochromatographic test for noroviruses genogroups I and II. J Virol Methods 2008;148:1–8.
39. Khamrin P, Nguyen TA, Phan TG, et al. Evaluation of immunochromatography and commercial enzyme-linked immunosorbent assay for rapid detection of norovirus antigen in stool samples. J Virol Methods 2008;147:360–3.
40. Derrington P, Schreiber F, Day S, et al. Norovirus Ridaquick: a new test for rapid diagnosis of norovirus. Pathology 2009;41:687–8.
41. Bruins MJ, Wolfhagen MJ, Schirm J, et al. Evaluation of a rapid immunochromatographic test for the detection of norovirus in stool samples. Eur J Clin Microbiol Infect Dis 2010;29:741–3.
42. Kirby A, Gurgel RQ, Dove W, et al. An evaluation of the RIDASCREEN and IDEIA enzyme immunoassays and the RIDAQUICK immunochromatographic test for the detection of norovirus in faecal specimens. J Clin Virol 2010;49:254–7.
43. Bruggink LD, Witlox KJ, Sameer R, et al. Evaluation of the RIDA®QUICK immunochromatographic norovirus detection assay using specimens from Australian gastroenteritis incidents. J Virol Methods 2011;173:121–6.
44. Geginat G, Kaiser D, Schrempf S. Evaluation of third-generation ELISA and a rapid immunochromatographic assay for the detection of norovirus infection in fecal samples from inpatients of a German tertiary care hospital. Eur J Clin Microbiol Infect Dis 2012;31:733–7.
45. Thongprachum A, Khamrin P, Tran DN, et al. Evaluation and comparison of the efficiency of immunochromatography methods for norovirus detection. Clin Lab 2012;58:489–93.
46. Sakamaki N, Ohiro Y, Ito M, et al. Bioluminescent enzyme immunoassay for the detection of norovirus capsid antigen. Clin Vaccine Immunol 2012;19:1949–54.
47. Ambert-Balay K, Pothier P. Evaluation of 4 immunochromatographic tests for rapid detection of norovirus in faecal samples. J Clin Virol 2013;56:194–8.
48. Shigemoto N, Tanizawa Y, Matsuo T, et al. Clinical evaluation of a bioluminescent enzyme immunoassay for detecting norovirus in fecal specimens from patients with acute gastroenteritis. J Med Virol 2014;86:1219–25.
49. Dunbar SA, Zhang H, Tang YW. Advanced techniques for detection and identification of microbial agents of gastroenteritis. Clin Lab Med 2013;33:527–52.
50. Rasool NB, Monroe SS, Glass RI. Determination of a universal nucleic acid extraction procedure for PCR detection of gastroenteritis viruses in faecal specimens. J Virol Methods 2002;100:1–16.
51. Al-Soud WA, Radstrom P. Purification and characterization of PCR-inhibitory components in blood cells. J Clin Microbiol 2001;39:485–93.
52. Jiang X, Wang J, Graham DY, et al. Detection of Norwalk virus in stool by polymerase chain reaction. J Clin Microbiol 1992;30:2529–34.
53. Mattison K, Grudeski E, Auk B, et al. Multicenter comparison of two norovirus ORF2-based genotyping protocols. J Clin Microbiol 2009;47:3927–32.
54. Kageyama T, Kojima S, Shinohara M, et al. Broadly reactive and highly sensitive assay for norwalk-like viruses based on real-time quantitative reverse transcription-PCR. J Clin Microbiol 2003;41:1548–57.
55. Pang XL, Preiksaitis JK, Lee B. Multiplex real time RT-PCR for the detection and quantitation of norovirus genogroups I and II in patients with acute gastroenteritis. J Clin Virol 2005;33:168–71.

56. Trujillo AA, McCaustland KA, Zheng DP, et al. Use of TaqMan real-time reverse transcription-PCR for rapid detection, quantification, and typing of norovirus. J Clin Microbiol 2006;44:1405–12.

57. Hoehne M, Schreier E. Detection of Norovirus genogroup I and II by multiplex real-time RT-PCR using a 3'-minor groove binder-DNA probe. BMC Infect Dis 2006. http://dx.doi.org/10.1186/1471-2334-6-69.

58. Jothikumar N, Lowther JA, Henshilwood K, et al. Rapid and sensitive detection of noroviruses by using TaqMan-based one-step reverse transcription-PCR assays and application to naturally contaminated shellfish samples. Appl Environ Microbiol 2005;71:1870–5.

59. Logan CL, O'Leary JJ, O'Sullivan N. Real-time reverse transcription PCR detection of norovirus, sapovirus and astrovirus as causative agents of acute viral gastroenteritis. J Virol Methods 2007;146:36–44.

60. Stals A, Baert L, Botteldoorn N, et al. Multiplex real-time RT-PCR for simultaneous detection of GI/GII noroviruses and murine norovirus 1. J Virol Methods 2009;161: 247–53.

61. Neesanant P, Sirinarumitr T, Chantakru S, et al. Optimization of one-step real-time reverse transcription-polymerase chain reaction assays for norovirus detection and molecular epidemiology of noroviruses in Thailand. J Virol Methods 2013;194:317–25.

62. Butot S, Le Guyader FS, Krol J, et al. Evaluation of various real-time RT-PCR assays for the detection and quantitation of human norovirus. J Virol Methods 2010; 167:90–4.

63. Moore C, Clark EM, Gallimore CI, et al. Evaluation of a broadly reactive nucleic acid sequence based amplification assay for the detection of noroviruses in faecal material. J Clin Virol 2004;29:290–6.

64. Notomi T, Okayama H, Masubuchi H, et al. Loop-mediated isothermal amplification of DNA. Nucleic Acids Res 2000;28:E63.

65. Iturriza-Gómara M, Xerry J, Gallimore CI, et al. Evaluation of the Loopamp (loop-mediated isothermal amplification) kit for detecting norovirus RNA in faecal samples. J Clin Virol 2008;42:389–93.

66. Yoda T, Suzuki Y, Yamazaki Y, et al. Application of a modified loop-mediated isothermal amplification kit for detecting norovirus genogroups I and II. J Med Virol 2009;81:2072–8.

67. Suzuki Y, Narimatsu S, Furukawa T, et al. Comparison of real-time reverse-transcription loop-mediated isothermal amplification and real-time reverse-transcription polymerase chain reaction for detection of noroviruses in municipal wastewater. J Biosci Bioeng 2011;112:369–72.

68. Navidad JF, Griswold DJ, Gradus MS, et al. Evaluation of Luminex xTAG gastrointestinal pathogen analyte-specific reagents for high-throughput, simultaneous detection of bacteria, viruses, and parasites of clinical and public health importance. J Clin Microbiol 2013;51:3018–24.

69. Mengelle C, Mansuy JM, Prere MF, et al. Simultaneous detection of gastrointestinal pathogens with a multiplex Luminex-based molecular assay in stool samples from diarrhoeic patients. Clin Microbiol Infect 2013;19:E458–65.

70. Claas E, Burnham CA, Mazulli T, et al. Performance of the xTAG® Gastrointestinal Pathogen Panel (GPP), a multiplex molecular assay for simultaneous detection of bacterial, viral and parasitic causes of infectious gastroenteritis. J Microbiol Biotechnol 2013;23:1041–5.

71. Khare R, Espy MJ, Cebelinski E, et al. Comparative evaluation of two commercial multiplex panels for detection of gastrointestinal pathogens by use of clinical stool specimens. J Clin Microbiol 2014;52:3667–73.

72. Hasing ME, Hazes B, Lee BE, et al. Detection and analysis of recombination in GII.4 norovirus strains causing gastroenteritis outbreaks in Alberta. Infect Genet Evol 2014;27:181–92.
73. Srivatsan A, Han Y, Peng J, et al. High-precision, whole-genome sequencing of laboratory strains facilitates genetic studies. PLoS Genet 2008;4:e1000139.
74. Rasmussen M, Li Y, Lindgreen S, et al. Ancient human genome sequence of an extinct Palaeo-Eskimo. Nature 2010;463:757–62.
75. Lo YM, Chiu RW. Next-generation sequencing of plasma/serum DNA: an emerging research and molecular diagnostic tool. Clin Chem 2009;55:607–8.
76. Wong TH, Dearlove BL, Hedge J, et al. Whole genome sequencing and de novo assembly identifies Sydney-like variant noroviruses and recombinants during the winter 2012/2013 outbreak in England. Virol J 2013;10:335.
77. Batty EM, Wong TH, Trebes A, et al. A modified RNA-Seq approach for whole genome sequencing of RNA viruses from faecal and blood samples. PLoS One 2013;8:e66129.
78. Kundu S, Lockwood J, Depledge DP, et al. Next-generation whole genome sequencing identifies the direction of norovirus transmission in linked patients. Clin Infect Dis 2013;57:407–14.
79. Cotten M, Petrova V, Phan MV, et al. Deep sequencing of norovirus genomes defines evolutionary patterns in an urban tropical setting. J Virol 2014;88: 11056–69.

# Rotavirus

Mathew D. Esona, PhD, Rashi Gautam, PhD*

## KEYWORDS

- Rotavirus • Acute gastroenteritis • Rotavirus vaccines • Rotarix® • RotaTeq®
- qRT-PCR • Multiplex assays • Next-generation sequencing

## KEY POINTS

- Rotavirus was discovered in 1973 and is the major cause of acute gastroenteritis (AGE) in children less than 5 years of age worldwide.
- Rotavirus infection causes watery diarrhea with vomiting and fever that can result in dehydration and death.
- Two live, attenuated oral vaccines, Rotarix® and RotaTeq®, are recommended by the World Health Organization for routine immunization of all infants.
- Rotavirus can be detected in stool samples by electron microscopy (EM) and serologic or molecular techniques, such as reverse transcription (RT)–polymerase chain reaction (PCR) and quantitative RT-PCR (qRT-PCR).
- Rotavirus can be simultaneously detected along with other enteric pathogens in stool samples by using multipathogen detection kits.
- Rotavirus strain characterization is performed by new sensitive, specific, and high-throughput molecular techniques, such as RT-PCR, followed by gel-based genotyping, qRT-PCR, Sanger sequencing, and next-generation sequencing (NGS).

## INTRODUCTION
### Historical Aspects of Rotavirus

Although infantile diarrhea or gastroenteritis of viral etiology has been a global problem since antiquity, the first human-associated rotavirus was discovered in 1973 and

Conflict of Interest Statement: The authors declare that they have no financial, professional, or personal conflicts of interest.
Disclaimer: The findings and conclusions in this report are those of the author(s) and do not necessarily represent the official position of the Centers for Disease Control and Prevention. Names of specific vendors, manufacturers, and products are included for public health and informational purposes; inclusion does not imply endorsement of the vendors, manufacturers, and products by the Centers for Disease Control and Prevention or the US Department of Health and Human Services.
Division of Viral Diseases, Gastroenteritis and Respiratory Viruses Laboratory Branch, Centers for Disease Control and Prevention, 1600 Clifton Road, Northeast, Mail Stop G04, Atlanta, GA 30333, USA
* Corresponding author.
E-mail address: ijs0@cdc.gov

reported by Bishop and coworkers in Australia.[1–4] The virus was visualized by EM in intestinal biopsy specimens and stools of children with acute gastroenteritis. Epidemiologic studies have indicated that rotaviruses are important agents of severe infantile diarrhea and are responsible for an estimated 35% to 50% of hospitalizations in young children and infants.[5] It is now known that infection with rotavirus is universal, with almost all children infected by 5 years of age.[6,7] Rotavirus is responsible for 20 to 60 deaths per year in the United States and an estimated 453,000 deaths from diarrhea worldwide.[8] To date, rotaviruses have been isolated from humans and many species of nonhuman mammals and birds.[5,6,9]

## Morphology and Structure of Rotavirus

### Morphology

Rotaviruses take their name from the Latin word *rota*, which means wheel. Intact rotavirus particles have a distinctive appearance of a well-defined rim, with short spikes radiating from a wide hub when observed by negative-stain EM. The intact virus is composed of a 3-capsid structure: an inner core, an intermediate capsid, and an outer capsid with short radiating spikes. Rotaviruses possess a double-stranded RNA (dsRNA), which is enclosed in the core structure. Three types of rotavirus particles are recognized under the EM (**Fig. 1**); these are (1) the complete infectious or triple-layered particles, (2) the double-layered particles, and (3) the core or single-layered particles.[6]

### Structure

Rotaviruses are nonenveloped dsRNA viruses with a segmented genome.[6,10,11] Each of the 11 gene segments codes for a single protein except for segment 11, which codes for 2 different nonstructural proteins (NSP5 and NSP6) in some strains (**Table 1**). Six of the gene segments encode viral structural proteins (VP1 to VP4, VP6, and VP7), which are integrated into the virion, and 5 gene segments encode for nonstructural proteins (NSP1, NSP2, NSP3, NSP4, and NSP5/NSP6).[6,10] The infectious rotavirus particle is composed of 3 concentric shells that encase 11 gene

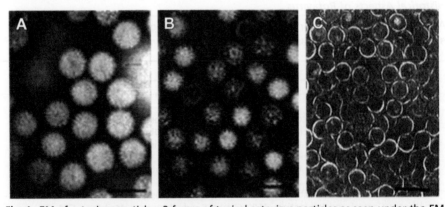

**Fig. 1.** EM of rotavirus particle—3 forms of typical rotavirus particles as seen under the EM after negative staining (*A–C*). (*A*) Complete infectious rotavirus particle, triple layered particle, double-shelled, 70-nm in diameter with wheel-shape appearance. (*B*) Double-layered particle, single-shelled, 55-nm in diameter with a circular bristled appearance. (*C*) Single-layered core particle, 37-nm in diameter and appears hexagonal under EM. (*From* Estes MK, Kapikian A. Rotaviruses. In: Knipe DM, Howley PM, eds. Fields virology, 5th edition. Philadelphia: Lippincott, Williams & Wilkins; 2007. p. 1924; with permission.)

**Table 1**
**Nucleotide percentage identity cutoff values defining genotypes for 11 rotavirus gene segments**

| Gene Product | Percentage Identity | Genotypes | Name of Genotypes |
|---|---|---|---|
| VP7 | 80 | 27G | Glycosylated |
| VP4 | 80 | 35P | Protease sensitive |
| VP6 | 85 | 16I | Inner capsid |
| VP1 | 83 | 9R | RNA-dependent RNA polymerase |
| VP2 | 84 | 9C | Core protein |
| VP3 | 81 | 8M | Methyltransferase |
| NSP1 | 79 | 16A | Interferon antagonist |
| NSP2 | 85 | 9N | NTPase |
| NSP3 | 85 | 12T | Translation enhancer |
| NSP4 | 85 | 14E | Enterotoxin |
| NSP5/NSP6[a] | 91 | 11H | Phosphoprotein |

[a] In some strains.

*Adapted from* Matthijnssens J, Ciarlet M, Rahman M, et al. Recommendations for the classification of group A rotaviruses using all 11 genomic RNA segments. Arch Virol 2008;153:1621–9; and Estes MK, Greenberg HB. Rotaviruses. In: Knipe DM, Howley PM, editors. Fields virology. Philadelphia: Kluwer/Lippincott, Williams and Wilkins; 2013. p. 1352.

segments and are referred to as triple-layered viruses. The virion consists of an inner VP2 protein layer surrounding the RNA segments and several molecules of VP1 and VP3 proteins,[12,13] a middle VP6 protein capsid, and an outer layer containing VP4 protein spikes embedded in a VP7 capsid. Both of the outer capsid proteins, VP7 and VP4, possess neutralization antigens and play important roles in virus entry and infection of target cells.[10] The majority of the outer capsid is formed of the VP7 proteins, which form the shell around the virion (**Fig. 2**).[14–16] The VP4 proteins form protease-activated spikes that project outward from the capsid for attachment. In the intestines, the presence of trypsin-like proteases cleave the VP4 protein into 2 polypeptides, VP8* and VP5*.[17,18] The VP8* forms the head of the VP4 spike, whereas the VP5* forms the stalk and base of the protein. Both proteins contain sequential neutralizing epitopes and surface-exposed neutralizing epitopes.[15,19–22]

### Rotavirus Classification and Nomenclature

Based on similarities between capsid structure, genome organization, and replication strategy, rotaviruses have been classified as a separate genus (*Rotavirus*) within the Reoviridae family.[6,10] Differences in the antigenic properties, gene sequences, and genome pattern serve as the basis for further classification within the genus; serogroups (groups), subgroups, serotypes and genotypes, and electropherotypes are distinguished.[6,10] The inner shell protein, VP6, is the group- and subgroup-specific antigen. There are at least 8 groups (designated A to H), 4 of which (groups A, B, C, and H) cause disease in humans. Among these 4, group A viruses (RVAs) are responsible for more than 90% of all infections in humans.[6,10] Within RVAs, 4 subgroups (SGs) are distinguished (SGI, SGII, SGI+II, and SG nonI-nonII) and are based on reactivity patterns with 2 subgroup-specific monoclonal antibodies (MAbs) directed to VP6.[23–26]

Serotype/genotype specificities are determined by the 2 outer capsid antigens, VP7 and VP4, and rotaviruses have been classified according to their VP7 and VP4 antigenic

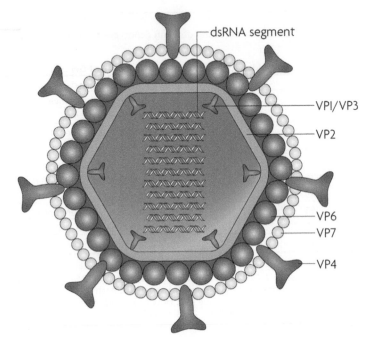

**Fig. 2.** A schematic diagram of rotavirus virion—the virion consists of an inner VP2 protein layer surrounding the RNA segments and several molecules of VP1 and VP3 proteins, a middle VP6 protein capsid, and an outer layer containing VP4 protein spikes embedded in a VP7 capsid. (*From* Angel J, Franco MA, Greenberg HB. Rotavirus vaccines: recent developments and future considerations. Nat Rev Microbiol 2007;5(7):531; with permission.)

properties into G and P types. The VP7 antigen determines the G (glycoprotein) serotypes/genotypes and the VP4 antigen determines the P (protease-sensitive) serotypes/genotypes. The use of the terms, serotype and genotype, depends on whether antigen-based detection methods (MAb-ELISA and cross-neutralization assay) or nucleic acid–based detection methods (nucleotide sequencing, RT-PCR, and oligonucleotide probe hybridization) are used.[6,10]

To date, RVAs of human and animals have been classified into at least 27 G and 37 P genotypes based on differences in their VP7 and VP4 gene sequences, respectively.[6,10,27,28] Currently, only 12 G and 15 P genotypes are known to infect humans.[6,10,29]

Rotaviruses can be classified into 2 major genome patterns (also called RNA profile or electropherotype [E-type]), which are designated as long or short profile, based on differences in the relative migration pattern of genome segments 10 and 11 in polyacrylamide gels. A large extent of pattern variability is seen, however, within the 2 major electropherotypes.[6,10]

Rotavirus classification methods have evolved primarily from antibody-based assays to genetic characterization and, recently, a new rotavirus classification scheme based on nucleotide sequence identity cutoff percentages for each of the 11 RVA genome segments was proposed by the Rotavirus Classification Working Group.[28] The new classification system assigns a genotype to each of the 11 rotavirus proteins as follows: Gx-P[x]-Ix-Rx-Cx-Mx-Ax-Nx-Tx-Ex-Hx for VP7-VP4-VP6-VP1-VP2-VP3-NSP1-NSP2-NSP3-NSP4-NSP5/6.[28] To date, at least 27 G, 37 P, 16 I, 9 R, 9 C,

8 M, 16 A, 9 N, 12 T, 15 E, and 11 H genotypes have been identified from humans and/or animals.[10]

## Replication

In the host, rotavirus replication is restricted to the gut, specifically in the cell cytoplasm of the host cell, and occurs within the viroplasms.[30] The triple-capsid protein coats make them resistant to the acidic environment of the stomach and the digestive enzymes in the gut. Once in the gut, rotavirus virions infect and enter enterocytes of the villi of the small intestine by a process known as endocytosis, leading to both functional and structural changes of the epithelium, and form a vesicle called an endosome.[31]

During rotavirus infection, mRNA for both protein biosynthesis and gene replication is produced. Packaging and replication of the rotavirus dsRNA genome takes place in cytoplasmic inclusion bodies (viroplasms) that are rich in viral RNA and protein.[32] Migration of the intermediates to the endoplasmic reticulum initiates a budding process that culminates in final virion assembly.[32]

## Pathogenesis

Rotavirus infection can result in either symptomatic or asymptomatic disease. Although rotavirus infection is mainly localized in the small intestine, extraintestinal (systemic) spread, although uncommon in immunocompetent persons, has been documented in many organs.[2,33] Rotavirus diarrhea pathogenesis depends on several host and viral factors, and both affect the outcome of the disease. The most evident host factor that affects the clinical outcome of the disease is age.[30] As a result of protection mediated primarily by transplacental transfer of maternal antibodies, children less than or equal to 3 months of age infected with rotavirus seldom have symptomatic disease,[34] except for immunocompromised children.[10] Reduction in the titer of maternal antibodies corresponds with the age of maximum exposure of children to rotavirus between the ages of 3 and 24 months.[30] Also, age at the time of inoculation has an impact on the severity of symptoms; for example, in newborns or interferon signaling–deficient mice, infection with rotavirus can result in biliary atresia.[10]

Irrespective of the host or viral factors associated with the disease, rotavirus diarrhea-inducing ability has been attributed to several different mechanisms, including malabsorption secondary to destruction of enterocytes or disruption of enterocyte absorptive functions, villus ischemia, enterotoxin activity and mobilization of intracellular fluid (calcium and chloride ion) secretion by NSP4, and activation of the enteric nervous and vascular systems that stimulate indirect secretion.[35–37]

## Epidemiology

### Occurrence, reservoir, and transmission of rotavirus
Rotaviruses are ubiquitous and infectious and occur throughout the world, with the reservoir being infected humans and nonhuman mammals. Although transmission of rotavirus of animal origin to humans is thought common, most strains do not lead to clinical illness.[10] Rotaviruses are generally transmitted by the fecal-oral route through direct or indirect spread, although contaminated food, water, and fomites are also involved in spread of the virus.[38–40]

Oral administration of rotavirus-positive stool material has been shown to induce diarrheal illness and viral shedding in adult volunteers.[10,41,42] Infected or symptomatic children start shedding rotaviruses in their stools before the onset of symptoms and may excrete more than $10^{10}$–$10^{11}$ rotavirus particles per gram of feces, with fewer than 100 particles required to infect new contacts.[43] Peak shedding typically occurs on day 3 of infection and declines after 7 days.[44] Approximately 5 days prior to onset of clinical symptoms, however, rotavirus can be detected in stools and shedding has been documented to persist in immunocompetent infants and children less than 5 years of age for several weeks.[45] The more severe the disease, the more prolonged is the period of shedding of rotavirus particles.[46]

### Seasonality of rotavirus infection

Rotavirus infections display a distinct seasonal pattern in temperate climates, with epidemic peaks occurring predominantly in the fall and winter months of the year. The seasonal nature of rotaviral infections is not universal and in countries with tropical climates, rotavirus disease seasonality is less defined, although sometimes an increase is noticed during the dry cold months of the year.[47–49] Rotavirus infection is predominantly seen among children 12 months old and older in temperate countries compared with younger children (≤6 months of age) in tropical countries.[47,50] The seasonality observed in temperate countries probably results from unfavorable conditions for transmission of rotavirus in the summer months, such as higher ambient temperatures, high relative humidity, and less crowding. The mechanism underlying this seasonal variation is unclear but involves a variety of factors, such as survival of virus in the environment, physiologic effects on the host, and level of crowding of susceptible children.[43]

### Clinical Manifestations

Rotavirus infections produce a range of responses in children that varies from subclinical infection to mild, watery diarrhea of limited duration to severe diarrhea with vomiting and fever that can result in dehydration with shock, electrolyte imbalance, and death.[10,43,51] Symptoms associated with rotavirus infection in both developed and developing settings are typically associated with a triad of vomiting, diarrhea, and fever.[52,53] Other clinical symptoms, such as irritability, lethargy, pharyngeal erythema, rhinitis, and palpable cervical lymph nodes, are also associated with the diarrhea.[54] The incubation period of rotavirus infections in young children is 24 to 78 hours after infection whereas in adults it is between 1 and 4 days.[43] On average, rotavirus infection lasts 3 to 7 days; however, more severe cases can last up to 14 days.[10,52] Rotavirus infection in infants and young children can lead to severe dehydration (10–20 bowel movements per day), electrolyte imbalance, and metabolic acidosis.[10] Rotavirus infection may last longer among children who are immunocompromised because of certain congenital immunodeficiency disorders.[10,53,55] Although rotavirus proteins and RNA have been detected in several organs, including body fluids such as blood and cerebrospinal fluid, the clinical significance of these findings is unknown.[56]

### Rotavirus Immunity

Rotavirus infections are ubiquitous and by the age of 5 most children have had more than 1 rotavirus infection. Children 3 months of age and younger, however, may not develop diarrhea symptoms when they are infected with rotavirus because they have transplacental maternal antibodies to protect them in the first few months of life.[34] Usually, the first infections are most severe and occur when circulating maternal rotavirus-specific immunoglobulin G is waning, typically at 3 to 12 months of age. Recovery from a first rotavirus infection usually does not lead to permanent immunity. Children from less developed countries have a higher risk of early rotavirus infection compared with those in developed countries.[57] After several rotavirus infections, children develop natural antibodies that protect them from symptoms of diarrhea when they are reinfected. Subsequent or recurrent rotavirus infections affect people of all ages and confer progressively more protection against severe disease.[53]

## Treatment, Control, and Prevention and Strain Distribution

### Treatment

Rotavirus cannot be treated with antibiotics or other drugs. The primary aim of the treatment is to replace fluids and electrolytes lost by vomiting and diarrhea. Mild rotavirus infections can be treated effectively in the same manner as other forms of diarrhea, by providing fluids and salts until the disease runs its course. Children with severe rotavirus diarrhea, however, urgently need intravenous fluids or they risk dying from dehydration.[6,10,58] In low-income countries, this type of urgent health care is often inaccessible or unreachable, making rotavirus prevention through vaccination critical.[59]

### Control and prevention

Rotaviruses are infectious and relatively resistant to inactivation by chemical disinfectants and antiseptics. The control and prevention of rotavirus infections are difficult because the virus is stable on environmental surfaces and is shed in high concentrations in the stool of infected patients.[43] Rotavirus particles are easily transmitted in hospital settings and day care facilities to susceptible hosts. Infection control measures, such as isolation of infected children; hand cleaning using agents containing alcohol to be used after contact with infected children; improvements in water quality, hygiene, and sanitation; and disinfecting environmental surfaces with appropriate detergents,[60,61] are important to prevent the spread of rotavirus infection. Based on the burden of rotavirus disease in many countries, rotavirus vaccination is considered the most cost-effective public health intervention in both developed and developing countries to reduce mortality and morbidity associated with rotavirus disease. The major goal of rotavirus vaccines is to prevent severe rotavirus gastroenteritis during the first 2 to 3 years of life when rotavirus disease impact is greatest.[43,62] Introducing rotavirus vaccines with other diarrhea prevention and treatment methods, such as oral rehydration therapy, zinc supplementation, exclusive breastfeeding, improved hygiene, water quality, sanitation, and nutrition, can significantly reduce child illnesses and deaths.[63]

In 1998, a rhesus-based tetravalent rotavirus vaccine known as Rotashield (Wyeth Pharmaceuticals, Collegeville, PA, USA)[5] was recommended by the US Advisory Committee on Immunization Practices for routine vaccination of children in the United States. The vaccine was administered to children at ages 2, 4, and 6 months.[64] After 1 year of Rotashield introduction into the US market, the vaccine was withdrawn because of its association with an elevated risk for intussusception.[65] At the time of its withdrawal, Rotashield had not been introduced in any other national vaccination program worldwide.[53] Currently, 2 live oral vaccines, Rotarix® developed by GlaxoSmithKline Biologicals (Rixensart, Belgium) and RotaTeq® by Merck (Blue Bell, Pennsylvania), are licensed in more than 100 countries for inclusion into routine immunization programs in the United States and other countries in Latin America, Europe, Africa, and Asia. Rotarix®, licensed in the United States in 2008, is given in 2 doses at ages 2 months and 4 months, whereas RotaTeq® (RV5), licensed in the United States in 2006, is given in 3 doses at ages 2 months, 4 months, and 6 months. Since rotavirus vaccine implementation, substantial reductions in rotavirus-associated disease burden have been reported.[8,66–68] In addition, studies have reported an 85% to 98% efficacy rate against severe rotavirus infection and a 74% to 87% efficacy rate against rotavirus infection of any severity.[53] Although the efficacy of both vaccines is high in developed countries, it is typically lower in developing countries.[8,69–71] Due to high rotavirus-associated mortality in developing countries, disease prevention and management through vaccination are a public health priority.[72]

### Rotavirus strain distribution: pre- and postvaccine introduction eras

In the postvaccination era, there has been decline in the strain prevalence and changes in the geographic distribution of circulating rotavirus strains. Also, strains that are not included in the current vaccines are present in certain parts of the world.[29,73] Although there are extensive geographic and temporal differences in rotavirus strain distribution in the pre- and postvaccination eras, 6 RVA strains (G1P[8], G2P[4], G3P[8], G4P[8], G9P[8], and G12P[8]) account for an estimated 80% to 90 % of all rotavirus infections globally.[29,73–76] Additionally, uncommon rotavirus strains associated with genotypes of animal origin (G5, G6, G8, G10, P[9], P[11], and P[14]) have been reported in humans worldwide.[77–79]

Although there are no direct evidences of vaccine selection pressure on circulating rotavirus strains, an increase in prevalence of G2P[4] rotavirus strains postvaccine introduction has been reported in the Americas, parts of Europe, and Australia.[80,81] Any unusual increase in any of the common RVA strains postvaccine introduction should, however, be investigated.

## ROTAVIRUS DIAGNOSTIC TESTING

Rapid identification of viruses associated with diarrhea is essential to ensure administration of the appropriate patient management and to control AGE outbreaks. Several diagnostic techniques have been developed to detect rotavirus in stool samples. These techniques include EM,[82] virus isolation in cell culture,[83,84] polyacrylamide gel electrophoresis (PAGE) of viral RNA segments,[85] enzyme immunoassays (EIAs),[86] passive particle agglutination tests,[87] immunochromatographic tests,[88] coupled RT-PCR,[89–92] and qRT-PCR.[93–95] Several multipathogen detection assays are commercially available to simultaneously detect various enteropathogens (viruses including rotavirus, bacteria, and parasites) causing gastroenteritis.[96,97] Several serologic and molecular techniques have been developed for rotavirus genotyping and strain characterization, including rotavirus serotyping,[92] dot blot hybridization,[98,99] RT-PCR followed by gel-based genotyping, real-time RT-PCR (qRT-PCR),[100–102] Sanger sequencing,[103,104] full-genome sequencing,[28] and NGS.[105–109] Traditional microbiological culture- and immunologic-based assays are time consuming, are laborious, and often lack diagnostic specificity and sensitivity. Molecular techniques are more sensitive and specific and are rapidly replacing conventional assays to detect and genotype rotavirus strains.

### Rotavirus Detection Assays

#### Electron microscopy

Direct EM examination of feces after negative staining with phosphotungstic acid is a highly specific method to detect rotavirus particles due to its characteristic morphologic appearance of a triple-layered virus with spikes (see **Fig. 1**).[82] Briefly, fecal samples are suspended in phosphate buffer saline and centrifuged. The final pellet is resuspended in Tris buffer and then negatively stained with phosphotungstic acid on fomvar-coated grids. The grids are then examined under an EM at high magnification ($\times 40,000$).[110] The threshold for detection of RVA by EM is approximately $10^7$ viral particles/mL of stool. EM, however, requires an expensive instrument, is too labor intensive for routine detection of rotavirus in large number of stool samples, and requires highly trained professionals. Various methods with higher throughput than EM are now available for the detection of rotaviruses in stool specimens.

### Cell culture isolation

Cultivation of rotavirus from clinical fecal specimens is achieved through the use of several primary cell types and continuous cell lines. Rotaviruses can be isolated in African green monkey kidney cells and continuous cell lines, including Rhesus monkey kidney (MA104) cells.[83] The virions can be purified from RV-infected cell lysate using cesium chloride gradients. Purified virus is analyzed by sodium dodecyl sulfate –PAGE to verify rotavirus recovery. Plaque assay can be performed to determine the viral titer in plaque-forming units per milliliter of virus based on the cytopathic effect caused by rotavirus in cultured cells.[84] Alternatively, fluorescence focus assay could be used to quantify rotavirus because it is a more rapid approach than the plaque assay.[83] This assay detects viral antigen through the use of polyclonal antibodies generated against intact virions that cross-react with several rotavirus strains and provide a strong fluorescence signal. The limit of rotavirus detection by this technique is $5 \times 10^2$ infectious units per mL of sample. Isolation and cultivation of human rotaviruses from clinical fecal specimens is difficult and adaptation to grow rotavirus in vitro typically requires multiple rounds of passage in primary cells. The efficiency of virus recovery from stool samples using cell culture is considerably lower. Diagnosis of rotavirus in stool samples using cell culture method is not performed routinely because it is time consuming, labor intensive, and prone to contamination.

### Polyacrylamide gel electrophoresis

Rotavirus nucleic acid segments can be visualized directly after extraction from virus particles by PAGE followed by silver staining.[85] After electrophoresis, human rotavirus groups A, B, and C have distinct patterns of gene-segment distribution according to size, designated as electropherotypes (**Fig. 3**). PAGE assay can simultaneously detect rotavirus in stool samples and provide information about the viral electropherotype. Human and animal RVAs possess 2 kinds of electropherotypes, long and short (see **Fig. 3**). A short electrophoretic pattern exhibits a larger segment 11 (encoding NSP5) that migrates more slowly and is located between gene segments 9 and 11 (see **Fig. 3**).[111] The sensitivity of PAGE assay is comparable to EM and ELISA but is labor intensive and time consuming, thus not routinely performed to detect rotavirus in stool samples today.

### Enzyme immunoassays

EIA is the most widely used method for rotavirus detection using broadly reactive antibodies against epitopes of VP6 shared among RVAs. EIA offers a simple, rapid, and highly sensitive method for routine laboratory diagnosis of rotavirus in stool specimens.[112] In EIA, rotavirus antigen is detected in a colorimetric reaction using solid-phase sandwich EIA format. The optical density can be easily recorded using a plate reader. EIAs are 10 to 100 times more sensitive than EM assays, but the sensitivity and specificity of EIAs are more variable. Several commercial EIA kits are available for routine laboratory detection of rotavirus antigen in stool specimens (**Table 2**). Using RT-PCR as the gold standard, 3 commercially available EIA kits, Premier Rotaclone (Meridian Bioscience, Cincinnati Ohio), ProSpecT (Oxoid, Basingstoke, Hampshire, United Kingdom), and RIDASCREEN (R-Biopharm AG, Darmstadt, Germany), were evaluated for rotavirus diagnostics in stool samples. Testing showed

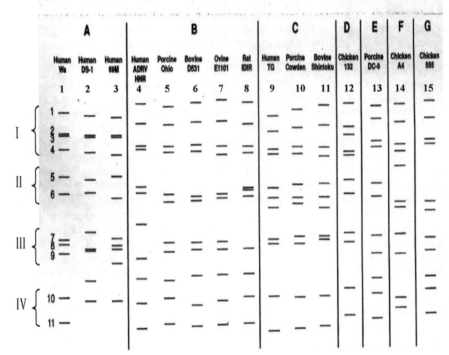

**Fig. 3.** Rotavirus detection by PAGE—PAGE gel showing differences in segment migration configuration of group A (lane 1—long electropherotype, and lanes 2 and 3—short electropherotype), group B (lanes 4, 5, 6, 7, and 8), group C (lanes 9, 10, and 11), group D (lane 12), group E (lane 13), group F (lane 14), and group G (lane 15) rotavirus electropherotypes. (*From* Kapikian AZ, Chanock RM. Rotaviruses. In: Knipe DM, Howley PM, et al, editors. Fields virology. Philadelphia: Lippincott Williams and Wilkins; 2001. p. 1790; with permission.)

that all 3 kits had comparable sensitivity and specificity and were thus suitable for routine rotavirus detection in stool samples.[113] The Premier Rotaclone kit is the only multiwell EIA kit approved by the US Food and Drug Administration (FDA) for in vitro diagnostic use.

### Passive particle agglutination tests

Latex agglutination is a rapid test in which latex particles coated with rotavirus antibodies react in the presence of rotavirus antigen to produce macroscopically visible aggregates. Various latex agglutination kits are commercially available for detecting rotavirus in stool samples, including, the Rotalex latex agglutination kit (Orion Diagnostica, Helsinki, Finland), the Slidex Rota-Kit (bioMérieux, Marcy-l'Etoile, France), the Pastorex Rotavirus (Biorad, Hercules, CA), the RotaScreen latex test (Mercia Diagnostics, Surrey, United Kingdom), Rotastat (Novamed Ltd, Jerusalem, Israel), Meritec-Rotavirus (Meridian Diagnostics, Cincinnati, Ohio), Virogen (Wampole Laboratories, Cranbury, New Jersey), and the Wellcome Latex test (Wellcome Diagnostics, Research Triangle Park, North Carolina).[87,110,112] The latex agglutination test for rotavirus antigen detection is direct, easy to perform, and more rapid than EM and EIAs and can be used in diagnostic laboratories, emergency rooms, and physicians'

**Table 2**
**List of enzyme immunoassay kits commercially available to detect group A rotavirus in stool samples**

| EIA Kits | Manufacturer | Antibody | Number of Tests/Kit | Reference |
|---|---|---|---|---|
| Premier Rotaclone | Meridian Bioscience, OH, USA | Monoclonal | 48 | Gautam et al,[113] 2013 |
| Pathfinder | Kallestad Laboratories, TX, USA | Monoclonal | 50 | Gerna et al,[147] 1987 |
| RIDASCREEN | R-Piopharm, Darmstadt, Germany | Monoclonal | 95 | Gautam et al,[113] 2013 |
| ProSpecT | Oxoid, Hampshire, UK | Polyclonal | 98 | Gautam et al,[113] 2013 |
| Rotavirus EIA | International Diagnostic Laboratories, Israel | Polyclonal | 32/96 | de Beer et al,[110] 1997 |
| Dako EIA | Dakopatts, Denmark | Polyclonal | — | de Beer et al,[110] 1997 |
| Rotazyme | Abbott Laboratories, IL, USA | Polyclonal | 50 | Dennehy et al,[112] 1988 |
| Rotazyme II | Abbott Laboratories, IL, USA | Polyclonal | 50 | Dennehy et al,[112] 1988 |
| TestPack Rotavirus | Abbott Laboratories, IL, USA | Monoclonal and polyclonal | — | Steele et al,[148] 1994 |
| Wellcozyme | Wellcome Diagnostics, NC, USA | Polyclonal | 96 | Dennehy et al,[112] 1988 |
| Fecal Rotavirus Antigen ELISA | Epitope Diagnostics, SD, USA | Monoclonal | 96 | — |

Data from Refs.[110,112,113,147,148]

offices. Although the latex agglutination test is the least complex method, it shows the least sensitivity and specificity compared with other diagnostic assays, including EM, ELISAs, and PAGE.

### Immunochromatographic tests

Immunochromatographic assays, also called lateral flow tests or strip tests, can be used for qualitative detection of rotavirus antigens in patient fecal samples. Immunochromatographic assays are based on the principle of sandwich immunochromatography where antibodies against RVA-specific VP6 protein are used to detect rotavirus antigen in stool samples. In immunochromatography strips, the rotavirus antigen present in the stool sample reacts with the antihuman antibody in the membrane strip first and then is captured by the recombinant antibody; appearance of a colored line in the test window indicates positive result. The immunochromatographic technique is rapid with high sensitivity and specificity compared with EIA, and latex agglutination assays and can be performed routinely in clinical laboratories. Several immunochromatographic kits, including IP-Rota V (Immuno Probe, Frederick, MD), Dipstick ROTA (Eiken Chemical, Eiken, Japan), Rota-Adeno (Sekisui Medical, Tokyo, Japan), SAS Rota Test (SA Scientific, San Diego, CA), and ASAN Easy Test Rota strip (ASAN Pharmaceutical, Seoul, Korea), are available commercially to rapidly detect rotavirus antigen in stool samples. Evaluation of 3 immunochromatographic test kits—IP-Rota V, Dipstick ROTA, and Rota-Adeno—and comparison with a reference RT-PCR method showed that all 3 kits were 88.7% to 97.2% sensitive and 93.3% to 100% specific.[88] The immunochromatographic tests have comparable sensitivity and specificity to EIA assays and are more sensitive and specific than latex agglutination tests.[114] Immunochromatographic tests can be used for rapid screening of RVA in fecal specimens.

### Reverse transcription–polymerase chain reaction

Combination of RT and PCR assays can detect rotavirus in stool samples at substantially lower concentration ($\times$1000 less) than those required for detection by EM and EIA.[89] RT-PCR is useful for verifying that RNA extracts contain intact rotavirus RNA. RT-PCR assays to detect rotavirus can be performed in either singleplex or multiplex format, in combination with gel electrophoresis, probe hybridization, or capturing real-time fluorescence. The rotavirus VP6 gene encodes a group-reactive protein and is highly conserved among all RVAs. VP6 gene–specific RT-PCR assay designed in the conserved region of the VP6 gene followed by gel electrophoresis is performed routinely to detect a wide range of rotavirus strains in stool samples.[89]

### Quantitative reverse transcription–polymerase chain reaction

qRT-PCR assays offer several advantages over traditional RT-PCR, including increased sensitivity, higher throughput, faster turnaround time, and quantification of viral loads. A variety of sensitive real-time RT-PCR methods have been developed for detection of RVA targeting the VP2,[115] VP4,[101,116] VP6,[46,117–119] VP7,[101] NSP3,[93,94,120–123] and NSP4[124] genes.

**Nonstructural protein3 assay for rotavirus detection** The 3′ end of NSP3 gene is a highly conserved region compared with other regions of the genome; thus, it is the best target for detection of a wide variety of RVA genotypes. Multiple qRT-PCR assays have targeted a highly conserved region near the 3′ end of the NSP3 gene.[93,120–122] One-step qRT-PCR assays have been developed for detection of the dsRNA RVA NSP3 gene using the recombinant thermostable *Thermus thermophilus* (r*Tth*) polymerase enzyme and validated on a large number of stool samples positive for rotavirus.[124] By using r*Tth* polymerase enzyme, the denaturation of an antecedent dsRNA step could be included in the thermal cycling program, thus reducing the possibility of sample cross-contamination and requiring less hands-on time. The sensitivity and specificity of NSP3 qRT-PCR assay were determined to be 100% and 86%, respectively, compared with conventional RT-PCR assay. The efficiency of the NSP3 qRT-PCR assay was determined to be 94% with a limit of detection of 1 copy (**Fig. 4**). Using a dsRNA transcript for NSP3 gene, the NSP3 qRT-PCR assay was made quantitative to determine the viral load in the samples. NSP3 qRT-PCR assay is a highly sensitive, specific, and quantitative tool to detect a broad spectrum of RVA genotypes in clinical stool, serum, or cerebrospinal fluid samples.

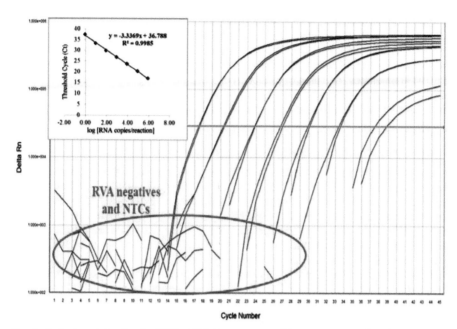

**Fig. 4.** Rotavirus detection by NSP3 qRT-PCR assay—amplification curves of 10-fold dilutions of RVA strain Wa dsRNA transcript using the NSP3 qRT-PCR assay and the linear relationship between Ct and log transcript copy number per reaction (*inset*). The graph showing the Ct value versus the log copy number was fitted with a regression line, and the slope for calculation of efficiency was obtained from the regression line. The Y-axis unit represents relative fluorescence, and Delta Rn refers to the fluorescence emission of a reaction minus the background fluorescence measured from early cycles of the real-time PCR run before a logarithmic increase in fluorescence. The fluorescent signals from RVA-negative samples and no-template controls (NTCs) are indicated by the red circle. (*From* Mijatovic-Rustempasic S, Tam KI, Kerin TK, et al. Sensitive and specific quantitative detection of rotavirus A by one-step real-time reverse transcription-PCR assay without antecedent double-stranded-RNA denaturation. J Clin Microbiol 2013;51(9):3049; with permission.)

**Rotavirus vaccines (Rotarix® and RotaTeq®) detection assays** Two live, attenuated oral vaccines, Rotarix® and RotaTeq®, provide protection against severe diarrhea caused by the major RVA serotypes in circulation and have reduced childhood AGE in both developed and developing countries.[125] Rotarix® and RotaTeq® are, however, live vaccines that can replicate in vaccinated individuals and are shed in feces postvaccination,[126,127] and RotaTeq® component strains can reassort with one another to produce reassortant strains causing gastroenteritis.[128] Reassortant strains derived from vaccine strains Rotarix®[129] and RotaTeq®[130,131] have been associated with AGE in vaccinated[128,132–135] and unvaccinated children.[136,137] RT-PCR reverse hybridization strip assays[138] and restriction endonuclease digest assays[139] have been developed to distinguish the Rotarix G1P[8] strain from wild-type G1P[8] strains. qRT-PCR assays have been developed to determine the in vitro infectious potency of RotaTeq® vaccine strains in Vero cells.[140] A dot blot Northern hybridization assay has been developed to detect RotaTeq® vaccine–derived strains circulating in the community.[134] qRT-PCR assays have been developed for vaccine-specific targets in the genome of Rotarix NSP2 gene, which has the highest degree of genetic dissimilarity between Rotarix® vaccine strain and other G1P[8] strains, and RotaTeq VP6 gene, which detects the bovine-WC3 backbone, and validated on sequence-confirmed stool samples from clinical and surveillance studies containing vaccine strains, wild-type RVA strains, and RVA-negative stools.[95] The Rotarix NSP2 qRT-PCR assay exhibits 100% sensitivity, 99% specificity, 94% efficiency, and limit of detection of 2 copies (**Fig. 5**).[95] The RotaTeq VP6 qRT-PCR assay exhibits 100% sensitivity, 98.6% specificity, 91% efficiency, and limit of detection of 1 copy (see **Fig. 5**).[95] Rotarix NSP2 and RotaTeq VP6 qRT-PCR assays are helpful in high-throughput screening of stool samples to determine the frequency of vaccine strain–associated AGE.

### Rotavirus Diagnosis by Multipathogen Diagnostic Assays

Several multipathogen diagnostic kits, including the FilmArray Gastrointestinal Panel (Biofire Diagnostics, Salt Lake City, UT), xTAG Gastrointestinal Pathogen Panel (GPP) (Luminex Corporation, Austin, TX), TaqMan Array Card (TAC) (Life Technologies, Carlsbad, CA), Seeplex Diarrhea ACE detection kit (Seegene, Seoul, Korea), FTD gastroenteritis kit (Fast Track Diagnostics, Junglinster, Luxembourg), RIDA GENE (R-BioPharm, Darmstadt, Germany), Faecal Pathogens A (AusDiagnostics, Bucks, United Kingdom), Enteric Pathogens (Nanosphere, Northbrook, IL), and Gastroenteritis Multiplex (Diagenode, Denville, NJ), are commercially available to support the rapid and accurate clinical diagnosis of pathogens causing human gastroenteritis (**Table 3**). These kits can be divided into 3 categories based on the molecular diagnostic technology they use to detect the pathogen. The TAC, Seeplex Diarrhea ACE detection kit, FTD gastroenteritis kit, RIDA GENE gastrointestinal kit, Gastroenteritis Multiplex, and Faecal Pathogens A kit are PCR-based kits (multiplex real-time PCR or RT-PCR) that allow the detection of enteric pathogens. The xTAG GPP kit is based on endpoint PCR array technology, including multiplex PCR followed by hybridization to bead-bound probes. The Enteric Pathogens kit and FilmArray Gastrointestinal Panel kit offer fully integrated platforms to generate "stool sample in to result out." A brief description of 8 multipathogen detection kits is in the reviews by Reddington and colleagues[96] and Gray and Coupland.[97] This article discusses the TAC method to simultaneously detect rotavirus along with various other enteropathogens causing gastroenteritis.

### TaqMan Array Card

The TAC system is a 384-well singleplex real-time PCR assay to detect 19 enteropathogens, including viruses, bacterias, protozoas, helminths, and 2 extrinsic controls to monitor extraction and amplification efficiency.[141] TAC cards can also provide information regarding rotavirus genotypes for VP7 and VP4 genes. Newly developed or published real-time assays (primers and probes) are spotted onto microfluidic cards. Fecal samples are spiked with extrinsic controls and RNA is extracted with QuickGene RNA tissue kit (Quest Biomedical, West Midlands, United Kingdom) and then mixed with AgPath-ID One Step RT-PCR Reagents (Life Technologies, Grand Island, New York) and loaded onto TAC cards and then the TAC card is inserted into a ViiA 7 instrument (Life Technologies, Carlsbad, CA). The results are reported in the units of median fluorescence intensity, which are compared with real-time PCR cycle threshold (Ct) values to calculate relative fluorescence intensity. The limits of detection of TAC assays are within a 10-fold difference from the cognate assays performed on plates. The TAC assays are 85% sensitive and 77% specific compared with conventional methods of enteropathogen detection, including microscopy, culture, and immunoassay.[141] The TAC assay allows fast, accurate, and quantitative detection of a broad spectrum of enteropathogens, including rotavirus, and is well suited for rotavirus diagnosis in clinical stool samples.

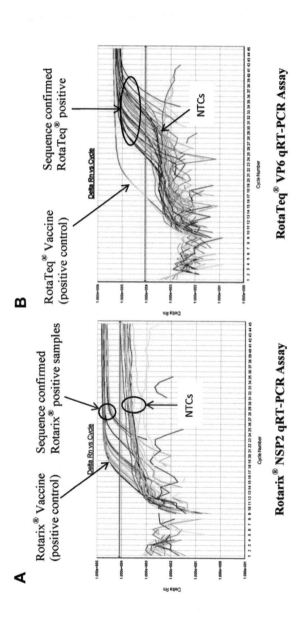

**Fig. 5.** Rotavirus vaccine strain detection by Rotarix NSP2 and RotaTeq VP6 qRT-PCR assays. (A) Amplification plot of Rotarix NSP2 qRT-PCR assay using sequence-confirmed Rotarix-positive stool samples. (B) Amplification plot of RotaTeq VP6 qRT-PCR assay using sequence-confirmed RotaTeq-positive stool samples. NTCs, no-template controls. (*From* Gautam R, Esona MD, Mijatovic-Rustempasic S, et al. Real-time RT-PCR assays to differentiate wild-type group A rotavirus strains from Rotarix(®) and RotaTeq(®) vaccine strains in stool samples. Hum Vaccin Immunother 2014;10(3):771, 774; with permission.)

**Table 3**
**List of commercially available multipathogen detection kits**

| Test System | Manufacturer | Regulatory Status | Technology | Automation | Detection | Number of Enteric Pathogens Detected | Turnaround Time | Reference |
|---|---|---|---|---|---|---|---|---|
| FilmArray Gastrointestinal Panel | Biofire Diagnostics, Salt Lake City, UT, USA | FDA approved | Nested-multiplex PCR | Automated | Endpoint melt curve analysis | 23 | ~1 h | Reddington et al,[96] 2014 |
| xTAG GPP | Luminex Corporation, Austin, TX, USA | FDA approved | Multiplex RT-PCR and hybridization | Semiautomated | Fluorescent-labeled bead array | 15 | ~5 h | Navidad et al,[149] 2013 |
| TAC | Life Technologies, Carlsbad, CA, USA | None | Singleplex real-time PCR | Semiautomated | Fluorescent labeled probe | 19 | ~4 h | Liu et al,[141] 2013 |
| Seeplex Diarrhea ACE detection | Seegene, Seoul, Korea | CE marked | Multiplex RT-PCR | Semiautomated | Auto-capillary electrophoresis device | 15 | ~10 h | Gray et al,[97] 2014 |
| FTD gastroenteritis kit | Fast Track Diagnostics, Junglinster, Luxembourg | None | Multiplex real-time PCR and RT-PCR | Semiautomated | Multiple fluorophore detection | 15 | ~6 h | McAuliffe et al,[150] 2013 |
| RIDA GENE | R-Biopharm, Darmstadt, Germany | CE marked | Multiplex real-time PCR and RT-PCR | Semiautomated | Multiple fluorophore detection | 3–4/ test kit | ~1.5 h | Coste et al,[151] 2013 |
| Faecal Pathogens A | AusDiagnostics, Bucks, UK | None | Intercalating dye detection | Semiautomated | Multiplex tandem PCR | 16 | ~3 h | Gray et al,[97] 2014 |
| Enteric Pathogens | Nanosphere, Northbrook, IL, USA | FDA approved | PCR hybridization to gold nanoparticle | Automated | Multiple fluorophore detection | 9 | ~2 h | Verigene,[152] 2014 |
| Gastroenteritis Multiplex | Diagenode, Denville, NJ, USA | None | Multiplex real-time PCR and RT-PCR | Semiautomated | Multiple fluorophore detection | 13 | — | Gray et al,[97] 2014 |

Data from Refs.[96,97,141,149–152]

## Rotavirus Strain Characterization and Genotyping Assays

Rotaviruses are classified based on the serologic characteristics or sequence diversity of the 2 outer capsid proteins, VP7 (glycosylated, G type) and VP4 (protease sensitive, P type), that elicit host-neutralizing antibodies. During rotavirus surveillance studies, both G and P serotypes/genotypes are monitored because they reassort independently from one another in vivo.[142]

### Rotavirus serotyping

G and P serotypes are defined by the reactivity of antibodies to the 2 outer capsid proteins, VP7 and VP4, respectively. Rotavirus serotyping can be performed by plaque reduction, tube neutralization, fluorescent focus reduction test, and MAb-ELISA.[90] Serologic classification of rotavirus by G and P typing ELISAs requires the presence of intact double-shelled virus particles in stool samples and serotype-specific neutralizing MAbs. MAbs specific for G and P serotypes are commercially available for characterizing RVA strains in fecal samples by ELISA.[92] Large-scale serotyping studies of rotaviruses in stool samples showed that serotypes G1, G2, G3, and G4 commonly cause gastroenteritis in children worldwide. Approximately 70% to 85% rotaviruses in stool samples are typeable by VP7-ELISA. P serotypes are not determined for most of the samples because fewer MAbs have been produced for VP4 protein than for VP7 protein. Similarly, using VP6-specific antibodies, rotavirus strains can be grouped as VP6 SGI that react with short electropherotype strains and VP6 SGII that react with long electropherotype strains. Some human rotavirus strains might react with both SGI and SGII MAbs or with neither type of MAb. Rotavirus strain characterization using serologic assay leaves 20% to 30% of the strains nontypeable because of insufficient numbers of intact virus particle present in stool samples, antigenic variation in common serotypes, or the presence of stool inhibitors. Due to low sensitivity and limited availability of MAbs, rotavirus serotyping assays are not routinely performed today to characterize rotavirus strains in stool samples.

### Dot blot hybridization

Dot blot hybridization assay is based on in situ hybridization of alkaline-phosphate conjugated oligonucleotide probes designed for different rotavirus serotypes to heat-denatured rotavirus RNA immobilized on a nitrocellulose membrane.[98,99] This method is highly specific and 10 to 100 times more sensitive than the ELISA assay but is not widely used for detection of rotaviruses because it is labor intensive and has a low-throughput format.

### Reverse transcription–polymerase chain reaction of viral structural protein7 and viral structural protein4 genes and gel-based genotyping

Rotavirus genotyping of VP4 (P genotype) and VP7 (G genotype) genes can be performed by RT-PCR using viral RNA extracted from fecal samples. RT-PCR assays use either 1-step or 2-step RT followed by an amplification approach to achieve increased sensitivity for the detection of RVA. P-genotyping RT-PCR is performed by seminested PCR in which the first-round PCR amplifies the whole length of VP4 gene, and the second round PCR is a multiplex reaction that includes oligonucleotide primers complementary to variable regions of (P[4], P[6], P[8], P[9], P[10], and P[11]) in the VP4 gene, which are highly distinct between different P types.[91] Similarly, G genotyping is performed by seminested PCR in which the first-round PCR amplifies the whole length of VP7 gene, and the second round PCR is a multiplex reaction that includes oligonucleotide primers complementary to 5 variable regions (G1, G2, G3, G4, and G9) in the VP7 gene that are distinct between

G types.[90,143] Seminested RT-PCR of VP4 and VP7 rotavirus genes can determine the rotavirus genotype by direct visualization of genotype-specific amplicons of different sizes by agarose gel electrophoresis (**Fig. 6**).[90,91] New genotyping assays are being developed to perform 1-step multiplex RT-PCR followed by agarose gel electrophoresis for genotyping of rotavirus VP4 (P[4], P[6], P[8], P[9], and P[10]) genes and VP7 (G1, G2, G3, G4, G9, and G12) and genes (Esona and colleagues, submitted for publication). This method is labor intensive but widely used for rotavirus genotyping in developing countries.

### Quantitative reverse transcription–polymerase chain reaction of viral structural protein7 and viral structural protein4 genes

Real-time RT-PCR assays are more sensitive and specific, have fast turnaround times, and can be performed in high-throughput formats. Multiplex qRT-PCR assays have been developed to genotype rotavirus VP4 and VP7 genes.[100–102] One-step multiplex qRT-PCR assay have been developed to detect and genotype rotavirus wild-type strains and vaccine strains (Rotarix® and RotaTeq®) in stool samples (Gautam and colleagues, unpublished data).

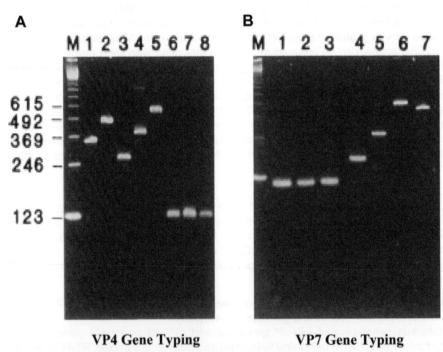

**VP4 Gene Typing**          **VP7 Gene Typing**

**Fig. 6.** RT-PCR and gel-based genotyping of rotavirus strains—(A) VP4 (P) gene typing—lanes: M, markers (123-bp ladder, marker molecular sizes are indicated on the left in base pairs); 1 to 5, products amplified from dsRNA from human rotavirus strains possessing P types 8 (lane 1, strain Wa), 4 (lane 2, strain DS-1), 6 (lane 3, strain M37), 9 (lane 4, strain K8), 10 (lane 5, strain 69M), and 11 (lane 6, strain 116E); 7 to 8, products from dsRNA extracted from culture adapted strains (lane 7, strain 113E; lane 8, strain 218D). (B) VP7 (G) gene typing. Lanes: M, markers (123-bp ladder); 1 to 3, products amplified from dsRNA of human rotavirus G serotype 9 (lane 1, strain116E; lane 2, strain F45; lane 3, strain WI61); 4 to 7, products amplified from samples possessing serotype GI to G4. (*From* Das BK, Gentsch JR, Cicirello HG, et al. Characterization of rotavirus strains from newborns in New Delhi, India. J Clin Microbiol 1994;32(7):1820; with permission.)

### Full-genome sequencing using Sanger dye-termination method

Sequence analysis is the most definitive method for confirmation of rotavirus detection and characterization of genotypes assigned by RT-PCR.[92] Rotavirus genotyping by RT-PCR may fail to identify the genotype in approximately 10% of cases in which a first-round PCR product is obtained but the second-round typing PCR does not reveal a specific type. Sequencing the first-round amplicons is necessary to genotype the virus from such samples. Since the 1990s, the most widely used method of automated DNA sequencing has been the Sanger dye-termination sequencing method, used in conjunction with gel-based or capillary array electrophoresis sequencers that use laser-induced fluorescence detection. For Sanger sequencing, most laboratories use BigDye Terminator v.3.1 Cycle Sequencing Kit and ABI sequencers (Applied Biosystems, Carlsbad, CA). Amplicons of rotavirus VP4 and VP7 genes are generated by RT-PCR amplification of viral RNA, as described previously.[91,143,144]

Previously, rotaviruses were classified based on the antigenicity of the 3 major capsid proteins: VP7 (G genotype), VP4 (P genotype), and VP6 (subgroups).[104] In April 2008, the Rotavirus Classification Working Group developed a nucleotide sequence–based complete genome classification system for RVAs to describe the genetic makeup of individual rotavirus strains. The nomenclature for the full-genome genotype of an RVA strain is now designated in the format Gx-P[x]-Ix-Rx-Cx-Mx-Ax-Nx-Tx-Ex-Hx, where each letter corresponds to a single gene encoding a viral protein (ie, VP7-VP4-VP6-VP1-VP2-VP3-NSP1-NSP2-NSP3-NSP4-NSP5/6, respectively) and x is the number that corresponds to the gene genotype.[28] Full-genome characterization of each rotavirus strain can be achieved by amplifying each gene segment using previously published RVA-specific consensus primers.[90–92] Additional primers can be designed using published consensus sequence for genes that fail to generate a complete open reading frame (ORF). For each gene, 5′ oligonucleotides with an M13 tail and 3′ oligonucleotides with an SP6 tail have been designed to obtain the end sequences of ORFs (Mijatovic and colleagues, unpublished data). Gene-specific PCR amplicons are excised from agarose gels and purified using the QIAquick Gel Extraction Kit (Qiagen, Valencia, CA). Cycle sequencing can be performed using the BigDye Terminator v.3.1 Cycle Sequencing mix. The amplicons generated by RT-PCR of rotavirus genes can be sequenced using an ABI 3130xl sequencer. The consensus sequences of each gene are compared with available RVA sequences in GenBank using nucleotide Basic Local Alignment Search Tool (BLAST) (http://blast.ncbi.nlm.nih.gov/Blast.cgi) or by submitting the sequences to an automated, online genotyping tool for group A rotaviruses — RotaC (http://rotac.regatools.be/)[145] for genotype characterization.

Full-genome classification of rotavirus strains provides understanding of the molecular epidemiology, evolutionary relationships among circulating RVA strains, and also the relatedness between animal and human RVA strains.

### Full-genome sequencing using sequence independent amplification and next-generation sequencing methods

Sequence-independent amplification of rotaviruses in combination with NGS technology provides high-throughput sequencing of all 11 rotavirus genes in a cost-effective and efficient way. NGS technology generates millions of sequences simultaneously from 1 sample.[146] There are many commercially available NGS platforms, such as the Roche 454 (Roche Diagnostic, Indianapolis, IN), Ion Torrent Personal Genome Machine (Life Technologies, Carlsbad, CA), SMRT (single-molecule, real-time) (Pacific Biosciences, Menlo Park, CA), and Illumina HiSeq and Illumina MiSeq (Illumina, San Diego, CA) sequencers. The sequencing technology in MiSeq relies on clustering and sequencing by synthesis using a fixed position on the flow cell rather than transport through a gel. For performing NGS, rotavirus dsRNA is extracted from the stool samples and libraries for NGS sequencing are constructed using reagents and kits specific for NGS instrument being used and by following manufacturer instructions. The quality and quantity of the library are assessed on Bioanalyzer (Agilent Technologies, Santa Clara, CA), LabChip (PerkinElmer, Waltham, MA), or Qubit 2.0 Fluorometer (Life Technologies, Carlsbad, CA) followed by sequencing on an NGS platform available using instrument-specific kits. Data analysis is performed by the reporter program integrated in the instrument to generate FASTQ formatted sequence data. Contigs are assembled from the obtained sequence reads using de novo assembly command in the CLC Genomics Workbench (CLC bio, Boston, MA). The assembled consensus sequences of each gene are used to query the available RVA nucleotide database in the GenBank using nucleotide BLAST or by submitting the sequences to RotaC[145] for genotype characterization. Finally, the complete genome for each sample is built from nucleotide sequences of 11 genome segments by MEGA version 5.0 software. Full-genome sequences of rotaviruses from stool samples have been obtained by using NGS technologies by several laboratories.[105–109]

## SELF-ASSESSMENT

1. The best method to reduce the disease burden caused by rotavirus-associated gastroenteritis is
   A. Good hygienic conditions
   B. Rotavirus vaccines
   C. Antiviral or other drugs
   D. Isolation of symptomatic patients
   E. Chemical inactivation of virus

2. The most widely used method for rotavirus detection is
   A. Cell culture isolation
   B. Polyacrylamide Gel electrophoresis
   C. Enzyme immunoassays
   D. Latex agglutination tests
   E. Electron Microscopy

3. Which technique is used for full-genome characterization of rotavirus strains?
   A. Serotyping using MAb-ELISA
   B. PAGE
   C. Quantitative (qRT-PCR) assays
   D. Next Generation Sequencing
   E. Dot blot hybridization

   ANSWERS

   Answer 1: B.
   Because rotavirus vaccines (Rotarix® and RotaTeq®) are the best strategy to decrease the burden associated with severe and fatal rotavirus diarrhea. Good hygienic condition does not reduce the prevalence or spread of RVA infection in both developed and developing countries. Antiviral or other drugs does not cure

rotavirus-related AGE. The only treatment is to replenish patients with fluids and electrolytes. Isolation of symptomatic patients only prevents spreading of rotavirus disease. Rotavirus is relatively resistant to chemicals and disinfectants.

Answer 2: C.

EIA is the most widely used method for rotavirus detection because it is a simple, rapid, and highly sensitive method for routine laboratory diagnosis of rotavirus in stool specimens. EIA kits use broadly reactive antibodies against epitopes of VP6 shared among RVAs. Detection of rotavirus in stool samples using cell culture method is not performed routinely because it is labor intensive, requires highly trained professionals, and is prone to contamination. PAGE is labor intensive and time consuming, thus is not routinely performed to detect rotavirus in stool samples. Latex agglutination test is the least complex method but it shows least sensitivity and specificity, thus is not routinely used for rotavirus detection. EM is too labor intensive for routine detection of rotavirus in large number of stool samples and requires expensive instrument and highly trained professionals.

Answer 3: D.

Sequence independent amplification followed by NGS provides sequences of all 11 rotavirus genes in a cost-effective manner. Serotyping using MAb-ELISA can only characterize VP4 and VP7 rotavirus genes. PAGE can only provide information about the rotavirus electropherotype (long or short). qRT-PCR assays have not been designed for all 11 rotavirus genes. Dot blot hybridization can only characterize rotavirus serotypes 1, 2, 3, and 4.

## ACKNOWLEDGMENTS

We wish to thank Dr Jon R. Gentsch, Dr Michael D. Bowen, and Ms Leanne Ward for their critical review of this article.

## REFERENCES

1. Bishop RF, Davidson GP, Holmes IH, et al. Virus particles in epithelial cells of duodenal mucosa from children with acute non-bacterial gastroenteritis. Lancet 1973;2(7841):1281–3.
2. Adams WR, Kraft LM. Epizootic diarrhea of infant mice: indentification of the etiologic agent. Science 1963;141(3578):359–60.
3. Malherbe H, Harwin R. The cytopathic effects of vervet monkey viruses. S Afr Med J 1963;37:407–11.
4. Mebus CA, Underdahl NR, Rhodes MB, et al. Further studies on neonatal calf diarrhea virus. Proc Annu Meet U S Anim Health Assoc 1969;73:97–9.
5. Kapikian AZ, Hoshino Y, Chanock RM. Rotaviruses. In: Knipe DM, Howley PM, et al, editors. Fields Virology. Philadelphia: Lippincott Williams and Wilkins; 2001. p. 1787–833.
6. Estes MK, Kapikian AZ. Rotaviruses. In: Fields BN, Knipe DM, Howley PM, et al, editors. Fields virology. Philadelphia: Lippincott Williams and Wilkins; 2007. p. 1917–57.
7. Parashar UD, Hummelman EG, Bresee JS, et al. Global illness and deaths caused by rotavirus disease in children. Emerg Infect Dis 2003;9(5): 565–72.
8. Tate JE, Burton AH, Boschi-Pinto C, et al. 2008 estimate of worldwide rotavirus-associated mortality in children younger than 5 years before the introduction of

universal rotavirus vaccination programmes: a systematic review and meta-analysis. Lancet Infect Dis 2012;12(2):136–41.

9. Nakagomi O, Nakagomi T. Interspecies transmission of rotaviruses studied from the perspective of genogroup. Microbiol Immunol 1993;37(5):337–48.

10. Estes MK, Greenberg HB. Rotaviruses. In: Knipe DM, Howley PM, et al, editors. Fields virology. Philadelphia: Kluwer/Lippincott, Williams and Wilkins; 2013. p. 1348–401.

11. McClain B, Settembre E, Temple BR, et al. X-ray crystal structure of the rotavirus inner capsid particle at 3.8 A resolution. J Mol Biol 2010;397(2): 587–99.

12. Liu M, Mattion NM, Estes MK. Rotavirus VP3 expressed in insect cells possesses guanylyltransferase activity. Virology 1992;188(1):77–84.

13. Lu X, McDonald SM, Tortorici MA, et al. Mechanism for coordinated RNA packaging and genome replication by rotavirus polymerase VP1. Structure 2008; 16(11):1678–88.

14. Aoki ST, Settembre EC, Trask SD, et al. Structure of rotavirus outer-layer protein VP7 bound with a neutralizing Fab. Science 2009;324(5933):1444–7.

15. Dormitzer PR, Sun ZY, Wagner G, et al. The rhesus rotavirus VP4 sialic acid binding domain has a galectin fold with a novel carbohydrate binding site. EMBO J 2002;21(5):885–97.

16. Malik J, Bhan MK, Ray P. Natural immunity to rotavirus infection in children. Indian J Biochem Biophys 2008;45(4):219–28.

17. Arias CF, Romero P, Alvarez V, et al. Trypsin activation pathway of rotavirus infectivity. J Virol 1996;70(9):5832–9.

18. Ruggeri FM, Greenberg HB. Antibodies to the trypsin cleavage peptide VP8 neutralize rotavirus by inhibiting binding of virions to target cells in culture. J Virol 1991;65(5):2211–9.

19. Dormitzer PR, Nason EB, Prasad BV, et al. Structural rearrangements in the membrane penetration protein of a non-enveloped virus. Nature 2004; 430(7003):1053–8.

20. Kovacs-Nolan J, Yoo D, Mine Y. Fine mapping of sequential neutralization epitopes- on the subunit protein VP8 of human rotavirus. Biochem J 2003; 376(Pt 1):269–75.

21. Larralde G, Li BG, Kapikian AZ, et al. Serotype-specific epitope(s) present on the VP8 subunit of rotavirus VP4 protein. J Virol 1991;65(6):3213–8.

22. Padilla-Noriega L, Fiore L, Rennels MB, et al. Humoral immune responses to VP4 and its cleavage products VP5* and VP8* in infants vaccinated with rhesus rotavirus. J Clin Microbiol 1992;30(6):1392–7.

23. Greenberg H, McAuliffe V, Valdesuso J, et al. Serological analysis of the subgroup protein of rotavirus, using monoclonal antibodies. Infect Immun 1983; 39(1):91–9.

24. Hoshino Y, Gorziglia M, Valdesuso J, et al. An equine rotavirus (FI-14 strain) which bears both subgroup I and subgroup II specificities on its VP6. Virology 1987;157(2):488–96.

25. Svensson L, Grahnquist L, Pettersson CA, et al. Detection of human rotaviruses which do not react with subgroup I- and II-specific monoclonal antibodies. J Clin Microbiol 1988;26(6):1238–40.

26. Taniguchi K, Urasawa T, Urasawa S, et al. Production of subgroup-specific monoclonal antibodies against human rotaviruses and their application to an enzyme-linked immunosorbent assay for subgroup determination. J Med Virol 1984;14(2):115–25.

27. Esona MD, Mijatovic-Rustempasic S, Conrardy C, et al. Reassortant group A rotavirus from straw-colored fruit bat (Eidolon helvum). Emerg Infect Dis 2010; 16(12):1844–52.
28. Matthijnssens J, Ciarlet M, McDonald SM, et al. Uniformity of rotavirus strain nomenclature proposed by the Rotavirus Classification Working Group (RCWG). Arch Virol 2011;156(8):1397–413.
29. Banyai K, László B, Duque J, et al. Systematic review of regional and temporal trends in global rotavirus strain diversity in the pre rotavirus vaccine era: insights for understanding the impact of rotavirus vaccination programs. Vaccine 2012; 30(Suppl 1):A122–30.
30. Greenberg HB, Estes MK. Rotaviruses: from pathogenesis to vaccination. Gastroenterology 2009;136(6):1939–51.
31. Greenberg HB, Clark HF, Offit PA. Rotavirus pathology and pathophysiology. Curr Top Microbiol Immunol 1994;185:255–83.
32. Patton JT, Silvestri LS, Tortorici MA, et al. Rotavirus genome replication and morphogenesis: role of the viroplasm. Curr Top Microbiol Immunol 2006;309: 169–87.
33. Kraft RO, Fry WJ. Operative technic of selective gastric vagotomy. Am J Surg 1963;105:423–35.
34. Ray PG, Kelkar SD, Walimbe AM, et al. Rotavirus immunoglobulin levels among Indian mothers of two socio-economic groups and occurrence of rotavirus infections among their infants up to six months. J Med Virol 2007;79(3):341–9.
35. Ball JM, Tian P, Zeng CQ, et al. Age-dependent diarrhea induced by a rotaviral nonstructural glycoprotein. Science 1996;272(5258):101–4.
36. Estes MK, Morris AP. A viral enterotoxin. A new mechanism of virus-induced pathogenesis. Adv Exp Med Biol 1999;473:73–82.
37. Lundgren O, Peregrin AT, Persson K, et al. Role of the enteric nervous system in the fluid and electrolyte secretion of rotavirus diarrhea. Science 2000;287(5452): 491–5.
38. Butz AM, Fosarelli P, Dick J, et al. Prevalence of rotavirus on high-risk fomites in day-care facilities. Pediatrics 1993;92(2):202–5.
39. Kiulia NM, Netshikweta R, Page NA, et al. The detection of enteric viruses in selected urban and rural river water and sewage in Kenya, with special reference to rotaviruses. J Appl Microbiol 2010;109(3):818–28.
40. van Zyl WB, Page NA, Grabow WO, et al. Molecular epidemiology of group A rotaviruses in water sources and selected raw vegetables in southern Africa. Appl Environ Microbiol 2006;72(7):4554–60.
41. Kapikian AZ, Wyatt RG, Levine MM, et al. Studies in volunteers with human rotaviruses. Dev Biol Stand 1983;53:209–18.
42. Kapikian AZ, Wyatt RG, Levine MM, et al. Oral administration of human rotavirus to volunteers: induction of illness and correlates of resistance. J Infect Dis 1983; 147(1):95–106.
43. Bishop RF. Natural history of human rotavirus infection. Arch Virol Suppl 1996; 12:119–28.
44. Vesikari T, Sarkkinen HK, Maki M. Quantitative aspects of rotavirus excretion in childhood diarrhoea. Acta Paediatr Scand 1981;70(5):717–21.
45. Richardson S, Grimwood K, Gorrell R, et al. Extended excretion of rotavirus after severe diarrhoea in young children. Lancet 1998;351(9119):1844–8.
46. Kang G, Iturriza-Gomara M, Wheeler JG, et al. Quantitation of group A rotavirus by real-time reverse-transcription-polymerase chain reaction: correlation with clinical severity in children in South India. J Med Virol 2004;73(1):118–22.

47. Armah GE, Mingle JA, Dodoo AK, et al. Seasonality of rotavirus infection in Ghana. Ann Trop Paediatr 1994;14(3):223–9.

48. Jagai JS, Sarkar R, Castronovo D, et al. Seasonality of rotavirus in South Asia: a meta-analysis approach assessing associations with temperature, precipitation, and vegetation index. PLoS One 2012;7(5):e38168.

49. Levy K, Hubbard AE, Eisenberg JN. Seasonality of rotavirus disease in the tropics: a systematic review and meta-analysis. Int J Epidemiol 2009;38(6): 1487–96.

50. Molbak K, Fischer-Perch TK, Mikkelsen CS. The estimation of mortality due to rotavirus infections in Sub-Saharan Africa. Vaccine 2001;19:393–5.

51. Carlson JA, Middleton PJ, Szymanski MT, et al. Fatal rotavirus gastroenteritis: an analysis of 21 cases. Am J Dis Child 1978;132(5):477–9.

52. Bernstein DI. Rotavirus overview. Pediatr Infect Dis J 2009;28(3 Suppl):S50–3.

53. Cortese MM, Parashar UD, Centers for Disease Control and Prevention (CDC). Prevention of rotavirus gastroenteritis among infants and children: recommendations of the Advisory Committee on Immunization Practices (ACIP). MMWR Recomm Rep 2009;58(RR-2):1–25.

54. Estes MK, Kang G, Zeng CQ, et al. Pathogenesis of rotavirus gastroenteritis. Novartis Found Symp 2001;238:82–96 [discussion: 96–100].

55. Yolken R, Wilde J. Assays for detecting human rotavirus. In: Kapikian AZ, editor. Viral infections of the gastrointestinal tract. New York: Marcel-Dekker; 1994. p. 251–78.

56. Blutt SE, Conner ME. Rotavirus: to the gut and beyond! Curr Opin Gastroenterol 2007;23(1):39–43.

57. Moon S, Wang Y, Dennehy P, et al. Antigenemia, RNAemia, and innate immunity in children with acute rotavirus diarrhea. FEMS Immunol Med Microbiol 2012; 64(3):382–91.

58. Atia AN, Buchman AL. Oral rehydration solutions in non-cholera diarrhea: a review. Am J Gastroenterol 2009;104(10):2596–604 [quiz: 2605].

59. World Health Organization. Rotavirus vaccine. Wkly Epidemiol Rec 2007;40: 285–95.

60. Dennehy PH. Transmission of rotavirus and other enteric pathogens in the home. Pediatr Infect Dis J 2000;19(10 Suppl):S103–5.

61. Ward RL, Bernstein DI, Knowlton DR, et al. Prevention of surface-to-human transmission of rotaviruses by treatment with disinfectant spray. J Clin Microbiol 1991;29(9):1991–6.

62. Velazquez FR, Matson DO, Calva JJ, et al. Rotavirus infections in infants as protection against subsequent infections. N Engl J Med 1996;335(14):1022–8.

63. Organization., W.H. and UNICEF. Ending preventable child deaths from pneumonia and diarrhoea by 2025: Proceedings of the integrated Global action plan for pneumonia and diarrhoea (GAPPD). 2013.

64. CDC. Rotavirus vaccine for the prevention of rotavirus gastroenteritis among children. MMWR Recomm Rep 1999;48(RR-2):1–20.

65. CDC. Withdrawal of rotavirus vaccine recommendation. MMWR Morb Mortal Wkly Rep 1999;48:1007.

66. Curns AT, Steiner CA, Barrett M, et al. Reduction in acute gastroenteritis hospitalizations among US children after introduction of rotavirus vaccine: analysis of hospital discharge data from 18 US states. J Infect Dis 2010;201(11): 1617–24.

67. Glass RI, Parashar UD, Bresee JS, et al. Rotavirus vaccines: current prospects and future challenges. Lancet 2006;368(9532):323–32.

68. Patel M, Pedreira C, De Oliveira LH, et al. Association between pentavalent rota-virus vaccine and severe rotavirus diarrhea among children in Nicaragua. JAMA 2009;301(21):2243–51.
69. Madhi SA, Kirsten M, Louw C, et al. Efficacy and immunogenicity of two or three dose rotavirus-vaccine regimen in South African children over two consecutive rotavirus-seasons: a randomized, double-blind, placebo-controlled trial. Vaccine 2012;30(Suppl 1):A44–51.
70. Seheri LM, Page NA, Mawela MP, et al. Rotavirus vaccination within the South African Expanded Programme on Immunisation. Vaccine 2012;30(Suppl 3): C14–20.
71. Steele AD, Neuzil KM, Cunliffe NA, et al. Human rotavirus vaccine Rotarix pro-vides protection against diverse circulating rotavirus strains in African infants: a randomized controlled trial. BMC Infect Dis 2012;12:213.
72. Neuzil KM, Armah GE, Parashar UD, et al. Rotavirus in Africa: shifting the focus to disease prevention. J Infect Dis 2010;202(Suppl):S1–4.
73. Doro R, Mihalov-Kovács E, Marton S, et al. Large-scale whole genome sequencing identifies country-wide spread of an emerging G9P[8] rotavirus strain in Hungary, 2012. Infect Genet Evol 2014;28:495–512.
74. Iturriza-Gomara M, Dallman T, Bányai K, et al. Rotavirus genotypes co-circulating in Europe between 2006 and 2009 as determined by EuroRotaNet, a pan-European collaborative strain surveillance network. Epidemiol Infect 2011;139(6):895–909.
75. Matthijnssens J, Bilcke J, Ciarlet M, et al. Rotavirus disease and vaccination: impact on genotype diversity. Future Microbiol 2009;4(10):1303–16.
76. Matthijnssens J, Heylen E, Zeller M, et al. Phylodynamic analyses of rotavirus genotypes G9 and G12 underscore their potential for swift global spread. Mol Biol Evol 2010;27(10):2431–6.
77. Desselberger U, Iturriza-Gomara M, Gray JJ. Rotavirus epidemiology and sur-veillance. Novartis Found Symp 2001;238:125–47 [discussion: 147–52].
78. Gentsch JR, Laird AR, Bielfelt B, et al. Serotype diversity and reassortment be-tween human and animal rotavirus strains: implications for rotavirus vaccine pro-grams. J Infect Dis 2005;192(Suppl 1):S146–59.
79. Santos N, Hoshino Y. Global distribution of rotavirus serotypes/genotypes and its implication for the development and implementation of an effective rotavirus vaccine. Rev Med Virol 2005;15(1):29–56.
80. Grimwood K, Kirkwood CD. Human rotavirus vaccines: too early for the strain to tell. Lancet 2008;371(9619):1144–5.
81. Matthijnssens J, Nakagomi O, Kirkwood CD, et al. Group A rotavirus univer-sal mass vaccination: how and to what extent will selective pressure influence prevalence of rotavirus genotypes? Expert Rev Vaccines 2012;11(11): 1347–54.
82. Flewett TH, Davies H, Bryden AS, et al. Diagnostic electron microscopy of faeces. II. Acute gastroenteritis associated with reovirus-like particles. J Clin Pathol 1974;27(8):608–14.
83. Ward RL, Knowlton DR, Pierce MJ. Efficiency of human rotavirus propagation in cell culture. J Clin Microbiol 1984;19(6):748–53.
84. Arnold M, Patton JT, McDonald SM. Culturing, storage, and quantification of ro-taviruses. Curr Protoc Microbiol 2009;15C:3.1–3.24.
85. Herring AJ, Inglis NF, Ojeh CK, et al. Rapid diagnosis of rotavirus infection by direct detection of viral nucleic acid in silver-stained polyacrylamide gels. J Clin Microbiol 1982;16(3):473–7.

86. Herrmann JE, Blacklow NR, Perron DM, et al. Enzyme immunoassay with mono-clonal antibodies for the detection of rotavirus in stool specimens. J Infect Dis 1985;152(4):830–2.

87. Cevenini R, Rumpianesi F, Mazzaracchio R, et al. Evaluation of a new latex agglutination test for detecting human rotavirus in faeces. J Infect 1983;7(2): 130–3.

88. Khamrin P, Tran DN, Chan-it W, et al. Comparison of the rapid methods for screening of group a rotavirus in stool samples. J Trop Pediatr 2011;57(5): 375–7.

89. Wilde J, Yolken R, Willoughby R, et al. Improved detection of rotavirus shedding by polymerase chain reaction. Lancet 1991;337(8737):323–6.

90. Gouvea V, Glass RI, Woods P, et al. Polymerase chain reaction amplification and typing of rotavirus nucleic acid from stool specimens. J Clin Microbiol 1990; 28(2):276–82.

91. Gentsch JR, Glass RI, Woods P, et al. Identification of group A rotavirus gene 4 types by polymerase chain reaction. J Clin Microbiol 1992;30(6):1365–73.

92. Gomara MI, Green J, Gray J. Methods of rotavirus detection, sero- and genotyp-ing, sequencing, and phylogenetic analysis. Methods Mol Med 2000;34: 189–216.

93. Freeman MM, Kerin T, Hull J, et al. Enhancement of detection and quantification of rotavirus in stool using a modified real-time RT-PCR assay. J Med Virol 2008; 80(8):1489–96.

94. Jothikumar N, Kang G, Hill VR. Broadly reactive TaqMan assay for real-time RT-PCR detection of rotavirus in clinical and environmental samples JIN2@cdc.gov. J Virol Methods 2009;155(2):126–31.

95. Gautam R, Esona MD, Mijatovic-Rustempasic S, et al. Real-time RT-PCR as-says to differentiate wild-type group A rotavirus strains from Rotarix® and RotaTeq® vaccine strains in stool samples. Hum Vaccin Immunother 2014; 10(3):767–77.

96. Reddington K, Tuite N, Minogue E, et al. A current overview of commercially available nucleic acid diagnostics approach to detectand identify human gastroenteritis pathogens. Biomol Det Quant 2014;1:3–7.

97. Gray J, Coupland LJ. The increasing application of multiplex nucleic acid detec-tion tests to the diagnosis of syndromic infections. Epidemiol Infect 2014;142: 1–11.

98. Yamakawa K, Oyamada H, Nakagomi O. Identification of rotaviruses by dot-blot hybridization using an alkaline phosphatase-conjugated synthetic oligonucleo-tide probe. Mol Cell Probes 1989;3(4):397–401.

99. Flores J, Green KY, Garcia D, et al. Dot hybridization assay for distinction of rota-virus serotypes. J Clin Microbiol 1989;27(1):29–34.

100. Podkolzin AT, Fenske EB, Abramycheva NY, et al. Hospital-based surveillance of rotavirus and other viral agents of diarrhea in children and adults in Russia, 2005–2007. J Infect Dis 2009;200(Suppl 1):S228–33.

101. Kottaridi C, Spathis AT, Ntova CK, et al. Evaluation of a multiplex real time reverse transcription PCR assay for the detection and quantitation of the most common human rotavirus genotypes. J Virol Methods 2012;180(1–2):49–53.

102. Liu J, Lurain K, Sobuz SU, et al. Molecular genotyping and quantitation assay for rotavirus surveillance. J Virol Methods 2014;213C:157–63.

103. Green KY, Sears JF, Taniguchi K, et al. Prediction of human rotavirus serotype by nucleotide sequence analysis of the VP7 protein gene. J Virol 1988;62(5): 1819–23.

104. Fischer TK, Gentsch JR. Rotavirus typing methods and algorithms. Rev Med Virol 2004;14(2):71–82.

105. Mlera L, Jere KC, van Dijk AA, et al. Determination of the whole-genome consensus sequence of the prototype DS-1 rotavirus using sequence-independent genome amplification and 454(R) pyrosequencing. J Virol Methods 2011;175(2):266–71.

106. Minami-Fukuda F, Nagai M, Takai H, et al. Detection of bovine group a rotavirus using rapid antigen detection kits, rt-PCR and next-generation DNA sequencing. J Vet Med Sci 2013;75(12):1651–5.

107. Masuda T, Nagai M, Yamasato H, et al. Identification of novel bovine group A rotavirus G15P[14] strain from epizootic diarrhea of adult cows by de novo sequencing using a next-generation sequencer. Vet Microbiol 2014;171(1–2):66–73.

108. Dennis FE, Fujii Y, Haga K, et al. Identification of novel Ghanaian G8P[6] human-bovine reassortant rotavirus strain by next generation sequencing. PLoS One 2014;9(6):e100699.

109. Libonati MH, Dennis AF, Ramani S, et al. Absence of genetic differences among G10P[11] rotaviruses associated with asymptomatic and symptomatic neonatal infections in V ellore, India. J Virol 2014;88(16):9060–71.

110. de Beer M, Peenze I, da Costa Mendes VM, et al. Comparison of electron microscopy, enzyme-linked immunosorbent assay and latex agglutination for the detection of bovine rotavirus in faeces. J S Afr Vet Assoc 1997;68(3):93–6.

111. Matsui SM, Mackow ER, Matsuno S, et al. Sequence analysis of gene 11 equivalents from "short" and "super short" strains of rotavirus. J Virol 1990;64(1):120–4.

112. Dennehy PH, Gauntlett DR, Tente WE. Comparison of nine commercial immuno assays for the detection of rotavirus in fecal specimens. J Clin Microbiol 1988;26(9):1630–4.

113. Gautam R, Lyde F, Esona MD, et al. Comparison of Premier Rotaclone(R), ProSpecT, and RIDASCREEN(R) rotavirus enzyme immunoassay kits for detection of rotavirus antigen in stool specimens. J Clin Virol 2013;58(1):292–4.

114. Lee SY, Hong JH, Lee SW, et al. Comparisons of latex agglutination, immunochromatography and enzyme immunoassay methods for the detection of rotavirus antigen. Korean J Lab Med 2007;27(6):437–41 [in Korean].

115. Gutierrez-Aguirre I, Steyer A, Boben J, et al. Sensitive detection of multiple rotavirus genotypes with a single reverse transcription-real-time quantitative PCR assay. J Clin Microbiol 2008;46(8):2547–54.

116. Min BS, Noh YJ, Shin JH, et al. Assessment of the quantitative real-time polymerase chain reaction using a cDNA standard for human group A rotavirus. J Virol Methods 2006;137(2):280–6.

117. Logan C, O'Leary JJ, O'Sullivan N. Real-time reverse transcription-PCR for detection of rotavirus and adenovirus as causative agents of acute viral gastroenteritis in children. J Clin Microbiol 2006;44(9):3189–95.

118. Nordgren J, Bucardo F, Svensson L, et al. Novel light-upon-extension real-time PCR assay for simultaneous detection, quantification, and genogrouping of group A rotavirus. J Clin Microbiol 2010;48(5):1859–65.

119. Schwarz BA, Bange R, Vahlenkamp TW, et al. Detection and quantitation of group A rotaviruses by competitive and real-time reverse transcription-polymerase chain reaction. J Virol Methods 2002;105(2):277–85.

120. Pang XL, Lee B, Boroumand N, et al. Increased detection of rotavirus using a real time reverse transcription-polymerase chain reaction (RT-PCR) assay in stool specimens from children with diarrhea. J Med Virol 2004;72(3):496–501.

121. Zeng SQ, Halkosalo A, Salminen M, et al. One-step quantitative RT-PCR for the detection of rotavirus in acute gastroenteritis. J Virol Methods 2008;153(2):238–40.

122. Pang X, Cao M, Zhang M, et al. Increased sensitivity for various rotavirus genotypes in stool specimens by amending three mismatched nucleotides in the forward primer of a real-time RT-PCR assay. J Virol Methods 2011;172(1–2):85–7.

123. Mijatovic-Rustempasic S, Tam KI, Kerin TK, et al. Sensitive and specific quantitative detection of rotavirus A by one-step real-time reverse transcription-PCR assay without antecedent double-stranded-RNA denaturation. J Clin Microbiol 2013;51(9):3047–54.

124. Adlhoch C, Kaiser M, Hoehne M, et al. Highly sensitive detection of the group A Rotavirus using Apolipoprotein H-coated ELISA plates compared to quantitative real-time PCR. Virol J 2011;8:63.

125. Patel MM, Tam KI, Kerin TK, et al. Real-world impact of rotavirus vaccination. Pediatr Infect Dis J 2011;30(1 Suppl):S1–5.

126. Anderson EJ. Rotavirus vaccines: viral shedding and risk of transmission. Lancet Infect Dis 2008;8(10):642–9.

127. Yen C, Jakob K, Esona MD, et al. Detection of fecal shedding of rotavirus vaccine in infants following their first dose of pentavalent rotavirus vaccine. Vaccine 2011;29(24):4151–5.

128. Bowen MD, Payne DC. Rotavirus vaccine-derived shedding and viral reassortants. Expert Rev Vaccines 2012;11(11):1311–4.

129. Rose TL, Marques da Silva MF, Goméz MM, et al. Evidence of vaccine-related reassortment of rotavirus, Brazil, 2008–2010. Emerg Infect Dis 2013;19(11):1843–6.

130. Patel NC, Hertel PM, Estes MK, et al. Vaccine-acquired rotavirus in infants with severe combined immunodeficiency. N Engl J Med 2010;362(4):314–9.

131. Werther RL, Crawford NW, Boniface K, et al. Rotavirus vaccine induced diarrhea in a child with severe combined immune deficiency. J Allergy Clin Immunol 2009;124(3):600.

132. Boom JA, Sahni LC, Payne DC, et al. Symptomatic infection and detection of vaccine and vaccine-reassortant rotavirus strains in 5 children: a case series. J Infect Dis 2012;206(8):1275–9.

133. Hemming M, Vesikari T. Vaccine-derived human-bovine double reassortant rotavirus in infants with acute gastroenteritis. Pediatr Infect Dis J 2012;31(9):992–4.

134. Donato CM, Ch'ng LS, Boniface KF, et al. Identification of strains of RotaTeq rotavirus vaccine in infants with gastroenteritis following routine vaccination. J Infect Dis 2012;206(3):377–83.

135. Bucardo F, Rippinger CM, Svensson L, et al. Vaccine-derived NSP2 segment in rotaviruses from vaccinated children with gastroenteritis in Nicaragua. Infect Genet Evol 2012;12(6):1282–94.

136. Payne DC, Edwards KM, Bowen MD, et al. Sibling transmission of vaccine-derived rotavirus (RotaTeq) associated with rotavirus gastroenteritis. Pediatrics 2010;125(2):e438–41.

137. Rivera L, Peña LM, Stainier I, et al. Horizontal transmission of a human rotavirus vaccine strain–a randomized, placebo-controlled study in twins. Vaccine 2011;29(51):9508–13.

138. van Doorn LJ, Kleter B, Hoefnagel E, et al. Detection and genotyping of human rotavirus VP4 and VP7 genes by reverse transcriptase PCR and reverse hybridization. J Clin Microbiol 2009;47(9):2704–12.

139. Rose TL, Miagostovich MP, Leite JP. Rotavirus A genotype G1P[8]: a novel method to distinguish wild-type strains from the Rotarix vaccine strain. Mem Inst Oswaldo Cruz 2010;105(8):1068–72.

140. Ranheim T, Mathis PK, Joelsson DB, et al. Development and application of a quantitative RT-PCR potency assay for a pentavalent rotavirus vaccine (Rota-Teq). J Virol Methods 2006;131(2):193–201.

141. Liu J, Gratz J, Amour C, et al. A laboratory-developed TaqMan Array Card for simultaneous detection of 19 enteropathogens. J Clin Microbiol 2013;51(2):472–80.

142. Hoshino Y, Sereno MM, Midthun K, et al. Independent segregation of two antigenic specificities (VP3 and VP7) involved in neutralization of rotavirus infectivity. Proc Natl Acad Sci U S A 1985;82(24):8701–4.

143. Das BK, Gentsch JR, Cicirello HG, et al. Characterization of rotavirus strains from newborns in New Delhi, India. J Clin Microbiol 1994;32(7):1820–2.

144. Iturriza-Gómara BI, Desselberger U, Gray J. Reassortment in vivo: driving force for diversity of human rotavirus strains isolated in the United Kingdom between 1995 and 1999. J Virol 2001;75(8):3696–705.

145. Maes P, Matthijnssens J, Rahman M, et al. RotaC: a web-based tool for the complete genome classification of group A rotaviruses. BMC Microbiol 2009;9:238.

146. Schuster SC. Next-generation sequencing transforms today's biology. Nat Methods 2008;5(1):16–8.

147. Gerna G, Sarasini A, Passarani N, et al. Comparative evaluation of a commercial enzyme-linked immunoassay and solid-phase immune electron microscopy for rotavirus detection in stool specimens. J Clin Microbiol 1987;25(6):1137–9.

148. Steele AD, Williams MM, Bos P, et al. Comparison of two rapid enzyme immunoassays with standard enzyme immunoassay and latex agglutination for the detection of human rotavirus in stools. J Diarrhoeal Dis Res 1994;12(2):117–20.

149. Navidad JF, Griswold DJ, Gradus MS, et al. Evaluation of Luminex xTAG gastrointestinal pathogen analyte-specific reagents for high-throughput, simultaneous detection of bacteria, viruses, and parasites of clinical and public health importance. J Clin Microbiol 2013;51(9):3018–24.

150. McAuliffe GN, Anderson TP, Stevens M, et al. Systematic application of multiplex PCR enhances the detection of bacteria, parasites, and viruses in stool samples. J Infect 2013;67(2):122–9.

151. Coste JF, Vuiblet V, Moustapha B, et al. Microbiological diagnosis of severe diarrhea in kidney transplant recipients by use of multiplex PCR assays. J Clin Microbiol 2013;51(6):1841–9.

152. Nanosphere. Verigene Platform. 2014. Available at: http://www.nanosphere.us/technology. Accessed April 25, 2014.

# Intestinal Amebae

Ibne Karim M. Ali, PhD

## KEYWORDS

- Amebiasis laboratory diagnosis • *Entamoeba histolytica* • *Entamoeba dispar*
- *Entamoeba moshkovskii* • *Entamoeba Bangladeshi* • Serology • Antigen detection
- Molecular detection

## KEY POINTS

- Among the 4 morphologically identical *Entamoeba* species that infect humans, *Entamoeba histolytica* unequivocally causes diseases; *Entamoeba dispar* is a harmless commensal; *Entamoeba moshkovskii* seems to be an emerging pathogen; and the pathogenicity of *Entamoeba bangladeshi* remains to be investigated.
- Species-specific detection of intestinal amebae is needed for appropriate treatment decisions as well as for understanding the true epidemiology and pathogenicity of these amebae.
- Antigen-based simple, reliable, and specific detection methods are needed for *E dispar, E moshkovskii*, and *E bangladeshi*.
- A molecular diagnostic test capable of detecting *E histolytica, E dispar, E moshkovskii*, and *E bangladeshi* simultaneously in clinical samples is needed.
- Next-generation sequencing of DNA from stool specimens is needed to identify potentially novel species of *Entamoeba* that may infect humans.

## INTRODUCTION

There are many species in the genus *Entamoeba* and at least 8 of them infect humans, namely *Entamoeba histolytica, Entamoeba dispar, Entamoeba coli, Entamoeba moshkovskii, Entamoeba hartmanni, Entamoeba polecki, Entamoeba gingivalis*, and

Conflicts of interest: The author has no conflicts of interest.

Search strategy and selection criteria: References for this article were identified through searches of PubMed, by use of the search terms "amebiasis," "*Entamoeba histolytica*," "*Entamoeba dispar*," "*Entamoeba moshkovskii*," "*Entamoeba bangladeshi*," "diagnosis," "molecular tools," and combinations of these terms. The search was mostly limited to English language articles that were published up to December 2014.

Disclaimer: The use of trade names is for identification only and does not imply the endorsement of the US Centers for Disease Control and Prevention (CDC). The findings and conclusions in this article are those of the author, and do not necessarily represent the official position of the CDC.

Division of Foodborne Waterborne and Environmental Diseases, National Center for Emerging and Zoonotic Infectious Diseases, Centers for Disease Control and Prevention, 1600 Clifton Road Northeast, Mailstop D-66, Atlanta, GA 30329, USA
*E-mail address:* xzn5@cdc.gov

*Entamoeba bangladeshi*. It is only *E histolytica* that has been universally recognized as a cause of intestinal and extraintestinal diseases in humans. *E polecki* has uninucleate cysts, whereas *E coli* cysts have eight nuclei. The size of the *E hartmanni* cysts and trophozoites is much smaller than those of *E histolytica*, although both have cysts with four nuclei. *E gingivalis*, a parasite of the human oral cavity, is a nonencysting species. As a result, as far as microscopic diagnosis of amebiasis is concerned, none of these species pose a problem for morphologic identification. However, four of the *Entamoeba* species that infect humans are morphologically indistinguishable: *E histolytica*, *E dispar*, *E moshkovskii*, and *E bangladeshi*.

*E histolytica*, the causative agent of amebiasis, is the second leading cause of mortality caused by an intestinal parasitic infection (after cryptosporidiosis). Amebiasis was responsible for a death toll of 55,500 people in 2010 worldwide.[1] However, not all *E histolytica* infections lead to disease in the host and at most 1 in 10 *E histolytica* infections progresses to development of clinical symptoms.[2] Nevertheless, *E histolytica* remains a significant source of morbidity and mortality in developing countries.[3] *E histolytica* infections have also been linked to childhood morbidities, growth stunting, and delayed cognitive development.[4–6]

*E dispar*, a nonpathogenic commensal species, is perhaps 10 times more common than *E histolytica* worldwide,[7] but local prevalences may vary significantly. Evidence is now building that a second member of the *Entamoeba* genus, *E moshkovskii*, is also associated with human disease.[8,9] It is intriguing to speculate that other *Entamoeba* species that do not apparently cause clinical diseases may still have a large impact on host microflora composition and indirectly affect health and wellness.[10]

This article discusses the tools commonly used for the diagnosis of intestinal amebiasis, their advantages and disadvantages, tools that are missing, and recent advancements in diagnostic techniques.

## ENTAMOEBA HISTOLYTICA

In 1875, Fedor Aleksandrovich Lösch first identified amebae in clinical samples from a case of fatal dysentery, reproduced the disease in dogs, and suggested the name *Amoeba coli* for this species.[11,12] In 1890, Osler first positively diagnosed a case of amebic liver abscess. One year later, Councilman and Lafleur, at Johns Hopkins Hospital, confirmed the pathologic role of amebae through studies on patients with dysentery and liver abscesses and introduced the terms amebic dysentery and amebic liver abscess. The organism was formally named *E histolytica* by Schaudinn in 1903.

## ENTAMOEBA DISPAR

As early as 1925, Brumpt suggested the existence of 2 morphologically identical species, one being pathogenic and the other not, and proposed the name *E dispar* for the nonpathogenic species. However, Brumpt's proposal was ignored for many years. Eventually, in 1993, 68 years after the original discovery of *E dispar*, biochemical, immunologic, and genetic evidence accumulated to suggest that *E histolytica* and *E dispar* are two different species. Following much debate, *E dispar* (which had previously been known as nonpathogenic *E histolytica*) was separated from *E histolytica* based on isoenzyme[13] and DNA sequence data,[14] and was accepted as a distinct species. Although *E dispar* is considered a harmless commensal organism, there are a few reports that suggest that *E dispar* may be capable of causing intestinal and extraintestinal diseases in humans and experimental animals.[15]

## ENTAMOEBA MOSHKOVSKII

*E moshkovskii*, which was mainly considered to be a free-living environmental ameba, is indistinguishable in both its cyst and trophozoite forms from *E histolytica* and *E dispar*. It was first discovered by Tshalaia[16] in 1941 in Moscow sewage. The first human case of *E moshkovskii* was reported in 1961, which was isolated from a resident of Laredo, Texas, and presented with diarrhea, weight loss, and epigastric pain.[17] *E moshkovskii* is osmotolerant, can be cultured at room temperature, and is resistant to emetine; all characteristics that distinguish it from *E histolytica* and *E dispar*.[17–20]

*E moshkovskii* seems to be ubiquitous in anoxic sediments. Although the early isolations of this species were from sewage, *E moshkovskii* can also be found in environments ranging from clean riverine sediments to brackish coastal pools.[18] In 2003, *E moshkovskii* was reported to be highly prevalent in Bangladeshi children.[9] Since then, human isolates of *E moshkovskii* have been reported from at least 13 other countries, including both resource-poor and resource-rich countries: the United States, Italy, South Africa, India, Australia, Pakistan, Iran, Tanzania, Turkey, Malaysia, Thailand, Tunisia, and the United Arab Emirates.[9,21–33] In most of these studies the ameba has not been associated with disease and was isolated from very few individuals. However, high prevalences of *E moshkovskii* were reported in some countries: 50% in Australia,[23] 24.9% and 15.6% in 2 different study populations in India,[34,35] 21.1% in Bangladesh,[9] 13.2% in Tanzania,[26] 13.2% in Pakistan,[24] and 5.2% in Iran.[25]

Although previous reports on the identification of *E moshkovskii* in fecal samples had not shown any association with clinical illness, recent studies from Bangladesh,[8,9] India,[34,35] and Pakistan[24] reported *E moshkovskii* in patients with gastrointestinal symptoms, such as diarrhea or dysentery, and with no other known pathogens, raising questions about the long-accepted status of this organism as nonpathogenic. Supporting an association with human disease, *E moshkovskii* has been shown to cause diarrhea and weight loss in experimental mice.[8] There is a need to include *E moshkovskii* in epidemiologic studies and diagnostic laboratories that deal with *E histolytica* and *E dispar* to better understand the global picture of *E moshkovskii* prevalence and pathogenicity.

## ENTAMOEBA BANGLADESHI

In 2010 to 2011, during analysis of feces from a disadvantaged Bangladeshi community that were positive for *Entamoeba* organisms by microscopy or culture but negative for *E histolytica*, *E dispar*, and *E moshkovskii* by polymerase chain reaction (PCR), a new species was identified using broad-specificity primers for the *Entamoeba* small subunit (SSU) ribosomal RNA (rRNA) gene sequences.[36,37] The new species was named *E bangladeshi*. Several *E bangladeshi* isolates were established in xenic culture. Surprisingly, they grow at 37°C as well as 25°C, a characteristic that they share with *E moshkovskii*. Axenization of this species has been unsuccessful to date. Under light microscopy, it has a similar appearance to *E histolytica*. However, a minor difference between *E bangladeshi* and *E histolytica* was observed using electron microscopy. The nucleus of *E bangladeshi* appears to be darker staining than that of *E histolytica*. Phylogenetically, based on SSU rRNA gene sequences, *E bangladeshi* is closer to *E histolytica* than *E moshkovskii*. Stool samples that were positive for *E bangladeshi* by PCR originated from both diarrheal and asymptomatic children. More studies are required to understand the epidemiology and potential pathogenicity of this novel species. Although *E bangladeshi* can grow at room temperature, it is yet to be determined whether it can live outside a host, like *E moshkovskii*. Also, the potential host range and environmental reservoirs of this parasite need to be investigated.

## PREVALENCE

*E histolytica* has a worldwide distribution. Infection with *E histolytica* usually occurs through the ingestion of ameba cysts in food or water, although an unusual route of infection is through oral/anal sex, where trophozoites can also be infectious. It remains a major public health problem in countries where sanitation and hygiene are poor. The worldwide prevalence of true *E histolytica* infection is not well understood because most published studies did not use *E histolytica*–specific diagnostic tools. In general, the prevalence of amebic infection is high in the Indian subcontinent, Africa, the Far East, and areas of South and Central America. In developing countries it depends largely on cultural habits, age, level of sanitation, crowding, and socioeconomic status. In developed countries, entamoeba infection is mostly caused by *E dispar* and is confined to certain groups of people: immigrants from or travelers to areas of endemicity, homosexual men, patients infected with immunodeficiency virus, and institutionalized populations.[12] However, in Japan, carriage of *E histolytica* is more common.[38] Similarly, in Australia infection with *E moshkovskii* is more common than with *E histolytica* or *E dispar*.[23] Case studies of patients with amebic colitis in Natal, South Africa, showed that there was a peak incidence of infection among children less than 14 years of age and a second increase in infection in adults greater than 40 years old.[7] Acuna-Soto and colleagues,[39] after reviewing all the published reports from 1929 to 1997, found that the male/female ratios for invasive intestinal amebiasis and asymptomatic carriage were 3.2:1 and 1:1, respectively. In Mexico, more than 8% of the population was reported in 1994 to be seropositive for *E histolytica*, and 1.3 million cases of intestinal amebiasis were reported in 1996.[40,41] In contrast, only 2970 symptomatic cases of amebiasis were reported in the United States in 1993 (when the population of the country was 258 million), and half of those cases were in immigrants from Mexico, South and Central America, Asia, and Pacific Islands.[42]

The reported prevalence of *E histolytica* using different diagnostic methods in 2014 publications is provided in **Tables 1** and **2**.

## CLINICAL MANIFESTATIONS

About 90% of all *E histolytica* infections remain asymptomatic. Invasive intestinal infection and amebic colitis are marked by loose stools containing blood and mucus. Complications of amebic colitis include perforation and secondary bacterial infection of ulcers and are associated with very high mortalities. Occasionally, chronic ulceration results in ameboma formation.

The most common form of extraintestinal amebiasis is the amebic liver abscess, which unless properly diagnosed and promptly treated is a potentially lethal disease. In areas of endemicity, amebic liver abscess is suspected in a patient with fever, weight loss, and right upper quadrant pain and tenderness.[43]

There are sporadic case reports of cerebral amebiasis,[44–46] which has an abrupt onset and rapid progression, almost always resulting in death. Infections of kidney,[47] heart,[48] lung,[49,50] appendix,[51] and skin[52,53] by *E histolytica* have also been reported.

## DIAGNOSIS OF INTESTINAL AMEBIASIS

Amebiasis has been defined by World Health Organization and Pan American Health Organization as the infection with *E histolytica* regardless of symptoms.[54] They recommended in 1997 that, "Optimally, *E histolytica* should be specifically identified and, if present, treated. If only *E dispar* is identified, treatment is unnecessary. If the infected person has gastrointestinal symptoms, other causes should be sought."[54] However, these

**Table 1**
**Advantages and disadvantages of different methods used in the diagnosis of amebiasis**

| Methods | Advantages | Disadvantages |
|---------|-----------|---------------|
| Microscopy | Simple, rapid, inexpensive | Nonspecific, insensitive, requires expertise, cannot be performed on frozen specimens |
| Culture | Visual observation of motile trophozoites; allows downstream analysis | Time consuming, insensitive, biased because it may facilitate the growth of the predominant species/strain or other organisms |
| Isoenzyme | Capable of differentiating between *E histolytica* and *E dispar* | Time consuming; labor intensive; insensitive; and depends on amebic culture growth, which is not always successful |
| Serology | Easy to perform, provides individual's past or present exposure to *E histolytica* | Unable to differentiate between an acute infection and a past infection; little diagnostic value, especially in the amebiasis-endemic areas; may give false-negative results in early infections |
| Antigen detection | Simple, rapid, allows specific detection of *E histolytica*; most suitable diagnostic technique for resource-poor nations where amebiasis is endemic | Does not work on formalin-fixed stools; less sensitive than PCR diagnosis |
| Conventional PCR | Sensitive, specific, works on broad specimen types | Contamination prone; sophisticated laboratory setup and expertise required; not suitable as a diagnostic test for resource-poor nations |
| Real-time PCR | Highly sensitive, highly specific, rapid, works on broad specimen types, does not require postanalysis of PCR amplicons | Sophisticated laboratory setup and expertise required; not suitable for resource-poor nations |

recommendations were made before the acceptance of *E moshkovskii* as a human ameba (and possibly a pathogen), as well as before the identification of *E bangladeshi* in asymptomatic and symptomatic children in Mirpur, Bangladesh. So, a review of these recommendations based on new findings is needed.

Different diagnostic methods have been used for the detection of *E histolytica* (**Fig. 1**). These methods have different levels of sensitivity and specificity. Advantages and disadvantages of some of the commonly used techniques for diagnosis of intestinal amebiasis are provided in **Table 1**.

## MICROSCOPY

The microscopic examination, often referred to as ova and parasite examination, remains the most widely used method of amebiasis diagnosis (see **Fig. 1**), especially in endemic areas, despite the severe limitations on sensitivity and specificity. For several reasons microscopy should not be the method of choice for the diagnosis of amebiasis. First, it requires expertise with knowledge of morphology of *Entamoeba*

**Table 2**
**Latest prevalence of *E histolytica* reported in 2014 (in PubMed) using different methods**

| Method | Prevalence[a] |
|---|---|
| Microscopy | Egypt: 22.2% among 194 patients with diarrhea and/or dysentery by microscopy (Ibrahim et al, 2014) |
| | Spain: 11.04%, 5.10%, 13.33%, and 11.11% among immigrant populations in Spain from sub-Saharan Africa, Latin America, Maghreb, and eastern Europe, respectively (Cobo et al, 2014) |
| | South Africa: 26.5% in patients with HIV/AIDS (Samie et al, 2014) |
| | Ethiopia: 5% among 340 randomly selected students from south eastern Ethiopia (Tulu et al, 2014) |
| | Ethiopia: 5.4% among diarrheal patients during 2007–2012 (Ramos et al, 2014) |
| | Ethiopia: 48.8% and 51.7% among prison and tobacco farm populations, respectively (Mamo 2014) |
| | Ethiopia: 40% among patients with HIV/AIDS on antiretroviral therapy at Adigrat hospital from northern Ethiopia (Mahmud et al, 2014) |
| | Cameroon: 15.93% among HIV-positive patients (Vouking et al, 2014) |
| | Iraq: 23.44% among children in Baghdad (Waqar et al, 2014) |
| | Pakistan: 2.9% among renal transplant patients (Raja et al, 2014) |
| | Nigeria: 5.7% in HIV-positive patients (Jegede et al, 2014) |
| | Malaysia: 18.6% among 2 indigenous subtribes (Lee et al, 2014) |
| | Malaysia: 14.1% among Orang Asli school children in rural Malaysia (Al-Delaimy et al, 2014) |
| | Malaysia: 1.8% overall prevalence among populations living in different communities (Sinniah et al, 2014) |
| | Brazil: 46.28% among asymptomatic children 2–10 y old from north eastern Brazil; however, these were negative by *E histolytica*–specific antigen detection ELISA, suggesting they are *E dispar/E moshkovskii/E bangladeshi* but not *E histolytica* (Silva et al, 2014) |
| | Brazil: 0.7% among 150 street food vendors from Paraná State, southern Brazil (Colli et al, 2014) |
| | Canada: only 63.7 cases per annum from Calgary Health Zone (Alberta) with a population of 1.2 million during 2006–2011 (Skappak et al, 2014) |
| | Turkey: 0.27% among 1466 appendectomy specimens (Yabanoglu et al, 2014) |
| | Nicaragua: 8.3% among 826 children with diarrhea after rotavirus vaccination (Becker-Dreps, 2014) |
| | Tanzania: 43% among people in communities living in Mwanza region, Tanzania (Barda et al, 2014) |
| | Nepal: 12.92% among 2005 combatants and their families from a hospital-based study in Mid-Western Regional Police Hospital (Paudel et al, 2014) |
| | Cambodia: 27.1% among 218 people and particularly in children (Schar et al, 2014) |
| | India: 21.8% among people living in low socioeconomic areas from Chennai South, India (Dhanabal et al, 2014) |
| | Jordan: 0.11% (1/901) among food handlers in hotels in the Dead Sea area, Jordan (Abdel-Dayem et al, 2014) |
| | Israel: 5.4%, 1.8%, and 8.8% among Bedouin, non-Ethiopian Jewish, and Ethiopian children aged <5 y, respectively. 19.4%, 6.0%, and 24.6% among Bedouin, non-Ethiopian Jewish, and Ethiopian children aged 5–19 y, respectively (Ben-Shimol et al, 2014) |
| | China: 1.4% among 369 pulmonary tuberculosis cases without HIV infection, and 2.2% in healthy controls in a rural county in China (Li et al, 2014) |

*(continued on next page)*

| Table 2 *(continued)* | |
|---|---|
| **Method** | **Prevalence[a]** |
| Serology | Kenya: 12.8% and 16.6% in Kwale and Mbita, respectively (Fujii et al, 2014) |
| | Japan: 11.3% (8 of 71) in asymptomatic Japanese individuals infected with HIV-1 who underwent colonoscopy for detection of diseases other than amebiasis at the AIDS Clinical Center, National Center for Global Health and Medicine, Tokyo, (Watanabe et al, 2014) |
| | Japan: 21.3% (277/1303) among asymptomatic individuals infected with HIV-1 attending AIDS Clinical Center, National Center for Global Health and Medicine, Tokyo, Japan (Watanabe et al, 2014) |
| | Haiti: 63.92% among Haitian children (Moss et al, 2014) |
| Antigen detection | Egypt: 3.6% *E histolytica* among 194 diarrhea and/or dysenteric patients by *E histolytica* II ELISA compared with 22.2% *Entamoeba* complex by microscopy (Ibrahim et al, 2014) |
| | Turkey: 25.1% of the microscopically parasite-positive diarrheal patients admitted into a hospital (Yildirim et al, 2014) |
| | India: 11.38% among diarrheal patients admitted into a hospital (Mohanty et al, 2014) |
| | Pakistan: 11.1%, 16.8%, and 28.3% among upper, middle, and low socioeconomic populations living in Lahore (Alam et al, 2014) |
| | Brazil: 3.1% among 1403 samples collected from students aged 6–14 y who were living in Divinópolis, Minas Gerais, Brazil (Pereira et al, 2014) |
| | Brazil: of the 24 (25%) samples that tested positive for the *Entamoeba* species by microscopy, only 2 (8.3%) tested positive for *E histolytica* by ELISA, and none tested positive by PCR (Carneiro Santos et al, 2014) |
| PCR | Iran: 1.9% *E histolytica* and 2.86% *E dispar* among 105 children with dysentery (Sharbatkhori et al, 2014) |
| | Korea: 0.9% *E histolytica* and 0.6% *E dispar* among 320 clinical samples submitted to Hanyang University during 2004–2011 (Choi et al, 2014) |
| Real-time PCR | Italy: 0.44% *E histolytica* and 7.61% *E dispar* among 8886 patients with clinically suspected parasitosis (Calderaro et al, 2014) |
| | [b]Taiwan: the average annual incidence of cases of *E histolytica* infections was 0.49, 0.42, and 9.26 for cases of local acquisition, travelers to countries of endemicity, and immigrants/foreign workers from endemic countries, respectively per 100,000 people (Leung et al, 2014) |
| | Denmark: no *E histolytica* and only 1.45% (2 of 138) *E dispar* among Danish primary care patients with irritable bowel syndrome (Engsbro et al, 2014) |

Case studies were not included in the prevalence data.

*Abbreviations:* AIDS, acquired immunodeficiency syndrome; ELISA, enzyme-linked immunosorbent assay; HIV, human immunodeficiency virus.

[a] Because of space limitations these references were not added to the Reference list.

[b] For all cases in the Taiwan study, at least 2 unambiguous results of 4 tests (stool microscopy, serologic tests, coproantigen ELISA, and real-time PCR for fecal samples) were available, and at least 2 test results were unambiguously positive for *E histolytica*.

species. Second, it is primarily a nonspecific method, because it cannot differentiate pathogenic *E histolytica* from nonpathogenic *E dispar*, *E moshkovskii*, or *E banglade-shi*. Third, it has a low (10%–60%) sensitivity.[55] Fourth, it requires immediate processing of fresh samples if trophozoites are the predominant forms of the parasite. Fifth, it is recommended that at least 3 consecutive stool samples collected within 10 days be checked to improve the chance of ameba detection because the amebae are not excreted in every stool.

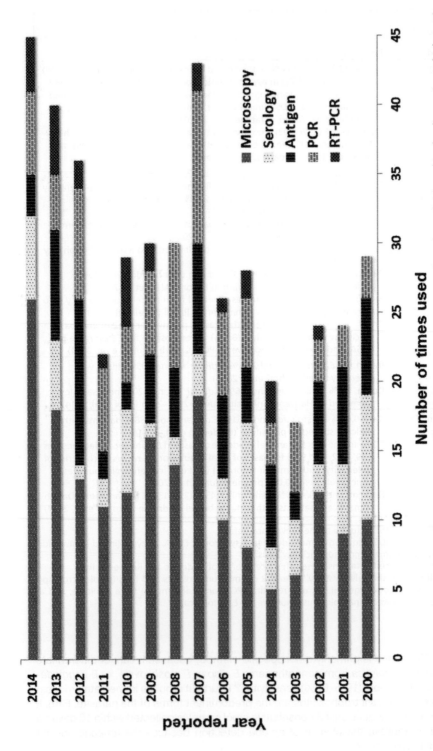

**Fig. 1.** Tools used to diagnose entamoeba infections during 2000 to 2014. Microscopy represents the sole method used in the diagnosis, and when microscopy was used in combination with other methods it was not included here. The other methods might have been used in combination except for microscopy. Data were obtained from PubMed search using the keywords "*Entamoeba*" and "diagnosis." In most cases, only articles written in English were selected. For 2014, articles published by December 8 were selected. RT-PCR, real-time PCR.

## CULTURE

Growth of amebae in culture is a difficult, labor-intensive, time-consuming, and often unsuccessful process. Most clinical laboratories do not culture *Entamoeba* species because of the associated difficulties and expense.

Three types of culture system are used for the cultivation of *Entamoeba* species: xenic cultivation, in which the ameba is grown in the presence of an undefined flora (mostly bacteria); monoxenic, in which the ameba is grown in the presence of another single species; and axenic, in which the ameba is grown in the absence of any other metabolizing cells. Stools are the main starting material for culture initiation, and in xenic cultures maintaining a balance between the requirements of the bacterial flora and the ameba is important.

Culture has poor diagnostic value because in humans several intestinal species of *Entamoeba* can be found that are sufficiently similar to cause diagnostic confusion, and all can grow in the same media. However, culture is an important research tool to grow amebae in large numbers to conduct other investigations. In addition, culture-derived isoenzyme analysis provided the first evidence that *E histolytica* comprised 2 separate species.[13]

## ISOENZYME ANALYSIS

Reeves and Bischoff[56] were the first investigators to use isoenzyme electrophoresis patterns to classify *Entamoeba* species. However, it was the seminal work of Sargeaunt and colleagues[13] that established the unique isoenzyme profiles (known as zymodemes) for *E histolytica* and *E dispar*. Four enzymes were used to profile their isoenzyme patterns, and isoenzyme analysis of cultured amebae was considered the gold standard for diagnosis of amebic infection before development of newer DNA-based techniques. However, a major disadvantage of isoenzyme analysis as a diagnostic method is that it depends on the growth of the amebae in culture, which is often unsuccessful.

## ANTIBODY DETECTION TESTS

Different serologic assays have been used to detect antibodies specific to *E histolytica*. Some of these tests developed using the crude antigens of *E histolytica* are commercially available. These tests showed greater than 90% sensitivity and specificity in various studies (reviewed by Fotedar and colleagues,[57] 2007). Serum antiamebic antibodies against *E histolytica* persist several years following an *E histolytica* infection.[58] In amebiasis-endemic countries, serologic tests are not useful for diagnostic purposes because of a high percentage of asymptomatic individuals already carrying antibodies specific to *E histolytica* and because the tests are unable to distinguish between a past and current infection.[2,41] However, amebic serologic tests are still useful in nonendemic countries where prior exposure to *E histolytica* is almost negligible.[59,60]

Recently Moss and colleagues[61] developed a high-throughput multiplex, bead-based serologic assay that can detect serologic response to multiple diarrhea-causing intestinal pathogens such as *Giardia intestinalis*, *Cryptosporidium parvum*, and *E histolytica*. However, there are still no serologic tests specific for other *Entamoeba* species such as *E moshkovskii* (an emerging pathogen), *E bangladeshi* (of unknown virulence), and *E dispar*.

## ANTIGEN DETECTION TESTS

Detection of amebic antigen directly in stool samples is a superior method to microscopy, culture, isoenzyme analysis, or antibody detection. It is more sensitive than microscopy or culture, less labor intensive than the isoenzyme analysis, and capable of detecting acute infections that serology cannot detect. Antigen detection enzyme-linked immunosorbent assay (ELISA) is a good diagnostic tool for resource-poor endemic countries because it is simple to perform, rapid, and does not require expertise or sophisticated instruments.

Several commercially available antigen detection ELISA tests are available for *E histolytica* and *E dispar* (**Table 3**). Some of the tests are specific for *E histolytica*, whereas others detect both *E histolytica* and *E dispar*. These tests showed 55% to 100% sensitivity, and 93% to 100% specificity compared with other established tests as detected in various different investigations (reviewed in Ref.[57]).

A major limitation of the current ELISA kits is that none of them works on formalin-fixed stool samples. In addition, several important ELISA tests are lacking. For example, no ELISA kits are available specifically to detect *E dispar*, *E moshkovskii*, or *E bangladeshi*. Since use of ELISA methods is more feasible than PCR in amebiasis-endemic, resource-poor nations, novel ELISAs are desirable that are capable of detecting each of the 4 morphologically identical *Entamoeba* species.

## POINT-OF-CARE TESTS

TechLab developed the first point-of-care (POC) test (popularly known as bedside tests, near-patient tests, and alternate-site tests) specific for *E histolytica* in 2006[62] based on the amebic adherence lectin. This test showed 97% sensitivity and

**Table 3**
**Commercially available antigen detection ELISA kits for diagnosis of *E histolytica***

| Name | Target | Ameba Specificity | Manufacturers | Detection Limit |
|---|---|---|---|---|
| TechLab *E histolytica* II | Gal/GalNac lectin | *E histolytica* | TechLab, Blacksburg, VA | 0.2–0.4 ng of lectin per well |
| Entamoeba CELISA-PATH | Gal/GalNac lectin | *E histolytica* | Cellabs Pty Ltd, Brookvale, Australia | 0.2–0.4 ng of lectin per well |
| Optimum S *E histolytica* antigen ELISA | SREHP | *E histolytica* | Merlin Diagnostika, Berheim-Hersel, Germany | Unknown |
| Triage parasite panel | 29-kDa surface antigen | *E histolytica/ E dispar*[a] | BIOSITE Diagnostics, San Diego, CA | Unknown |
| ProSpecT *E histolytica* microplate assay | EHSA | *E histolytica/ E dispar* | REMEL Inc, Lenexa, KS | 40 ng/mL of *E histolytica*–specific antigen |
| *E histolytica/ E dispar* | Unknown | *E histolytica/ E dispar* | IVD Research, Carlsbad, CA | Unknown |
| R-Biopharm Ridascreen Entamoeba test | Gal/GalNac lectin | *E histolytica/ E dispar* | Darmstadt, Germany | 17 *E histolytica* or 595 *E dispar* per well[b] |

*Abbreviations:* EHSA, *E histolytica*–specific antigen (targeted using polyclonal antibodies); SREHP, serine-rich *E histolytica* protein.
[a] The Triage parasite panel also detects *G lamblia* (target: alpha-1-giardin) and C. parvum (target: disulfide isomerase) in addition to *E histolytica/E dispar*.
[b] According to the manufacturer.

100% specificity compared with the standard *E histolytica* II ELISA antigen detection method (TechLab). However, compared with real-time PCR the POC test was approximately 80% sensitive. Verkerke and colleagues[63] evaluated the next-generation TechLab *E. HISTOLYTICA* QUIK CHEK POC test to detect amebic antigen in fecal samples from 2 independent study populations in South Africa and Bangladesh. They compared the performance of this POC test with the commercially available ProSpecT *E histolytica* microplate assay (Remel) and the *E histolytica* II ELISA (TechLab), using unfixed frozen stool samples. Compared with the *E histolytica* II ELISA, the *E. HISTOLYTICA* QUIK CHEK showed 98.0% sensitivity and 100% specificity. Compared with the ProSpecT microplate assay the *E. HISTOLYTICA* QUIK CHEK showed 97.0% sensitivity and 100% specificity. One major limitation of the existing POC tests is that they are all directed toward trophozoite-specific proteins. As a result, their efficacy in detecting *E histolytica* in stool specimens that contain only the cyst form of the parasite is not well established.

## POLYMERASE CHAIN REACTION–BASED DIAGNOSTIC TESTS

Since the formal separation of *E histolytica* (pathogenic *E histolytica*) from *E dispar* (nonpathogenic *E histolytica*) several PCR-based diagnostic tests have been developed. These tests have advantages compared with the other tests such as microscopy, culture, isoenzyme analysis, serology, and antigen detection. PCR-based assays are highly sensitive, and some of these tests can detect as little as a single ameba in clinical specimens. Several PCR-based tests are specific at the species level. However, one major limitation is that these PCR-based assays are still mostly limited to research laboratories and clinical laboratories in developed countries because the facilities to conduct DNA-based tests are lacking in resource-limited countries.

For *E histolytica*, DNA has been extracted from axenic and xenic cultures, stools, liver aspirated pus, blood, tissue, saliva, urine, and formalin-preserved biopsy or autopsy samples. For the most part, extraction of DNA from axenic and xenic cultures of *Entamoeba* species is not a problem because of the presence of high number of organisms and largely inhibitor-free environment. As a result, almost any DNA extraction protocol works with the cultured organisms.

## STOOL SAMPLES

Stool is the predominant specimen type for the diagnosis of intestinal amebiasis. Although easily obtainable, stool samples are among the most complex biological samples for PCR diagnosis for 2 main reasons. First, amebae may not be excreted in every stool of the infected individual, requiring checking of at least 3 consecutive stools. Second, PCR inhibitors may be present in stool samples and are generally copurified during extraction if additional steps are not implemented. Optimization of DNA extraction is therefore a crucial first step to achieve success in PCR.

Other challenges associated with stool samples include storage and transportation of stools. Although the cyst form of the parasite is stable, the trophozoite form is not and may disintegrate rapidly outside the host environment. If only the trophozoite form is excreted in the stool, the processing of a sample should begin almost immediately (or within an hour or so of production) or stools should be stored appropriately. If only the cyst form is excreted in the stool, which may be the case for most asymptomatically infected individuals, appropriate steps should be included in the DNA extraction procedure to break open the rigid cyst wall of the parasite. This process is usually achieved by (1) freezing (at $-20°C$ or lower temperature) and thawing of stool samples multiple times in presence of protease inhibitors, (2) enzymatic degradation of the cyst wall, or (3) using commercial kits such as the QIAamp Stool DNA Mini Kit.[64]

## DNA EXTRACTION

Several DNA extraction kits are now available commercially that offer isolation of PCR-quality pathogen DNA directly from stool samples. In amebiasis, the most widely and successfully used method is the QIAamp Stool DNA Mini Kit (Qiagen).[65–71] The extraction procedure is rapid and can be performed within 2 to 3 hours. However, several groups have reported further improvement of the QIAamp DNA extraction procedure. Kebede and colleagues[72] prewashed stools with phosphate-buffered saline, resuspended in polyvinylpolypyrrolidone, heated, and then treated with proteinase-K before processing with the Qiagen kit. Pinar and colleagues[73] described an improvement of the QIAamp DNA extraction procedure for isolation of DNA before real-time PCR by including an overnight incubation step with proteinase K and sodium dodecyl sulfate. The modification led to a 3-log improvement of the detection limit from 5000 copies/mL to only 5 copies/mL of target DNAs in the starting stool sample. Cnops and Esbroeck[74] showed that freezing of stool samples before DNA extraction improves the real-time PCR detection. Other commercially available kits are XTRAX DNA extraction kit (Gull Laboratories, Salt Lake City, UT),[65] the Extract MasterFaecal DNA extraction kit (Epicenter Biotechnologies, Madison, WI), and the Genomic DNA Prep Plus kit (A&A Biotechnology, Poland).[75]

Recently, the extraction of DNA from stool samples using the QIAamp DNA Stool Mini Kit has been automated on the QIAcube machine from the same manufacturer. However, the high price of this machine and associated maintenance costs prevent its use in amebiasis-endemic resource-poor countries. There are several other automated DNA isolation systems available. However, it seems that none of the automated systems have yet been used for *Entamoeba* DNA isolation.

## CONVENTIONAL POLYMERASE CHAIN REACTION

In 1992, at least 3 groups independently developed and used PCR for the detection of *E histolytica*.[76–78] Romero and colleagues[76] used repetitive sequences to detect and differentiate between *E histolytica* and *E dispar* using DNA from reference culture organisms. The PCR products were verified using nonradioactive probes. The PCR results showed excellent correlation with the isoenzyme data. Cruz-Reyes and colleagues[78] used ribosomal gene sequences in their PCR and probes to detect and differentiate between *E histolytica* and *E dispar*, again using DNA from cultured organisms. Tachibana and colleagues[77] were the first to use PCR on amebic liver abscess (ALA) pus fluid, using primers specific for a gene encoding a 30-kDa protein of *E histolytica*.

Acuna-Soto and colleagues[79] first used PCR in epidemiologic studies. They studied 201 randomly selected formalin-fixed stool samples from people living in a rural community in Mexico, of which 25 (12%) were microscopically positive for *E histolytica*. PCR positively detected 21 of the 25 microscope-positive samples, plus an additional 3 microscope-negative samples. According to PCR results, 14 individuals were infected with both species, 9 with *E histolytica*, and the remaining individual was infected with *E dispar*. Later, Rivera and colleagues[80] developed a simple and rapid DNA isolation method for formalin-fixed stool specimens and applied it to a panel of 72 randomly selected stool samples from the Philippines. In sharp contrast with the data of Acuna-Soto and colleagues[79] in Mexico, Rivera and colleagues[80] found that 19 of their samples were positive by PCR, and all of these were *E dispar*. These two data sets showed the first molecular-based evidence that variation in the prevalence of *E histolytica* and *E dispar* exists between different geographic areas.

Ali and colleagues[9] first developed a nested PCR based on SSU ribosomal DNA (rDNA) sequence of *E moshkovskii* to detect this organism directly on the stool DNA. The identity of the amplified products was verified using restriction endonuclease digestion. Using this PCR it was shown for the first time that *E moshkovskii* was highly prevalent in children in Mirpur, Bangladesh. Before this study *E moshkovskii* was considered primarily to be a free-living ameba. The same PCR was used to detect *E moshkovskii* in human infections in other countries.

A list of different PCRs used in the detection of *E histolytica*, *E dispar*, and *E moshkovskii* is provided in **Table 4**.

## *Real-time Polymerase Chain Reaction*

The first development and use of a real-time PCR for *E histolytica* detection was by Blessmann and colleagues.[81] They used LightCycler probes for detection of *E histolytica* and *E dispar*, and incorporated a touch-down PCR strategy to increase the specificity. The PCR had a detection limit of 0.1 cells per gram of feces for both *E histolytica* and *E dispar*. Since then there have been at least 31 additional reports (up to December 31, 2014) using a real-time PCR for detection of *E histolytica*. These real-time PCRs used primers (and probes) that are located almost exclusively in the SSU rDNA genes of the *Entamoeba* species. The most widely used real-time PCR was TaqMan. Some of the real-time PCRs targeted only *E histolytica*, or *E histolytica* plus *E dispar*. However, since the recognition of the high prevalence of *E moshkovskii* in humans, 2 real-time PCRs have been developed to detect *E histolytica*, *E dispar*, and *E moshkovskii* in stool specimens.[30,31] There is currently no real-time PCR to detect *E bangladeshi*.

In 2004, Verweij and colleagues[82] developed a TaqMan real-time PCR for simultaneous detection of *E histolytica* and 2 other diarrhea-causing parasites, *Cryptosporidium* and *Giardia* species. The triplex PCR to detect *E histolytica*, *Cryptosporidium*, and *Giardia* species has also been used by several other groups.[83–86] It is also commercially available in kit format (Fast-Track Diagnostics Ltd, Malta). Nazeer and colleagues[87] added *E dispar* to the panel of diarrhea-causing pathogens and developed a new tetraplex TaqMan real-time PCR. This PCR may prove helpful in finding any association of *E dispar* with the diarrhea or dysentery in the infected individuals. In addition, 5-plex or even 8-plex real-time PCRs are now available for detection of intestinal pathogens, including *E histolytica*. These multiplex PCRs showed excellent sensitivity and specificity for the detection of *E histolytica* in stool samples.

Recently, Stark and colleagues[88] evaluated a commercially available EasyScreen enteric parasite detection real-time PCR kit (Genetic Signatures, Sydney, Australia) for the detection of *Entamoeba* spp, *Blastocystis* spp, *Cryptosporidium* spp, *Dientamoeba fragilis*, and *G intestinalis* from clinical stool samples. The kit was rapid, and showed 92% to 100% sensitivity and 100% specificity in detecting these 5 clinically important human parasites compared with individual PCRs. However, one major limitation of this kit is that it uses a broad-spectrum *Entamoeba* primer that does not differentiate between pathogenic and nonpathogenic *Entamoeba* species.

A list of real-time PCRs used in the detection of *E histolytica*, *E dispar*, and *E moshkovskii* with primer and probe sequences is provided in **Table 5**.

**Table 4**
Primers used for conventional PCR for E histolytica, E dispar, and E moshkovskii

| PCR Assay | Gene Target or Name[a] | Primer Name | Primer Sequence (5'→3') | References[b] |
|---|---|---|---|---|
| Singleplex | M17 | P1-S17[c] | GCAACTAGTGTAGTTA | Gomes et al, 1999; Tannich and Burchard, 1991; Zaman et al, 2000 |
| | | P1-AS20[c] | CCTCCAAGATATGTTTAAC | |
| | 30-kDa protein | P11[c] | GGAGGAGTAGGAAAGTTGAC | Haghighi et al, 2002; Myjak et al, 2000; Pinheiro et al, 2004; Rivera et al, 2006; Rivera et al, 1998; Rivera et al, 1996; Sanuki et al, 1997; Tachibana et al, 2001; Tachibana et al, 2000; Tachibana et al, 1992; Tachibana et al, 1991; Zaman et al, 2000; Zindrou et al, 2001; Dagci et al; 2007 |
| | | P12[c] | TTCTTGCAATTCCTGCTTCGA | |
| | | P13[d] | AGGAGGAGTAGGAAAATTAGG | |
| | | P14[d] | TTCTTGAAACTCCTGTTTCTAC | |
| | DNA highly repetitive sequences | EHP1[c] | TCAAAATGGTCGTCGTCTAGGC | Romero et al, 1992 |
| | | EHP2[c] | CAGTTAGAAATTATTGTACTTTGTA | |
| | | EHNP1[d] | GGATCCTCCAAAAAATAAAGT | |
| | | EHNP2[d] | CCACAGAACGATATTGGATACC | |
| | SSU rRNA | Psp F[c] | GGCCAATTCATTCAATGAATTGAG | Clark and Diamond, 1992; Lebbad and Svard, 2005; Leiva et al, 2006; Moran et al, 2005; Moran et al, 2005; Myjak et al, 1997; Myjak et al, 2000; Ramos et al, 2005; Ramos et al, 2000; Verweij et al, 2000 |
| | | Psp R[c] | CTCAGATCTAGAAACAATGCTTCTC | |
| | | NPspF[d] | GGCCAATTTATGTAAGTAAATTGAG | |
| | | NPspR[d] | CTTGGATTTAGAAACAATGTTTCTTC | |
| | | P1[c] | TCAAAATGGTCGTCGTCTAGGC | Acuna-Soto et al, 1993; Aguirre et al, 1995; Britten et al, 1997; Zaman et al, 2000 |
| | | P2[c] | CAGTTAGAAATTATTGTACTTTGTA | |
| | | NP1[d] | GGATCCTCCAAAAAATAAAGTT | |
| | | NP2[d] | ATGATCATAGGTTATAGCAAGACA | |
| | | RD5[e] | GGAAGCTTATCTGGTTGATCCTGCCAGTA | Ramos et al, 2005; Zaman et al, 2000 |
| | | RD3[e] | GGGATCCTGATCCTTCCGCAGGTTCACCTAC | |
| | | Eh5[c] | GTACAAATGGCCAATTCATCAATG | Heckendorn et al, 2002; Troll et al, 1997; Fotedar et al, 2007; Stark et al, 2008 |
| | | Eh3[c] | CTCAGATCTAGAAACAATGCTTCTCT | |
| | | Ed5[d] | GTACAAAGTGGCCAATTTATGTAAGT | |
| | | Ed5[d] | ACTTGGATTTAGAAACAATGTTTCTTC | |
| | | EH1[c] | GTACAAAATGGCCAATTCATTCAATG | Gonin and Trudel, 2003; Ben Ayed et al, 2008 |
| | | ED1[d] | TACAAAGTGGCCAATTTATGTAAGTA | |
| | | EHD2[e] | ACTACCAACTGATTGATAGATCAG | |
| | Hemolysin gene (HLY6) LSU rRNA | EH6F[c] | GACCTCTCCAATATCCTGT | Zindrou et al, 2001 |
| | | Eh6R[c] | GCAGAGAAGTACTGTGAAGG | |
| | 30-kDa protein | HF[e] | AAGAAATTGATATTAATGAATATA | Hooshyar et al, 2004 |
| | | HR[e] | ATCTTCCAATTCCATCATCAT | |

| | Gene | Primer | Sequence | References |
|---|---|---|---|---|
| **Duplex** | Cysteine proteinase | Ehcp6F[c] | GTTGCTGCTGAAGAAACTTG | Freitas et al, 2004 |
| | | Ehcp6R[c] | GTACCATAACCAACTACTGC | |
| | Actin gene | Act3F[e] | GGGACGATATGGAAAAGATC | |
| | | Act5R[e] | CAAGTCTAAGAATAGCA TGTG | |
| **Nested** | SSU rRNA | EH1[c] | GTACAAAATGGCCAATTCATTCAATG | Calderaro et al, 2006; Gonin and Trudel, 2003; Zeyrek et al, 2013 |
| | | ED1[d] | TACAAAGTGGCCAATTTATGTAAGTA | |
| | | EHD 2[e] | ACTACCAACTGATTGATAGATCAG | |
| | SSU rRNA | EH-1[e] | TTTGTATTAGTACAAA | Ayeh-Kumi et al, 2001; Haque et al, 1998; Katzwinkel-Wladarsch et al, 1994; Zaman et al, 2000; Zindrou et al, 2001; Beck et al, 2008; Khairnar et al, 2007; Azian et al, 2006; Samie et al, 2006 |
| | | EH-2[e] | GTA(A/G)TATTGATATACT | |
| | | EHP-1[c] | AATGGCCAATTCATTCAATG | |
| | | EHP-2[c] | TCTAGAAACAATGCTTCTCT | |
| | | EHN-1[d] | AGTGGCCAATTTATGTAAGT | |
| | | EHN-2[d] | TTTAGAAACAATGTTTCTTC | |
| | SSU rRNA | E1[e] | TGCTGTGATTAAAAGCT | Evangelopoulos et al, 2000; Evangelopoulos et al, 2001; Paglia and Visca, 2004; Goni et al, 2012 |
| | | E2[e] | TTAACTATTTCAATCTCGG | |
| | | Eh-L[c] | ACATTTTGAAGACTTTATGTAAGTA | |
| | | Eh-R[c] | CAGATCTAGAAACAATGCTTCTCT | |
| | | Ed-L[d] | GTTAGTTATCTAATTTCGATTAGAA | |
| | | Ed-R[d] | ACACCACTACTATCCCTACC | |
| | SSU rRNA | Outer 1F[e] | GAAATTCAGATGTACAAAGA | Hung et al, 2005 |
| | | Outer 1R[e] | CAGAATCCTAGAATTTCAC | |
| | | Eh1[c] | AAGCATTGTTCTAGATCTG | |
| | | Eh2[c] | CACGTTAAAAGAGGTCTAAC | |
| | | Ed1[d] | AAACATTGTTTCTAAATCCA | |
| | | Ed2[d] | ACCACTTACTATCCCTACC | |
| | SSU rRNA | Em-1[f] | CTCTTCACGGGAGTGCG | Ali et al, 2003; Fotedar et al, 2007/8?; Parija and Khairnar, 2005; Solaymani-Mohammadi et al, 2006; Beck et al, 2008; Stark et al, 2008; Khairnar et al, 2007 |
| | | Em-2[f] | TCGTTAGTTTCATTACCT | |
| | | nEm-1[f] | GAATAAGGATGGTATGAC | |
| | | nEm-2[f] | AAGTGGAGTTAACCACCT | |

(continued on next page)

**Table 4**
*(continued)*

| PCR Assay | Gene Target or Name[a] | Primer Name | Primer Sequence (5'→3') | References[b] |
|---|---|---|---|---|
| Multiplex | SSU rRNA | EntaF[g] | ATGCACGAGAGCGAAAGCAT | Hamzah et al, 2006; Sharbatkhori et al, 2014; Kheirandish et al, 2011, Nazemalhosseini et al, 2010; Hawash 2014; Lopez et al, 2012; Nazemalhosseini et al, 2010 |
| | | EhR[c] | GATCTAGAAACAATGCTTCTCT | |
| | | EdR[d] | CACCACTTACTATCCCTACC | |
| | | EmR[f] | TGACCGGAGCCAGAGACAT | |
| | SSU rRNA | EhP1[c] | CGATTTCCCAGTTAGAAATTA | Nunez et al, 2001; Gomes et al, 2014; Santos et al, 2007 |
| | | EhP2[c] | CAAAATGGTCGTCGTCTAGGC | |
| | | EdP1[d] | ATGGTGAGGTTGTAGCAGAGA | |
| | | EdP2[d] | CGATATTGGATACCTAGTACT | |
| | SSU rRNA | EH-1[c] | AAGCATTGTTTCTAGATCTGAG | Khairnar and Parija, 2007; Parija and Khairnar, 2007; Ngui et al, 2012; Yakoob et al, 2012 |
| | | EH-2[c] | AAGAGGTCTAACCGAAATTAG | |
| | | Mos-1[f] | GAAACCAAGAGTTCACAAC | |
| | | Mos-2[f] | CAATATAAGGCTTGGATGAT | |
| | | ED-1[d] | TCTAATTTCGATTAGAACTCT | |
| | | ED-2[d] | TCCCTACCTATTAGACATAGC | |
| | SSU rRNA | Eg-SS-F1[g] | TGTGATTAAAACGCTCGTAGTTGAA | Foo et al, 2012 |
| | | Eg-SS-CR1[g] | CTCGTTCGTTACCGGAATTAACC | |
| | | Eh-SS-F1[c] | GAAGCATTGTTTCTAGATCTGA | |
| | | Ed-SS-F7[d] | AATGCTGAGGAGATGTCAGTT | |
| | SSU rRNA | P1 5'[c] | ATGCACGAGAGCGAAAGCAT | Singh et al, 2011 |
| | | P2 5'[c] | GATCTAGAAACAATGCTTCTCT | |
| | SSU rRNA | E1[e] | TAGGATGAAACTGCGGACGGT | Intarapuk et al, 2009 |
| | | E2[e] | AGCCTTGTGACCATACTCCC | |
| | SSU rRNA | Ehf[c] | AACAGTAATAGTTTCTTGGTTAGTAAAA | Solaymani-Mohammadi et al, 2008; Solaymani-Mohammadi et al, 2007 |
| | | Ehr[c] | CTTAGAATGTCATTTCTCAATTCAT | |

*Abbreviation:* LSU, large subunit.

[a] For simplicity, primers to amplify polymorphic genes (eg, SREHP, chitinase, and transfer RNA array-linked short tandem repeat loci) used by some investigators were not included in this table.

[b] Because of space limitations most of these references were not added to the Reference list, except for some that have been discussed in the relevant parts of the article, and referenced appropriately.

[c] Specific for *E histolytica*.

[d] Specific for *E dispar*.

[e] Common for *E histolytica* and *E dispar*.

[f] Specific for *E moshkovskii*.

[g] *Entamoeba* species broad-spectrum.

**Table 5**
**Real-time PCR primer and probe information**

| Assay Type | Gene Target[a] | Primer or Probe | Sequence (5'→3') | References[b] |
|---|---|---|---|---|
| LightCycler | SSU rDNA | Eh-S26C[c] | GTACAAAATGGCCAATTCATTCAACG | Blessmann et al, 2002, Calderaro et al, 2006, Qvarnstrom et al, 2005; Vianna et al, 2009 |
| | | Ed-27 C[d] | GTACAAAGTGGCCAATTATGTAAGCA | |
| | | Eh-Ed-AS25[e] | GAATTGATTTTACTCAACTCTAGAG | |
| | | Eh/Ed-24LC-Red 640[e] | LC-Red-640-TCGAACCCCAATTCCTCGTTATCCp | |
| | | Eh-Ed-25-F[e] | FL-GCCATCTGTAAAGCTCCCTCCGAX | |
| TaqMan | SSU rDNA | Eh-d-239F[c] | ATTGTCGTGGCATCCTAACTCA | Kebede et al, 2004, Qvarnstrom et al, 2005, Verweij et al, 2004, Verweij et al, 2003; Frickmann et al, 2013; Stark et al, 2014; Wessels et al, 2014; Hartmeyer et al, 2013; Nazeer et al, 2013; Gutiérrez-Cisneros et al, 2010; Cnops and Esbroeck 2010; Bruijnesteijn van Coppenraet et al, 2009; ten Hove et al, 2009; ten Hove et al, 2007 |
| | | Ehd-88R[d] | GCGGACGGCTCATTATAACA | |
| | | Histolytica-96T[c] | VIC-TCATTGAATGAATTGGCCATTT-MGB (nonfluorescent quencher) | |
| | | Dispar-96T[d] | FAM-TTACTTACCATAAAATTGGCCACTTTG-nonfluorescent quencher | |
| TaqMan | SSU rDNA | Eh-196F[c] | AAATGGCCAATTCATTCAATGA | Desoubeaux et al, 2014 |
| | | Eh-294R[c] | CATTGGTTACTTGTTAAACACTGTGTG | |
| | | Eh-245[c] | FAM-AGGATGCCACGACAA-NFQ | |
| TaqMan (duplex) | SSU rDNA | Ehd-239F[e] | ATTGTCGTGGCATCCTAACTCA | Verweij et al, 2004/2003; Visser et al, 2006; Frickmann et al, 2013; Stark et al, 2014; Stark et al, 2011 |
| | | Ehd-88R[e] | GCGGACGGCTCATTATAACA | |
| | | Histolytica-96T[c] | VIC-TCATTGAATGAATTGGCCATTT- nonfluorescent quencher | |
| | | dispar-96T[d] | FAM-TTA CTT ACA TAA ATT GGC CAC TTTG-nonfluorescent quencher | |
| SYBER green | SSU rDNA | PSP5[c] | GGCCAATTCATTCAATGAATTGAG | Qvarnstrom et al, 2005 |
| | | PSP3[c] | CTCAGATCTAGAAACAATGCTTCTC | |
| | | NPSP5[d] | GGCCAATTTATGTAAGTAAATTGAG | |
| | | NPSP3[d] | CTTGGATTTAGAAACAATGTTTCTTC | |

(continued on next page)

**Table 5 (continued)**

| Assay Type | Gene Target[a] | Primer or Probe | Sequence (5′→3′) | References[b] |
|---|---|---|---|---|
| Molecular beacon | SSU rDNA | Ehf[c] | AACAGTAATAGTTTCTTTGGTTAGTAAAA | Roy et al, 2005 |
| | | Ehr[c] | CTTAGAAATGTCATTTCTCAATTCAT | |
| | | Molecular beacon probe[c] | Texas Red-GCGAGC-ATTAGTACAAAATGGCCAATTCATTCA-GCTCGC-dR Elle | |
| LightCycler (multiplex real-time PCR) | SSU rDNA | EhdmF[f] | CGAAAGCATTTCACTCAACTG | Hamzah et al, 2010 |
| | | EhdmR[f] | TCCCCCTGAAGTCCATAAACTC | |
| | | Ehdm-FL[f] | 5′FluoresceinLabel-ACT ATA AAC gAT gTC AAC CAA ggA TTg gAT gAAA-FITC-3′ | |
| | | Ehd-640[e] | 5′LCRed640-TCA gAT gTA CAA AgA TAg AgA AgT ATT gTT TCTA-phosphate-3′ | |
| | | Em-705[g] | 5′LCRed705-AAg AAA TTC gCg gAT gAA gAA ACA TTg TTT-phosphate-3′ | |
| TaqMan | SSU rDNA | Eh-f[c] | AACAGTAATAGTTTCTTTGGTTAGTAAAA | Haque et al, 2010 |
| | | Eh-r[c] | CTTAGAAATGTCATTTCTCAATTCAT | |
| | | Eh-YYT[c] | 5′YYT-ATT AGT ACA AAC TGG CCA ATT CAT TCA-Eclipse3′ | |
| TaqMan | SREPH gene | Histolytica-50F[c] | CATTAAAAATGGTGAGGTTCTTAGGAA | Qvarnstrom et al, 2005, Verweij et al, 2003, Verweij et al, 2003 |
| | | Histolytica-132R[c] | TGGTCGTCTAGGCAAAATATT | |
| | | Histolytica-78T[c] | FAM-TTGACCAATTACACCGTTGATTTTCGGA-Eclipse Dark quencher | |
| | | Dispar-1F[d] | GGATCCTCCAAAAAATAAAGTTTATCA | |
| | | Dispar-137R[d] | ATCACAGAACGATATTGGATACCTAGTA | |
| | | Dispar-33[d] | HEX-UGGUGAGGUUGUAGCAGAGAUAUUAAAU-TAMRA | |

| Multiplex SYBR Green | Tandem repeats in extrachromosomal circular rDNA | EhP1[c] EhP2[c] EdP1[d] EdP2[d] | CGATTTCCCAGTTAGAAATTA CAAAATGGTCGTCGTCTAGGC ATGGTGAGGTTGTAGCAGAGA CGATATTGGATACCTAGTACT | Gomes et al, 2014 |
|---|---|---|---|---|
| Multiplex tandem real-time PCR | Pxr[a] | Not available | Not available | Stark et al, 2011 |
| Artus (Hamburg, Germany) real-time LC-PCR kit[h] | Unknown[a] | Not available | Not available | Furrows et al, 2004 |

*Abbreviation:* LC, LightCycler.

[a] Gene target is not disclosed because of licensing issues.
[b] Because of space limitations most of these references were not added to the Reference list except for some that have been discussed in the relevant sections of the article, and referenced appropriately.
[c] Specific for *E histolytica.*
[d] Specific for *E dispar.*
[e] Common for *E histolytica* and *E dispar.*
[f] Common for *E histolytica, E dispar,* and *E moshkovskii.*
[g] Specific for *E moshkovskii.*
[h] Discontinued.

## COMPARISON OF DIAGNOSTIC METHODS

Several studies have used more than 1 diagnostic tool to detect entamoeba infections and compared their efficiencies with each other. Some of these study findings have already been mentioned, whereas others are briefly discussed later.

Qvarnstrom and colleagues[89] compared 3 real-time PCRs for *E histolytica* and *E dispar* based on SSU rRNA gene sequences (one was an SYBR Green real-time PCR and the others were TaqMan real-time PCRs). They used ameba-spiked stools and a modified FastDNA method (Q-Biogene, CA) for isolation of DNA followed by removal of potential PCR inhibitors using the QIAquick PCR purification kit (Qiagen, CA). The SYBR Green real-time PCR, which had a target amplification size of 877 bp for *E histolytica* and 878 bp for *E dispar*, showed an average detection limit of 17 amebae per milliliter of stool compared with 119 amebae per milliliter for corresponding conventional PCR. Both LightCycler real-time PCR (target amplification sizes 307 bp for *E histolytica* and 231 bp for *E dispar*), and TaqMan real-time PCR (target amplification sizes 231 bp for both *E histolytica* and *E dispar*) showed a detection limit of fewer than 5 amebae per milliliter of stool. However, the LightCycler real-time PCR was more expensive than the TaqMan, and also LightCycler seemed to give an *E dispar* false-positive signal even with the cultured *E histolytica* DNA, suggesting that the TaqMan real-time PCR was superior to the others for diagnostic purposes.

Visser and colleagues[90] compared the TechLab *Entamoeba* (designed to detect both *E histolytica* and *E dispar* antigen) and *E histolytica* II (designed to detect *E histolytica* specifically) tests with a TaqMan real-time PCR[91] using clinical samples from the Netherlands and Belgium. Compared with real-time PCR, the TechLab *Entamoeba* and the *E histolytica* II tests showed only 59% and 71% sensitivities, but 98% and 100% specificities, respectively. The investigators concluded that, in nonendemic countries, the TechLab ELISA tests were not suitable because of poor sensitivities. In contrast, Solaymani-Mohammadi and colleagues[92] found that the TechLab *E histolytica* II ELISA showed 100% correlation in detecting *E histolytica* in Iranian asymptomatic cyst passers compared with an SSU rDNA-based nested PCR.

Beck and colleagues[26] used an SSU rDNA-based PCR and the TechLab antigen detection ELISA to detect *E histolytica*, *E dispar*, and *E moshkovskii* infections in patients from Tanzania suspected or positive for human immunodeficiency virus (HIV). The PCR and ELISA results revealed that *E histolytica* was present in 4% (5 of 118) by ELISA, whereas *E dispar* and *E moshkovskii* were each detected by PCR in 13% (18 of 136) of individuals. However, neither *E moshkovskii* nor *E dispar* infections showed any association with the diarrheal status of the patients.

Overall, conventional or real-time PCRs perform better than antigen detection ELISA tests. Multiple pathogens can be detected in PCR assays with species-level specificity. PCR assays are more sensitive and specific than antigen detection ELISA tests. However, there are several potential limitations for PCR becoming readily available in resource-poor nations where amebiasis is endemic. For example, (1) the PCR instrument, its maintenance, and the reagent costs are high; (2) PCR laboratory setup requires substantially more space than an ELISA assay; (3) PCR assays require expertise to run, troubleshoot, and interpret the data; and (4) conventional PCR is highly prone to contamination.

## RECENT ADVANCEMENT IN THE *ENTAMOEBA HISTOLYTICA* DIAGNOSIS

Several novel techniques have been developed recently for the diagnosis of *E histolytica*. Some of the most promising ones are briefly discussed here.

## SINGLE-CHAIN FRAGMENT-VARIABLE PROBES

The single-chain fragment-variable (scFv) proteins are antibodylike molecules that can be expressed on the surface of *Saccharomyces cerevisiae*. An advanced antigen detection assay has been developed for *E histolytica* using whole yeast cells expressing scFv,[93] which could detect as little as 310 pM cognate cyst antigen, which was comparable with the sensitivity of a monoclonal antibody (mAb)–based ELISA. However, the whole-cell yeast scFv molecules are insoluble, often too large for diagnostic application, and they need a labeled secondary antibody to detect the specific antigen. Recently, the same group of investigators further improved the system by using a cell-wall fragments of selected scFv clones,[94] and then made it a label-free antigen detection system.[95] This method is rapid and far more cost-effective than that of mAb production in mice, and shows promise as an effective alternative to traditional mAbs.

## LUMINEX ASSAY

Luminex is a high-throughput bead-based multiplex system in which beads are internally labeled with fluorescent dyes to produce a specific spectral identifier. In DNA-based Luminex assays, oligonucleotides are conjugated to the surface of beads to capture pathogen DNA amplified during PCR. The Luminex technology enables up to 500 proteins or DNA sequences to be detected in a single assay using very small sample volumes.

In 2011, Taniuchi and colleagues[85] first developed a Luminex-based assay to simultaneously detect several major intestinal parasites, including *E histolytica* The Luminex protozoa assay showed a limit of detection of 10 *E histolytica* trophozoites in 200 mg of stool, identical to that of the parent real-time PCR assays. Another group reported successful development of a Luminex test for simultaneous detection of 5 intestinal parasites: *E histolytica*, *E dispar*, *E moshkovskii*, *E coli*, and *E hartmanni*.[96] Wessels and colleagues[97] developed a multiplex Luminex Gastrointestinal Pathogen Panel (xTAG GPP) capable of detecting 15 of the most common gastrointestinal pathogens or toxins, including *E histolytica*. The advantage of the Luminex method is that it provides a sensitive diagnostic screen for a large panel of pathogens simultaneously. However, a major limitation of this method is that it requires sophisticated instruments that are most often absent in amebiasis-endemic countries, limiting its use to research laboratories.

## LOOP-MEDIATED ISOTHERMAL AMPLIFICATION

Loop-mediated isothermal amplification (LAMP) is a single-tube technique for the amplification of DNA using a constant temperature.[98] During LAMP amplification, an increasing quantity of magnesium pyrophosphate is produced in solution as the reaction proceeds as a byproduct of amplification. Detection of amplification product can be determined via photometry for turbidity caused by increased magnesium pyrophosphate, and can be seen with the naked eye. Moreover, SYBR Green dye may be used to detect the amplification products. Also, in-tube detection of DNA amplification has been possible using manganese-loaded calcein, which starts fluorescing on conjugation of manganese and pyrophosphate during DNA synthesis.[99] Real-time detection has also been possible using intercalating dyes such as SYTO 9.[100]

The major advantages of LAMP are its simplicity and low cost. In LAMP, the target sequence is amplified using multiple sets of different primers to identify distinct regions on the target gene, which adds high specificity. A major disadvantage of LAMP is its lower versatility because the amplification products are generally not suitable for cloning or other molecular biology applications that are generally possible with PCR. Liang and colleagues[101] developed a LAMP assay for E histolytica, and compared its performance with that of a nested PCR based on the SSU rRNA gene of E histolytica. Both tests could detect as little as 1 ameba per reaction using culture DNA. In general, a LAMP assay has some added advantages compared with a traditional PCR assay. For example, it is (1) rapid, (2) simple, (3) sensitive, (4) specific, (5) more cost-effective, and (6) it does not require postamplification manipulation to detect the end results, which minimizes contamination issues.

## TAQMAN ARRAY CARD

Life Technologies developed a high-throughput TaqMan Array Card (TAC) platform enabling spatial multiplexing of up to 384 targets to perform simultaneous real-time PCR reactions without the need for robots or multichannel pipettors to load samples. Liu and colleagues[102] used the TAC platform for simultaneous detection of 19 of the most common diarrhea-causing enteropathogens: 5 viruses, 9 bacteria, and 5 parasites, including E histolytica. The accuracy of TAC was evaluated using 109 clinical stool specimens from Haydon, Tanzania, and from Mirpur, Bangladesh. Compared with the DNA-Luminex assays[85] TAC displayed 98% sensitivity and 96% specificity for E histolytica. Overall, TAC has a shorter turnaround time than conventional PCR; it is accurate, and it allows quantitative detection of multiple pathogens. TAC is thus well suited for surveillance or clinical investigations. One major limitation of TAC is that repeat assays are expensive because all the targets in the card must be run even though only a few targets need further investigation. In addition, TAC is not feasible in resource-poor developing countries because of the expensive setup and maintenance costs.

## BROAD-SPECTRUM ENTAMOEBA POLYMERASE CHAIN REACTION COUPLED WITH PYROSEQUENCING

Stensvold and colleagues[103] developed a new tool using a single-round PCR coupled to pyrosequencing for the detection and differentiation of members of the Entamoeba complex. The single-round PCR before pyrosequencing was designed to amplify a 252-bp region of E histolytica, E dispar, and E moshkovskii containing species-specific single-nucleotide polymorphisms to be detected by pyrosequencing for speciation. The results of this new technique on 102 stool-derived DNA samples from patients screened for enteric parasites from Sweden, Denmark, and the Netherlands were compared with those of a duplex real-time PCR for detection of E histolytica and E dispar, and a conventional PCR for detection of E moshkovskii. No E moshkovskii was detected by pyrosequencing, but 1 sample was positive by conventional PCR. Other than this, pyrosequencing, real-time PCR, and conventional PCR showed complete agreement in detection of 17 E histolytica, 86 E dispar, and 1 mixed infection with both species in those stool samples. The new technique has the potential to detect novel species of Entamoeba directly in stool-derived DNA without prior need of cultivation.

## SUMMARY AND FUTURE DIRECTION

There is a pressing need for newer diagnostic test options to replace the ova and parasite examination. Such tests should preferably detect most, if not all, pathogens commonly identified microscopically. Multiplexed PCR has the potential to meet this need. However, only 1 such assay has been approved by the US Food and

Drug Administration to date: the highly multiplexed Luminex xTAG GPP, which detects *Giardia* and *Cryptosporidium* in addition to numerous bacterial and viral targets. Such molecular assays, depending on their design, may require a laboratory with proficiency in molecular testing, which would limit their use to major academic hospitals and reference laboratories. Alternatively, sample-to-answer solutions, which provide direct diagnosis from unprocessed samples, such as the BioFire Diagnostics FilmArray platform, could be used in virtually any laboratory setting.

For the detection of intestinal amebae, several crucial tools are lacking. Existing antigen detection ELISA tests have been designed to detect proteins expressed predominantly in the trophozoite form of *E histolytica*. Because cysts are the predominant form of the parasite excreted in asymptomatically infected individuals, cyst-directed or stage-neutral tests (ie, tests that work for both stages) are needed. Some of the TechLab *E histolytica* II ELISA failures could be caused by the presence of only (or predominantly) the cyst form of the parasite in the samples tested because the TechLab *E histolytica* II ELISA detects lectin antigen expressed predominantly in the trophozoite surface.

No species-specific exclusive antigen detection ELISA or POC tests are currently available to detect *E dispar*, *E moshkovskii*, or *E bangladeshi*. Development of these tests is important to understand the epidemiology and pathogenicity of these amebae. Also, simple ELISA or POC tests, as opposed to PCRs, are more feasible in the resource-poor countries where these amebae are generally thought to be endemic. Furthermore, the cost of development of these tests could be substantially reduced if clinicians could use yeast-scFv affinity reagents as opposed to expensive and time-consuming monoclonal antibodies.

Highly multiplex Luminex assays may prove useful in detecting multiple pathogens, but mostly in the research or diagnostic laboratories in resource-rich countries. An alternative to conventional or real-time PCR would be the LAMP assay for resource-poor countries.

Although there is no controversy surrounding the pathogenicity of *E histolytica*, some genotypes seem to be more virulent than others. Some genotypes even seem to be associated with the asymptomatic status of infected individuals.[104] However, reliable methods to classify *E histolytica* genotypes according to their virulence do not exist. As a result, it remains unclear why ~90% of *E histolytica* infections remain asymptomatic. If carefully conducted future studies show that certain genotypes of *E histolytica* are inherently nonpathogenic, then clinical diagnosis should include approaches to detect and differentiate among *E histolytica* genotypes to help physicians in making correct treatment decisions.

Next-generation sequencing (NGS) approaches will be highly useful in the future to discover novel pathogens directly in the stool samples. This approach will prove important for species and strains that are not usually associated with diseases in humans. This approach would also be important to eliminate the bias introduced by growing pathogens in culture, or to identify strains and species that cannot be cultured at present. With significant decreases in the cost, and ever-increasing sensitivity and coverage, it is tempting to speculate that NGS will dictate the diagnostic needs and priorities in the future.

## SELF-ASSESSMENT

1. Amebiasis occurs through the ingestion of which of the following?
   a. Cysts of *E dispar*
   b. Trophozoites of *E histolytica*

c. Cysts of *E histolytica*
d. Cysts of both *E bangladeshi* and *E moshkovskii*
e. Cysts of any intestinal amebae
2. Which of the following can grow at room temperature?
    a. *E dispar* and *E moshkovskii*
    b. *E moshkovskii* and *E bangladeshi*
    c. *E histolytica* only
    d. *E bangladeshi* only
    e. All of the above
3. Which of the following approaches would more likely identify novel pathogens?
    a. Microscopy and culture
    b. Antigen or antibody detection
    c. PCR
    d. NGS
    e. LAMP

ANSWERS

1.a. Incorrect. Amebiasis has been defined as being infection with *E histolytica*
  b. Incorrect. Although *E histolytica* is the causative agent of amebiasis, it is the cyst form of the parasite that is resistance to the acidic pH of stomach, and when ingested, withstands the acidic environment and can colonize in the intestine, whereas the trophozoite form of amebae is disrupted in the stomach.
  c. **Correct**. Only the cyst form of *E histolytica* when ingested can colonize in the intestine and cause amebiasis.
  d. Incorrect. Amebiasis has been defined as being infection with *E histolytica*.
  e. Incorrect. Amebiasis has been defined as being infection with *E histolytica*.
2.a. Incorrect. *E dispar* does not grow at room temperature.
  b. **Correct**. Both *E moshkovskii* and *E bangladeshi* can grow at room temperature.
  c. Incorrect. *E histolytica* does not grow at room temperature.
  d. Incorrect. *E moshkovskii* can also grow at room temperature.
  e. Incorrect. Only *E moshkovskii* and *E bangladeshi* can grow at room temperature.
3.a. Incorrect. Morphologically identical different species of organisms exist, and not all organisms are expected to grow in culture.
  b. Incorrect. Both techniques are too specific to detect a novel species.
  c. Incorrect. PCR is generally too specific to detect a novel species.
  d. **Correct**. NGS has the potential to detect a novel species.
  e. Incorrect. The LAMP technique is too specific to detect a novel species.

## ACKNOWLEDGMENTS

The author would like to thank Dr C. Graham Clark, London School of Hygiene and Tropical Medicine, United Kingdom, for critical reading of the article, and for providing constructive comments and suggestions.

## REFERENCES

1. Lozano R, Naghavi M, Foreman K, et al. Global and regional mortality from 235 causes of death for 20 age groups in 1990 and 2010: a systematic analysis for the Global Burden of Disease Study 2010. Lancet 2012;380:2095–128.
2. Gathiram V, Jackson TF. A longitudinal study of asymptomatic carriers of pathogenic zymodemes of *Entamoeba histolytica*. S Afr Med J 1987;72:669–72.
3. Stanley SL Jr. Amebiasis. Lancet 2003;361:1025–34.

4. Tarleton JL, Haque R, Mondal D, et al. Cognitive effects of diarrhea, malnutrition, and *Entamoeba histolytica* infection on school age children in Dhaka, Bangladesh. Am J Trop Med Hyg 2006;74:475–81.
5. Petri WA Jr, Mondal D, Peterson KM, et al. Association of malnutrition with amebiasis. Nutr Rev 2009;67(Suppl 2):S207–15.
6. Mondal D, Minak J, Alam M, et al. Contribution of enteric infection, altered intestinal barrier function, and maternal malnutrition to infant malnutrition in Bangladesh. Clin Infect Dis 2012;54:185–92.
7. Gathiram V, Jackson TF. Frequency distribution of *Entamoeba histolytica* zymodemes in a rural South African population. Lancet 1985;1:719–21.
8. Shimokawa C, Kabir M, Taniuchi M, et al. *Entamoeba moshkovskii* is associated with diarrhea in infants and causes diarrhea and colitis in mice. J Infect Dis 2012;206:744–51.
9. Ali IK, Hossain MB, Roy S, et al. *Entamoeba moshkovskii* infections in children, Bangladesh. Emerg Infect Dis 2003;9:580–4.
10. Everard A, Lazarevic V, Gaïa N, et al. Microbiome of prebiotic-treated mice reveals novel targets involved in host response during obesity. ISME J 2014;8:2116–30.
11. Martinez Palomo A. The Spanish republicans and health research in Mexico. Gac Med Mex 1993;129:92–5.
12. Petri WA Jr. Recent advances in amebiasis. Crit Rev Clin Lab Sci 1996;33:1–37.
13. Sargeaunt PG, Williams JE, Grene JD. The differentiation of invasive and non-invasive *Entamoeba histolytica* by isoenzyme electrophoresis. Trans R Soc Trop Med Hyg 1978;72:519–21.
14. Diamond LS, Clark CG. A redescription of *Entamoeba histolytica* Schaudinn, 1903 (Emended Walker, 1911) separating it from *Entamoeba dispar* Brumpt, 1925. J Eukaryot Microbiol 1993;40:340–4.
15. Dolabella SS, Serrano-Luna J, Navarro-García F, et al. Amebic liver abscess production by Entamoeba dispar. Ann Hepatol 2012;11:107–17.
16. Tshalaia LE. On a species of *Entamoeba* detected in sewage effluents. Med Parazit (Moscow) 1941;10:244–52.
17. Dreyer DA. Growth of a strain of *Entamoeba histolytica* at room temperature. Tex Rep Biol Med 1961;19:393–6.
18. Clark CG, Diamond LS. Intraspecific variation and phylogenetic relationships in the genus *Entamoeba* as revealed by riboprinting. J Eukaryot Microbiol 1997;44:142–54.
19. Entner N, Most H. Genetics of *Entamoeba*: characterization of two new parasitic strains which grow at room temperature (and at 37 Degrees C). J Protozool 1965;12:10–3.
20. Richards CS, Goldman M, Cannon LT. Cultivation of *Entamoeba* histolytica and *Entamoeba histolytica*-like strains at reduced temperature and behavior of the amebae in diluted media. Am J Trop Med Hyg 1966;15:648–55.
21. Clark CG, Diamond LS. The Laredo strain and other '*Entamoeba histolytica*-like' amoebae are *Entamoeba moshkovskii*. Mol Biochem Parasitol 1991;46:11–8.
22. Haque R, Ali IK, Clark CG, et al. A case report of *Entamoeba moshkovskii* infection in a Bangladeshi child. Parasitol Int 1998;47:201–2.
23. Fotedar R, Stark D, Marriott D, et al. *Entamoeba moshkovskii* infections in Sydney, Australia. Eur J Clin Microbiol Infect Dis 2008;27:133–7.
24. Yakoob J, Abbas Z, Beg MA, et al. *Entamoeba* species associated with chronic diarrhoea in Pakistan. Epidemiol Infect 2012;140:323–8.

25. Nazemalhosseini Mojarad E, Nochi Z, Sahebekhtiari N, et al. Discrimination of *Entamoeba moshkovskii* in patients with gastrointestinal disorders by single-round PCR. Jap J Infect Dis 2010;63:136–8.

26. Beck DL, Doğan N, Maro V, et al. High prevalence of *Entamoeba moshkovskii* in a Tanzanian HIV population. Acta Trop 2008;107:48–9.

27. Tanyuksel M, Ulukanligil M, Guclu Z, et al. Two cases of rarely recognized infection with *Entamoeba moshkovskii*. Am J Trop Med Hyg 2007;76:723–4.

28. Ngui R, Angal L, Fakhrurrazi SA, et al. Differentiating *Entamoeba histolytica*, *Entamoeba dispar* and *Entamoeba moshkovskii* using nested polymerase chain reaction (PCR) in rural communities in Malaysia. Parasit Vectors 2012;5:187.

29. Anuar TS, Al-Mekhlafi HM, Ghani MK, et al. First molecular identification of *Entamoeba moshkovskii* in Malaysia. Parasitology 2012;139:1521–5.

30. Lau YL, Anthony C, Fakhrurrazi SA, et al. Real-time PCR assay in differentiating *Entamoeba histolytica*, *Entamoeba dispar*, and *Entamoeba moshkovskii* infections in Orang Asli settlements in Malaysia. Parasit Vectors 2013;6:250.

31. Hamzah Z, Petmitr S, Mungthin M, et al. Development of multiplex real-time polymerase chain reaction for detection of *Entamoeba histolytica*, *Entamoeba dispar*, and *Entamoeba moshkovskii* in clinical specimens. Am J Trop Med Hyg 2010;83:909–13.

32. Ayed SB, Aoun K, Maamouri N, et al. First molecular identification of *Entamoeba moshkovskii* in human stool samples in Tunisia. Am J Trop Med Hyg 2008;79:706–7.

33. ElBakri A, Samie A, Ezzedine S, et al. Differential detection of *Entamoeba histolytica*, *Entamoeba dispar* and *Entamoeba moshkovskii* in fecal samples by nested PCR in the United Arab Emirates (UAE). Acta Parasitol 2013;58:185–90.

34. Parija SC, Khairnar K. *Entamoeba moshkovskii* and *Entamoeba dispar*-associated infections in Pondicherry, India. J Health Popul Nutr 2005;23:292–5.

35. Khairnar K, Parija SC. A novel nested multiplex polymerase chain reaction (PCR) assay for differential detection of *Entamoeba histolytica*, *E. moshkovskii* and *E. dispar* DNA in stool samples. BMC Microbiol 2007;7:47.

36. Stensvold CR, Lebbad M, Victory EL, et al. Increased sampling reveals novel lineages of *Entamoeba*: consequences of genetic diversity and host specificity for taxonomy and molecular detection. Protist 2011;162:525–41.

37. Royer TL, Gilchrist C, Kabir M, et al. *Entamoeba bangladeshi* nov. sp., Bangladesh. Emerg Infect Dis 2012;18:1543–5.

38. Martínez-Palomo A. 2nd edition. Parasitic amebas of the intestinal tract, vol. 3. San Diego, CA: Academic Press; 1993. p. 65–141.

39. Acuna-Soto R, Maguire JH, Wirth DF. Gender distribution in asymptomatic and invasive amebiasis. Am J Gastroenterol 2000;95:1277–83.

40. Anonymous. Health in the Americas. Washington, DC: Pan American Health Organization, Mexico; 1998. p. 357–78.

41. Caballero-Salcedo A, Viveros-Rogel M, Salvatierra B, et al. Seroepidemiology of amebiasis in Mexico. Am J Trop Med Hyg 1994;50:412–9.

42. Centers for Disease Control and Prevention (CDC). Summary of notifiable diseases, United States, 1993. MMWR Morb Mortal Wkly Rep 1994;42:i–xvii, 1–73.

43. Haque R, Mollah NU, Ali IK, et al. Diagnosis of amebic liver abscess and intestinal infection with the TechLab *Entamoeba histolytica* II antigen detection and antibody tests. J Clin Microbiol 2000;38:3235–9.

44. Hughes FB, Faehnle ST, Simon JL. Multiple cerebral abscesses complicating hepatopulmonary amebiasis. J Pediatr 1975;86:95–6.

45. Solaymani-Mohammadi S, Lam MM, Zunt JR, et al. *Entamoeba histolytica* encephalitis diagnosed by PCR of cerebrospinal fluid. Trans R Soc Trop Med Hyg 2007;101:311–3.
46. Sundaram C, Prasad BC, Bhaskar G, et al. Brain abscess due to *Entamoeba histolytica*. J Assoc Physicians India 2004;52:251–2.
47. Ramakrishnan AS, Ratnasabapathy PM, Natanasabapathy R, et al. An amebic liver abscess presenting as a space occupying lesion of the right kidney. Am Surg 1971;37:756–8.
48. Mehta AB, Mehta BC, Balse SL, et al. Amebic abscess of myocardium; a case report. Indian J Med Sci 1968;22:720–2.
49. Hara A, Hirose Y, Mori H, et al. Cytopathologic and genetic diagnosis of pulmonary amebiasis: a case report. Acta Cytol 2004;48:547–50.
50. Lichtenstein A, Kondo AT, Visvesvara GS, et al. Pulmonary amebiasis presenting as superior vena cava syndrome. Thorax 2005;60:350–2.
51. Ramdial PK, Madiba TE, Kharwa S, et al. Isolated amebic appendicitis. Virchows Arch 2002;441:63–8.
52. Kroft EB, Warris A, Jansen LE, et al. A Dutchman from Mali with a perianal ulcer caused by cutaneous amebiasis. Ned Tijdschr Geneeskd 2005;149:308–11.
53. Magana M, Magana ML, Alcantara A, et al. Histopathology of cutaneous amebiasis. Am J Dermatopathol 2004;26:280–4.
54. Anonymous. World Health Organization/Pan American Health Organization/UNESCO report of a consultation of experts on amebiasis. Wkly Epidemiol Rec 1997;72:97–9.
55. Huston CD, Haque R, Petri W, et al. Molecular-based diagnosis of *Entamoeba histolytica* infection. Expert Rev Mol Med 1999;1999:1–11.
56. Reeves RE, Bischoff JM. Classification of *Entamoeba* species by means of electrophoretic properties of amebal enzymes. J Parasitol 1968;54:594–600.
57. Fotedar R, Stark D, Beebe N, et al. Laboratory diagnostic techniques for *Entamoeba* species. Clin Microbiol Rev 2007;20:511–32 Table of contents.
58. Abd-Alla MD, Jackson TG, Ravdin JI. Serum IgM antibody response to the galactose-inhibitable adherence lectin of *Entamoeba histolytica*. Am J Trop Med Hyg 1998;59:431–4.
59. Ohnishi K, Murata M. Present characteristics of symptomatic amebiasis due to *Entamoeba histolytica* in the east-southeast area of Tokyo. Epidemiol Infect 1997;119:363–7.
60. Weinke T, Scherer W, Neuber U, et al. Clinical features and management of amebic liver abscess. Experience from 29 patients. Klin Wochenschr 1989;67:415–20.
61. Moss DM, Priest JW, Hamlin K, et al. Longitudinal evaluation of enteric protozoa in Haitian children by stool exam and multiplex serologic assay. Am J Trop Med Hyg 2014;90:653–60.
62. Leo M, Haque R, Kabir M, et al. Evaluation of *Entamoeba histolytica* antigen and antibody point-of-care tests for the rapid diagnosis of amebiasis. J Clin Microbiol 2006;44:4569–71.
63. Verkerke HP, Hanbury B, Siddique A, et al. Multisite clinical evaluation of a rapid test for *Entamoeba histolytica* in stool. J Clin Microbiol 2015;53:493–7.
64. ElBakri A, Samie A, Ezzedine S, et al. Genetic variability of the Serine-Rich *Entamoeba histolytica* protein gene in clinical isolates from the United Arab Emirates. Trop Biomed 2014;31:370–7.
65. Evangelopoulos A, Spanakos G, Patsoula E, et al. A nested, multiplex, PCR assay for the simultaneous detection and differentiation of *Entamoeba histolytica* and *Entamoeba dispar* in faeces. Ann Trop Med Parasitol 2000;94:233–40.

66. Freitas MA, Vianna EN, Martins AS, et al. A single step duplex PCR to distinguish *Entamoeba histolytica* from *Entamoeba dispar.* Parasitology 2004;128:625–8.
67. Gonin P, Trudel L. Detection and differentiation of *Entamoeba histolytica* and *Entamoeba dispar* isolates in clinical samples by PCR and enzyme-linked immunosorbent assay. J Clin Microbiol 2003;41:237–41.
68. Heckendorn F, N'Goran EK, Felger I, et al. Species-specific field testing of *Entamoeba* spp. in an area of high endemicity. Trans R Soc Trop Med Hyg 2002;96:521–8.
69. Paglia MG, Visca P. An improved PCR-based method for detection and differentiation of *Entamoeba histolytica* and *Entamoeba dispar* in formalin-fixed stools. Acta Trop 2004;92:273–7.
70. Verweij JJ, van Lieshout L, Blotkamp C, et al. Differentiation of *Entamoeba histolytica* and *Entamoeba dispar* using PCR-SHELA and comparison of antibody response. Arch Med Res 2000;31:S44–6.
71. Verweij JJ, Blotkamp J, Brienen EA, et al. Differentiation of *Entamoeba histolytica* and *Entamoeba dispar* cysts using polymerase chain reaction on DNA isolated from faeces with spin columns. Eur J Clin Microbiol Infect Dis 2000;19: 358–61.
72. Kebede A, Verweij JJ, Endeshaw T, et al. The use of real-time PCR to identify *Entamoeba histolytica* and *E. dispar* infections in prisoners and primary-school children in Ethiopia. Ann Trop Med Parasitol 2004;98:43–8.
73. Pinar A, Akyon Y, Alp A, et al. [Adaptation of a sensitive DNA extraction method for detection of *Entamoeba histolytica* by real-time polymerase chain reaction]. Mikrobiyol Bul 2010;44:453–9.
74. Cnops L, Esbroeck MV. Freezing of stool samples improves real-time PCR detection of *Entamoeba dispar* and *Entamoeba histolytica.* J Microbiol Methods 2010;80:310–2.
75. Myjak P, Kur J, Pietkiewicz H. Usefulness of new DNA extraction procedure for PCR technique in species identification of *Entamoeba* isolates. Wiad Parazytol 1997;43:163–70.
76. Romero JL, Descoteaux S, Reed S, et al. Use of polymerase chain reaction and nonradioactive DNA probes to diagnose *Entamoeba histolytica* in clinical samples. Arch Med Res 1992;23:277–9.
77. Tachibana H, Kobayashi S, Okuzawa E, et al. Detection of pathogenic *Entamoeba histolytica* DNA in liver abscess fluid by polymerase chain reaction. Int J Parasitol 1992;22:1193–6.
78. Cruz-Reyes JA, Spice WM, Rehman T, et al. Ribosomal DNA sequences in the differentiation of pathogenic and non-pathogenic isolates of *Entamoeba histolytica.* Parasitology 1992;104(Pt 2):239–46.
79. Acuna-Soto R, Samuelson J, De Girolami P, et al. Application of the polymerase chain reaction to the epidemiology of pathogenic and nonpathogenic *Entamoeba histolytica.* Am J Trop Med Hyg 1993;48:58–70.
80. Rivera WL, Tachibana H, Silva-Tahat MR, et al. Differentiation of *Entamoeba histolytica* and *E. dispar* DNA from cysts present in stool specimens by polymerase chain reaction: its field application in the Philippines. Parasitol Res 1996;82:585–9.
81. Blessmann J, Buss H, Nu PA, et al. Real-time PCR for detection and differentiation of *Entamoeba histolytica* and *Entamoeba dispar* in fecal samples. J Clin Microbiol 2002;40:4413–7.
82. Verweij JJ, Blangé RA, Templeton K, et al. Simultaneous detection of *Entamoeba histolytica, Giardia lamblia,* and *Cryptosporidium parvum* in fecal samples by using multiplex real-time PCR. J Clin Microbiol 2004;42:1220–3.

83. McAuliffe GN, Anderson TP, Stevens M, et al. Systematic application of multiplex PCR enhances the detection of bacteria, parasites, and viruses in stool samples. J Infect 2013;67:122–9.

84. Soonawala D, van Lieshout L, den Boer MA, et al. Post-travel screening of asymptomatic long-term travelers to the tropics for intestinal parasites using molecular diagnostics. Am J Trop Med Hyg 2014;90:835–9.

85. Taniuchi M, Verweij JJ, Noor Z, et al. High throughput multiplex PCR and probe-based detection with Luminex beads for seven intestinal parasites. Am J Trop Med Hyg 2011;84:332–7.

86. Van Lint P, Rossen JW, Vermeiren S, et al. Detection of *Giardia lamblia*, *Cryptosporidium* spp. and *Entamoeba histolytica* in clinical stool samples by using multiplex real-time PCR after automated DNA isolation. Acta Clin Belg 2013; 68:188–92.

87. Nazeer JT, El Sayed Khalifa K, von Thien H, et al. Use of multiplex real-time PCR for detection of common diarrhea causing protozoan parasites in Egypt. Parasitol Res 2013;112:595–601.

88. Stark D, Roberts T, Ellis JT, et al. Evaluation of the EasyScreen enteric parasite detection kit for the detection of *Blastocystis* spp., *Cryptosporidium* spp., *Dientamoeba fragilis*, *Entamoeba* complex, and *Giardia intestinalis* from clinical stool samples. Diagn Microbiol Infect Dis 2014;78:149–52.

89. Qvarnstrom Y, James C, Xayavong M, et al. Comparison of real-time PCR protocols for differential laboratory diagnosis of amebiasis. J Clin Microbiol 2005; 43:5491–7.

90. Visser LG, Verweij JJ, Van Esbroeck M, et al. Diagnostic methods for differentiation of *Entamoeba histolytica* and *Entamoeba dispar* in carriers: performance and clinical implications in a non-endemic setting. Int J Med Microbiol 2006; 296:397–403.

91. Verweij JJ, Laeijendecker D, Brienen EA, et al. Detection and identification of *Entamoeba* species in stool samples by a reverse line hybridization assay. J Clin Microbiol 2003;41:5041–5.

92. Solaymani-Mohammadi S, Rezaian M, Babaei Z, et al. Comparison of a stool antigen detection kit and PCR for diagnosis of *Entamoeba histolytica* and *Entamoeba dispar* infections in asymptomatic cyst passers in Iran. J Clin Microbiol 2006;44:2258–61.

93. Gray SA, Weigel KM, Ali IK, et al. Toward low-cost affinity reagents: lyophilized yeast-scFv probes specific for pathogen antigens. PLoS One 2012;7: e32042.

94. Grewal YS, Shiddiky MJ, Gray SA, et al. Label-free electrochemical detection of an *Entamoeba histolytica* antigen using cell-free yeast-scFv probes. Chem Commun (Camb) 2013;49:1551–3.

95. Grewal YS, Shiddiky MJ, Spadafora LJ, et al. Nano-yeast-scFv probes on screen-printed gold electrodes for detection of *Entamoeba histolytica* antigens in a biological matrix. Biosens Bioelectron 2014;55:417–22.

96. Santos HL, Bandyopadhyay K, Bandea R, et al. LUMINEX(R): a new technology for the simultaneous identification of five *Entamoeba* spp. commonly found in human stools. Parasit Vectors 2013;6:69.

97. Wessels E, Rusman LG, van Bussel, et al. Added value of multiplex Luminex gastrointestinal pathogen panel (xTAG(R) GPP) testing in the diagnosis of infectious gastroenteritis. Clin Microbiol Infect 2014;20:O182–7.

98. Notomi T, Okayama H, Masubuchi H, et al. Loop-mediated isothermal amplification of DNA. Nucleic Acids Res 2000;28:E63.

99. Tomita N, Mori Y, Kanda H, et al. Loop-mediated isothermal amplification (LAMP) of gene sequences and simple visual detection of products. Nat Protoc 2008;3:877–82.
100. Njiru ZK, Mikosza AS, Armstrong T, et al. Loop-mediated isothermal amplification (LAMP) method for rapid detection of *Trypanosoma brucei* rhodesiense. PLoS Neg Trop Dis 2008;2:e147.
101. Liang SY, Chan YH, Hsia KT, et al. Development of loop-mediated isothermal amplification assay for detection of *Entamoeba histolytica*. J Clin Microbiol 2009;47:1892–5.
102. Liu J, Gratz J, Amour C, et al. A laboratory-developed TaqMan Array Card for simultaneous detection of 19 enteropathogens. J Clin Microbiol 2013;51: 472–80.
103. Stensvold CR, Lebbad M, Verweij JJ, et al. Identification and delineation of members of the *Entamoeba* complex by pyrosequencing. Mol Cell Probes 2010;24:403–6.
104. Ali IK, Mondal U, Roy S, et al. Evidence for a link between parasite genotype and outcome of infection with *Entamoeba histolytica*. J Clin Microbiol 2007;45: 285–9.

# Infections by Intestinal Coccidia and *Giardia duodenalis*

Vitaliano A. Cama, DVM, PhD[a],*, Blaine A. Mathison, BS[b]

## KEYWORDS

- *Cryptosporidium* • *Cyclospora cayetanensis* • *Giardia duodenalis*
- *Cystoisospora belli* • Human enteric coccidian

## KEY POINTS

- Sample collection and preservation are important steps, and examination of 3 specimens from different days increases the accuracy of diagnosis.
- *Giardia* can be detected by light microscopy during ova-and-parasite (O&P) examination, antigen detection methods (laboratory and rapid diagnostic devices), or fluorescent microscopy.
- *Cryptosporidium* and *Cyclospora* are not easily detectable by O&P examination, and parasite-specific tests must be requested, such as modified acid-fast (MAF) microscopy. For *Cryptosporidium*, there are antigen detection assays (laboratory or rapid diagnostic devices) or antibody-based fluorescent microscopy. Properly equipped fluorescent microscopes can be used in research laboratories for confirmation of *Cyclospora*, as this parasite autofluoresces with the appropriate excitation wavelength.
- *Cystoisospora* can be detected by light microscopy, and confirmation is accomplished through morphometric characteristics of samples that have been stained with safranin or acid-fast stain and also by autofluorescence.

## INTRODUCTION

The protozoa, as typically delineated in public health, are a nonmonophyletic conglomerate of unicellular eukaryotic organisms that are characterized by having animallike affinities. Most protozoa that infect the human enteric tract are characterized by having an environmentally stable stage such as a cyst or oocyst. Cysts and

Disclosure: The authors have nothing to disclose.
[a] Division of Parasitic Diseases and Malaria, Centers for Disease Control and Prevention, MS D-65, Atlanta, GA 30341, USA; [b] Division of Parasitic Diseases and Malaria, Centers for Disease Control and Prevention, MS D-64, Atlanta, GA 30341, USA
* Corresponding author.
*E-mail address:* VCama@cdc.gov

oocysts confer protection from environmental factors, allowing these parasites to infect other susceptible hosts through either the water or food-borne routes.

There are several parasitic protozoa that can cause enteric infections in humans, the focus here being *Cryptosporidium* spp, *Cyclospora cayetanensis, Giardia duodenalis* (syn. *Giardia lamblia, Giardia intestinalis*), and *Cystoisospora belli* (previously *Isospora belli*). Infections are usually characterized by gastrointestinal clinical manifestations that may include diarrhea, vomiting, abdominal cramps, and general malaise.[1,2] Three of these protozoa, *Cryptosporidium, Cyclospora,* and *Cystoisospora,* were previously classified as coccidian parasites because of their intracellular location (these parasite infect enterocytes) and a complex life cycle that includes asexual (meronts) and sexual (microgametocytes and macrogametocytes) reproductive stages.[3] *Giardia* is a flagellate, does not invade epithelial cells, and reproduces only asexually by binary fission.

The classification of eukaryotic parasites is in frequent revision because of modern systematics that incorporate bioinformatic data and cladistics classification into the traditional morphometric-based taxonomy. As of 2012, the formerly known coccidians are classified in the subgroup Apicomplexa, with *Cyclospora* and *Cystoisospora* being classified as Eimeriorinas (the sporozoites, which are the infective stages, are always enclosed in sporocysts within an oocyst) and *Cryptosporidium* grouped alone as a single clade (oocysts without sporocysts, containing 4 naked sporozoites).[4]

These parasites produce resistant stages (cysts in *Giardia,*[5] oocysts in the coccidia), which are released into the environment. The excretion intensity of these parasites can vary significantly, from very high to low, and can be sporadic.[6] Therefore, the diagnostic success of a single stool sample can be suboptimal.[7] It is currently recommended to test 3 samples,[8] ideally collected every other day, over a period of at least 1 week.[9]

Samples have to be properly preserved to assure success of the assays to be conducted. The most widely used method relies on a 2-vial collection system with sodium acetate-acetic acid-formalin (SAF); 10% buffered formalin; polyvinyl alcohol (PVA) containing fixatives such as mercury, zinc, or copper (Zn PVA, Cu PVA); or Schaudinn fluid. However, there is a trend to minimize the use of formalin (because of toxicity) and mercury (environmental impact)[10]; however, those alternatives may not always have high parasite recovery rates and not are always compatible with immunoassays.[7]

See Appendix 1 for laboratory procedures for the microscopic detection of coccidian parasites (*Cryptosporidium* spp, *C cayetanensis,* and *C belli*).

## *CRYPTOSPORIDIUM* SPP

The genus *Cryptosporidium* was first described in 1910 by Tyzzer,[11] who in 1912 also described *Cryptosporidium parvum* in the small intestine of mice.[12] For several decades, human cryptosporidiosis was considered a benign self-resolving infection that was caused by *C parvum.*[13] This parasite was considered to have the potential to infect a broad range of mammalian species. With the advent of the human immunodeficiency virus (HIV)/AIDS epidemic, cryptosporidiosis became an important infection, where immunocompromised patients developed nonretractable life-threatening diarrhea.[14,15] Cryptosporidiosis was classified as opportunistic infection and also as an AIDS-defining illness.[16] Given its public health importance, numerous studies were conducted to better understand its pathogenesis, transmission routes, therapeutic approaches, and disease-prevention strategies. The renewed interest led to important discoveries that highlighted the importance of the immune system, more specifically CD4 cells, in the clearance of infections.[17,18] It was also confirmed that its primary route of transmission was waterborne and that people with immune deficiencies other than HIV were also at risk of severe disease.[19,20]

Data from studies using DNA-based methods started to provide evidence that not all isolates of *Cryptosporidium* previously identified as *C parvum* had the same DNA signatures.[21] Further studies showed that the parasites previously described as *C parvum* may actually encompass several species that were morphologically identical; however, DNA data showed distinct genetic signatures and epidemiologic and biological data showed that several isolates had defined host specificities.[22]

Differences in DNA patterns between human and animal isolates were reported using whole DNA extracts[21] and further substantiated using polymerase chain reaction (PCR)-amplified regions of the 18s small subunit ribosomal RNA gene.[22–24] The systematic use of DNA-based methods, in conjunction with biological and epidemiologic studies, have led to a major revision of the genus *Cryptosporidium*.[25–28]

At present, there are 26 different species of *Cryptosporidium*.[29] The species most frequently detected in humans are *Cryptosporidium hominis*, an anthroponotic parasite (infecting only humans), and *C parvum*, a zoonotic species. It should be noted that *C parvum* is most frequently detected in weaned calves but not in heifers or older cattle.[30] These 2 species of *Cryptosporidium* have different epidemiologic distributions. Both parasites are frequent in European countries, whereas *C parvum* has been the species more frequently reported in the Middle East. In the United States, other industrialized nations, and other developing countries, *C hominis* is the parasite most frequently detected in people. Species less frequently reported are *Cryptosporidium ubiquitum* (previously described as cervine genotype) mainly in industrialized nations, *Cryptosporidium canis* and *Cryptosporidium felis* in nonindustrialized countries, and *Cryptosporidium cuniculus*, primarily in the United Kingdom. Other species with limited number of cases reported are *Cryptosporidium meleagridis*, *Cryptosporidium viatorum*, *Cryptosporidium suis*, *Cryptosporidium muris*, *Cryptosporidium fayeri*, *Cryptosporidium andersoni*, *Cryptosporidium bovis*, *Cryptosporidium tyzzeri*, *Cryptosporidium erinacei*, *Cryptosporidium scrofarum*, and *Cryptosporidium xiaoi*.[31]

### Life Cycle and Biology

The latest classification of eukaryotic organisms places *Cryptosporidium* in its own clade, which is outside the Coccidia proper.[4] *Cryptosporidium* spp are morphologically characterized by the presence of an attachment feeder organelle, location in the host's cells (intracellular, but extracytoplasmic), presence of 2 functional types of oocysts (thin and thick walled), presence of a gamontlike extracellular stage, and lack of sporocysts, microphyles, and polar granules.[32–35]

Only 1 host is required for *Cryptosporidium* to complete its life cycle. Fully sporulated, thick-walled oocysts are shed in the feces. Unlike other intestinal coccidia, oocysts of *Cryptosporidium* spp are immediately infective when shed from the host. Infection occurs after the ingestion of oocysts in fecal-contaminated food, water, and fomites. After ingestion by a suitable host, oocysts excyst in the small intestine, releasing sporozoites. The sporozoites parasitize the epithelial cells of the intestinal tract and produce a parasitophorous vacuole located between the host cell's cytoplasm and cell membrane. This unique intracellular but extracytoplasmatic location allows the parasite to derive nutrients via a feeder organelle.

Within the parasitophorous vacuole, sporozoites undergo asexual cycles of merogony. Mature meronts rupture from the infected host cell and take 1 of 2 pathways. Type I meronts give rise to merozoites that perpetuate the asexual cycle in the surrounding host cells. Type II meronts give rise to merozoites that initiate the sexual cycle by producing microgametes (males) or macrogametes (females). Fertilization of macrogametes by microgametes results in the formation of zygotes. Zygotes differentiate into 4 sporozoites and develop a cyst wall, becoming oocysts. Thin-walled oocysts rupture in the lumen of the intestine and perpetuate autoinfection, whereas thick-walled oocysts are shed in stool where they are immediately infectious to a susceptible host.[36,37]

## Epidemiology

Cryptosporidiosis is ubiquitous and is reported worldwide. It is primarily transmitted through the waterborne route[38]; however, food-borne[39–41] or direct-contact transmission can also occur.[42–44] Overall, the frequency of cryptosporidiosis has shown distinct patterns between areas with high endemicity, mainly associated with other enteropathogens, and areas with low endemicity, mainly from industrialized countries, where infections are usually in low levels. There are some patterns for seasonality. For example, in European countries and New Zealand, *C hominis* was more frequently detected in fall, whereas *C parvum* was more frequently reported in spring.[45]

In areas of high endemicity, first cryptosporidial infections usually occur in young children, mainly by age 2 years. Most first infections are symptomatic, primarily associated with diarrhea. Detectable infections decrease with age, and cases of cryptosporidiosis are highly infrequent in children. Meanwhile, the adults living in the same settings usually do not have detectable cryptosporidiosis. Some seasonal trends have been reported.[1]

In industrialized nations, infections have been reported in people of all ages. Cryptosporidiosis in the United States is a reportable disease. The number of cases is consistently greater during the summer months, when outbreaks associated with the use of recreational waters are reported, and more frequently among children aged 1 to 9 years, followed by young adults (aged about 25–39 years).[46–48] Food-borne outbreaks have been associated with the consumption of raw or undercooked foods[49] or unpasteurized drinks.[50]

## Clinical Manifestations

Immunocompetent people and children usually present short-term, self-limited watery diarrhea that may be accompanied with nausea and vomiting, which can lead to dehydration.[1,51] People with immune deficiencies, especially with low CD4+ counts ($<140/mm^3$)[17] may present chronic and debilitating disease, which can lead to life-threatening syndromes.[52]

## Treatment

Multiple drugs or immunotherapeutic compounds have been developed or tested for the treatment of human cryptosporidiosis. Very few of these compounds have shown therapeutic efficacy. Rehydration through the oral route is the most widely used intervention. Thus far, only nitazoxanide has been approved by the US Food and Drug Administration (FDA) for the treatment of *Cryptosporidium* infections in people.[53] This product has shown to shorten the duration of diarrhea and parasite excretion, although it is not highly efficacious in the treatment of cryptosporidiosis in people with immune deficiencies.[54] In people with HIV infections and low CD4 counts, the preferred treatment and preventative measure would be the administration of highly active antiretroviral therapies (HAART). Relapses are frequent when patients discontinue HAART.

## Diagnosis

### Microscopy

*Cryptosporidium* spp are not readily detected by routine O&P testing such as formalin-ethyl acetate (FEA) concentration or trichrome staining.[9] Visualization of oocysts require special staining, such as Kinyoun MAF, Zieh-Neelsen acid-fast, or safranin (**Fig. 1**). *Cryptosporidium* may also be detected by the aurimine O stain used for mycobacteria. Direct fluorescent antibody (DFA) microscopy kits are also helpful for detection and specimen screening. Unlike several other coccidians, *Cryptosporidium* spp do not autofluoresce under ultraviolet (UV) light.[7,9,55]

### Antigen detection and rapid/point-of-care diagnosis

These assays are based on the detection of parasite antigens that can be detected in stool specimens. They have the advantage of simplicity and not requiring specialized trained personnel, and several products are already approved for clinical diagnosis (**Table 1**).[56] Disadvantages are that the species identification or quantification of parasite loads is not possible.

### Molecular diagnosis

DNA-based methods are primarily used for species identification and molecular typing. PCR and PCR-related methods have been developed for the detection and identification of species within *Cryptosporidium* spp. Several protocols for PCR detection of *Cryptosporidium* DNA have been made available; however, none of these methods has received approval from FDA or for use of the European Conformity (CE) logo. These protocols allow the identification of *Cryptosporidium* that are of public health importance. Methods using PCR amplification followed by restriction fragment length polymorphism have been developed for the detection and differentiation of *Cryptosporidium* at the species level. Most of these techniques are based on the amplification of the small-subunit (SSU) rRNA gene.[57] There are other PCR-based protocols that have been designed for the detection and differentiation of *C parvum* and *C hominis*, the 2 most frequent species affecting humans. However, these protocols cannot detect or differentiate other *Cryptosporidium* spp or genotypes.[45]

Subtype analyses, which are based on PCR amplification followed by DNA sequence analysis, is a powerful tool for outbreak investigations. Several subtyping tools have also been developed to characterize the diversity within *C parvum* or *C hominis*.[45] This method is based on the sequence polymorphism of the GP-60 locus (also known as gp15/45/60, gp40/15), which has shown to be a robust tool in outbreak investigations.[44]

## CYCLOSPORA CAYETANENSIS

This coccidian parasite was described in 1993.[2] It is recognized as an important cause of food-borne outbreaks, both in the United States as well as in other industrialized nations. The name *C cayetanensis* was first proposed in 1992; however, previous studies reported organisms that later have been considered to be similar to *Cyclospora*.[58] However, earlier reports hypothesized that those new organisms could belong to a new species of *Isospora*.[58]

In 1993, the description of oocysts, which after sporulation had 2 clearly defined sporocysts, each with 2 sporozoites, led to the organism's classification as *Cyclospora* and to the species name *C cayetanensis*. The genus *Cyclospora* is currently placed among the Eimeriorina.[4,59] Molecular data suggest that *Cyclospora* may actually belong nestled within the genus *Eimeria*.[60,61] At present, *C cayetanensis* is the only

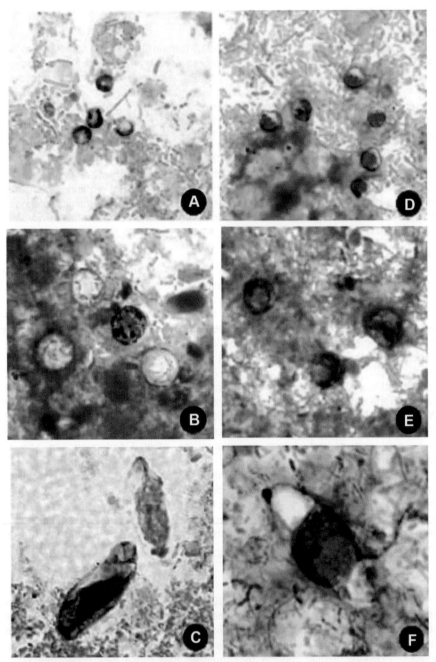

**Fig. 1.** Comparison of (*A, D*) *Cryptosporidium* spp, (*B, E*) *Cyclospora cayetanensis*, and (*C, F*) *Cystoisospora belli* stained with modified acid-fast and safranin stains, original magnification × 1000. (Public domain images, *courtesy of* DPDx, Centers for Disease Control and Prevention, Atlanta, USA).

**Table 1**

Commercial diagnostic assays for the detection of protozoa, either approved by the FDA or registered for selling in the European Union, having the CE seal of European Conformity or *Conformité Européenne*

| Product Name | Manufacturer, Country | Sensitivity (%) | Specificity (%) | Approval |
|---|---|---|---|---|
| **1.A. *Cryptosporidium*** | | | | |
| **A. Immunofluorescence assays** | | | | |
| Crypto-Cel IF Test | Celllabs, AUS | 100 | 100 | FDA/CE |
| **B. Enzyme immunoassays** | | | | |
| *Cryptosporidium* II TEST(direct Ag/ spectrophotometric/visual) | Alere/Techlab, Inc USA | 97 | 100 | FDA |
| Prospect *Cryptosporidium* Rapid Assay | Thermo Fisher Scientific/REMEL, USA | 100 | No data | FDA |
| RIDASCREEN *Cryptosporidium*[a] | R-Biopharm, Germany | 100 | 97.3 | CE |
| PARA-TEC *Cryptosporidium* | Medical Chemical Corporation, USA | 100 | 100 | CE |
| **C. Immunochromatographic/point-of-care assays** | | | | |
| UNI-GOLD *Cryptosporidium* | Trinity Biotech, Ireland/USA | 100 | 100 | FDA/CE |
| XPECT *Cryptosporidium* LATERAL FLOW ASSAY, MODEL 2451020 | Thermo Scientific REMEL, USA | 96.4 | 98.3 | FDA |
| *Cryptosporidium* Fecal ELISA Test | Cortez Diagnostics, USA | 100 | 100 | FDA[a]/CE |
| Crypto-Strip C-1005 (CRYPTO UNI-STRIP, CRYPTO-CIT)[a] | Coris BioConcept, Belgium | 95.7 | 100 | CE |
| RIDA Quick *Cryptosporidium* (dipstick or cassette)[a] | R-Biopharm, Germany | 93.8 | 100 | CE |
| CRYPTO (card and blister formats)[a] | CerTest Biotec, Spain | 99 | 99 | CE |
| Stick Crypto[a] | Operon, Spain | 79.3 | 99.5 | CE |
| **D. PCR-based assays** | | | | |
| KHCRYP (real-time PCR) | CEERAM S.A.S., France | No data | No data | CE |
| **1.B. *Giardia duodenalis*** | | | | |
| **A. Immunofluorescent assays** | | | | |
| *Giardia*-Cel IF Test | Celllabs, Australia | 90.3 | 100 | FDA/CE |

(continued on next page)

**Table 1**
*(continued)*

| Product Name | Manufacturer, Country | Sensitivity (%) | Specificity (%) | Approval |
|---|---|---|---|---|
| **B. Enzyme immunoassays (antigen detection)** | | | | |
| *Giardia lamblia* ANTIGEN DETECTION MICROWELL ELISA | Ivd Research, Inc USA | 100 | 100 | FDA |
| TechLab *Giardia* II TEST | Techlab Inc/Alere USA | 100 | 100 | FDA |
| *Giardia* ELISA kit | Cortez Diagnostics, USA | 100 | 100 | FDA[a]/CE |
| ProSpecT *Giardia* Microplate Assay (direct Ag/spectrophotometric/visual) | Thermo Fisher Scientific/REMEL, USA | 97 | No data | FDA |
| ProSpecT *Giardia* EZ Microplate Assay | Thermo Fisher Scientific/REMEL, USA | 97 | No data | FDA |
| RIDASCREEN *Giardia*[a] | R-Biopharm, Germany | 100 | 99.60 | CE |
| PARA-TEC *Giardia lamblia* | Medical Chemical Corporation, USA | 85 | 97.9 | CE |
| **C. Immunochromatographic/point-of-care diagnostics** | | | | |
| Uni-Gold *Giardia* | Trinity Biotech, Ireland | 100 | 100 | CE |
| Stick *Giardia*[a] | Operon, Spain | 93.8 | 98.9 | CE |
| *Giardia lamblia* (*Giardia*)[a] | CerTest Biotec, Spain | 97 | 99 | CE |
| *Giardia* (dipstick and cassete) | Coris BioConcept, Belgium | 96.3 | 97.8 | CE |
| **D. Molecular assays** | | | | |
| *Giardia* Test Kit KHGIAR | CEERAM S.A.S., France | No data | No data | CE |
| **1.C. Dual detection: *Cryptosporidium* spp (C) and *Giardia duodenalis*(G)** | | | | |
| **A. Immunofluorescent microscopy assays** | | | | |
| Crypto/Giardia-Cel IF Test | Cellabs, Australia | 100 | 100 | FDA/CE |
| MERIFLUOR *Cryptosporidium*/*Giardia* | Meridian Biosciences, USA | 100 | 100 | FDA |
| PARA-TECT *Cryptosporidium*/*Giardia* DFA 75Test Kit | Medical Chemical Corporation, USA | 100 | 100 | CE |
| IVD Crypto/Giardia DFA | IVD Research, Inc, USA | 100 | 100 | FDA |

**B. Enzyme immunoassays (antigen detection)**

| Test | Manufacturer | | | Approval |
|---|---|---|---|---|
| *Giardia/Cryptosporidium* QUIK CHEK test | Techlab Inc/Alere, USA | C-100, G-98.9 | C-99.8, G-100 | FDA |
| *Giardia/Cryptosporidium* CHEK | Techlab Inc/Alere, USA | 97.6 | 100 | FDA |
| Crypto/Giardia Ag Combo ELISA kit | Cortez Diagnostics, USA | 99 | 100 | CE/FDA[a] |
| ProSpecT *Giardia/Crypto* (spectrophotometric) | Thermo Fisher Scientific, USA | 100 | 95 | FDA |
| **C. Immunochromatographic/point-of-care assays** | | | | |
| XPECT *Giardia/Cryptosporidium* | Thermo Scientific REMEL, USA | C-96.4, G-95.8 | C-98.5, G-98.5 | FDA |
| Biosite Triage Parasite Panel | Alere/Biosite Incorporated, USA | C-91.4, G-95.1 | C-98.2, G-88.4 | FDA |
| ColorPAC *Giardia/Cryptosporidium* Rapid Assay | Becton Dickinson, USA | C-97.3, G-100 | C-100, G-100 | FDA |
| Crypto/Giardia Duo-Strip[a] | Coris BioConcept, Belgium | C-95.7, G-96.3 | C-100, G-97.8 | CE |
| ImmunoCard STAT! *Cryptosporidium/Giardia* Rapid Assay | Meridian Bioscience, USA | C-97.3, G-100 | C-100, G-100 | CE |
| RIDA Quick *Cryptosporidium/Giardia* Combi (dipstick or cassette)[a] | R-Biopharm, Germany | C-93.8, G-100 | C-100, G-95.2 | CE |
| RIDAQuick[b] *Cryptosporidium/Giardial Entamoeba* Combi (dipstick or cassette)[a] | R-Biopharm, Germany | C-83, G-91.9 | C-93.3, G-99.5 | CE |
| CRYPTO-GIARDIA (card and blister)[a] | CerTest Biotec, Spain | C-99, G-97 | C-99, G-99 | CE |
| CRYPTO-GIARDIA-ENTAMOEBA[a,b] | CerTest Biotec, Spain | C-99, G-97 | C-99, G-99 | CE |
| Stick Crypto-Giardia[a] | Operon, Spain | C-79.3, G-93.8 | C-99.5, G-98.9 | CE |
| **1.D. Molecular assays for detection of multiple enteric pathogens** | | | | |
| Film Array Instrument[c] | Biofire Diagnostics, USA | | | FDA/CE |
| xTAG Gastrointestinal Panel (GPP)[d] | Luminex, USA | C-100, G-100 Cyclospora-100 | C-99.6, G-99.5 Cyclospora-100 | FDA/CE |

[a] Not available in the United States.
[b] Also for *Entamoeba* spp.
[c] Multiplex assay including bacterial and viral pathogens.
[d] Multiplex assay including the protozoa *Cyclospora cayetanensis*, plus bacterial and viral pathogens.
*Data from* Catalog of cleared and approved medical device information from FDA. Database of approved in-vitro diagnostic devices. 2014. Accessed October 20, 2014.

species known to infect humans. Three other species are known to infect nonhuman primates, all parasites of monkeys in Africa.[62]

## Biology

*Cyclospora cayetanensis* (*Cyclospora*) is an anthroponotic parasite. Attempts to infect other animal species have proved unsuccessful[63]; thus, there is no animal model to better understand its biology. The live stages of *Cyclospora* were described from jejunal biopsies.[64] Infections start when a susceptible person ingests sporulated oocysts, a stage that is environmentally resistant. Oocysts are broken in the upper gastrointestinal tract because of partial digestion with gastric juices and digestive enzymes, leading to the release of the 2 internal cysts, called sporocysts, each with 2 infectious stages called sporozoites. On their release in the small intestine, the sporozoites infect epithelial cells where they transform into merozoites and replicate asexually, also infecting other enterocytes. After asexual replications, the merozoites differentiate into sexual stages called microgametocytes and macrogametocytes. New oocysts are formed as result of sexual reproduction between the microgametocytes and macrogametocytes. Unsporulated (and therefore noninfectious) oocysts are eventually released into the environment. Sporulation occurs in the environment. The precise factors that cause sporulation are not known, but it is estimated that it occurs in about 2 weeks.[2,65]

## Epidemiology

*Cyclospora* infections have been reported in several areas of the world. It is endemic mainly in nonindustrialized nations, whereas sporadic reports associated with outbreaks have been frequently reported in industrialized countries.[66] In endemic settings, cyclosporiasis is more frequent in children between the ages of 2 and 5 years, showing a marked seasonal pattern.[67] For example, in Nepal, there were higher rates of infection during the summer and rainy seasons,[68] whereas in Peru, most cases were detected between December and May, which are warmer months but without rain.[67]

In industrialized nations, cyclosporiasis has been more frequently reported in the summer months and most outbreaks have been traced back to imported fresh products. In the 1990s, most reported outbreaks in the United States were linked to imported berries. This trend has changed, and during the past 14 years, most outbreaks have been linked to leafy greens consumed raw, such as basil and herbs.

## Clinical Manifestations and Treatment

Gastrointestinal manifestations associated with cyclosporiasis include diarrhea, fatigue, and abdominal cramps, which are most likely reported between 1 and 2 weeks after infection. The duration of the patent period and the severity of symptoms are different between people living in endemic and nonendemic areas. Infections in endemic settings occur mainly in children older than 2 years and are almost never detected after 10 years of age. In these cases, infections may resolve spontaneously, and as high as 50% of infected people may not show any clinical symptoms. It seems that immunity plays a significant role.

In industrialized nations, where the parasite is not endemic, most people are likely to be naive and infections are almost always symptomatic, lasting 1 to 2 weeks or more. The main symptom is diarrhea, which persists if untreated.[69] Other symptoms are general malaise, lack of energy, loss of appetite, mild fever, nausea, flatulence, and abdominal cramps.[67,70]

In the case of people with deficits in their immune system, there are anecdotal reports of infections with a longer duration, although cyclosporiasis is not considered an opportunistic infection in HIV-infected people.[71] Treatment is highly effective and is based on the administration of sulfamethoxazole trimethoprim (TMP/SMX) orally, twice daily for 7 to 10 days.[72] However, no specific treatment is recommended for people who are allergic to sulfa drugs.[55]

## Diagnostic Testing

### Microscopy

As with other coccidia, *C cayetanensis* is not easily detected with traditional O&P procedures such as FEA concentration and trichrome stain.[55] Oocysts can be better visualized in FEA concentrates if viewed under differential interference contrast or phase contrast microscopy.[2,65] Oocysts can be more easily detected with permanent staining methods such as safranin or MAF staining. Oocysts stain red with both stains; however, characteristic nonuniform staining is observed with MAF and unstained oocysts are usually white and are referred to as ghost forms (see **Fig. 1**). In the case of safranin, oocysts stain more uniformly.[55]

Another characteristic of *C cayetanensis* is the autofluorescence of the oocyst wall under UV light, using excitation filters of 330 to 365 nm and less intense autofluorescense with filters of 450 to 490 nm.[2,9,65] Autofluorescence plus morphometric characteristics are helpful when detecting *Cyclospora* (**Fig. 2**). There are currently no DFA or molecular procedures that are approved by the FDA for routine clinical diagnosis of cyclosporiasis.

## CYSTOISOSPORA BELLI (PREVIOUSLY ISOSPORA BELLI)
### Biology and Taxonomy

*Cystoisospora belli* is placed among the Eimeriorina along with *Cyclospora*.[4] For several decades, *C belli* was placed in the genus *Isospora* until morphologic and molecular data were used to support its proper classification in the genus *Cystoisospora*.[73,74] This genus now includes all previously classified *Isospora* spp that infect mammals, whereas *Isospora* contains only parasites that infect passeriform birds.[74]

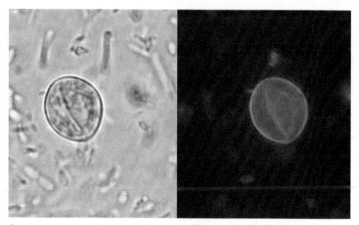

**Fig. 2.** *Cyclospora cayetanensis* oocyst viewed under normal light (*left*) and ultraviolet light (*right*) in an unstained wet mount. (Original magnification × 1000). (*Courtesy of* DPDx, Centers for Disease Control and Prevention, Atlanta, USA).

## Life Cycle and Biology

*Cystoisospora belli* is known to infect only humans and requires only the one host for completion of its life cycle, although paratenic hosts may be involved.[75] Typically, partially sporulated oocysts containing 1 (rarely 2) sporoblast are shed in feces. In the environment, the sporoblast divides into 2 sporoblasts, each of which secretes a cell wall to become sporocysts. After sporulation, each sporocyst contains 4 sporozoites. Humans become infected after ingestion of fully sporulated oocysts, through contaminated food, water, and fomites. On ingestion, the sporocysts excyst in the small intestine and release the sporozoites, which invade the host epithelial cells. The sporozoites undergo asexual replication called schizogony. Mature schizonts rupture, releasing merozoites that parasitize surrounding epithelial cells, perpetuating asexual multiplication. Eventually, multinucleate meronts are formed and sexual stages develop. Macrogametocytes are fertilized by microgametocytes resulting in formation of the oocyst, which can persist in the environment for several weeks or months.[55,75,76]

## Epidemiology

*Cystoisospora belli* has a worldwide distribution; however, several studies from AIDS patients with diarrhea have shown a higher prevalence of cystoisosporiasis among people from tropical or subtropical areas.[77–79]

## Clinical Manifestations and Treatment

In immunocompetent people, *C belli* has been associated with diarrhea, usually lasting 6 to 10 days, and infections self-resolving in 2 to 3 weeks, although intermittent shedding may continue for an additional 2 to –3 weeks. Severe symptoms were reported among people with immunocompromised systems, which can lead to life-threatening chronic profuse diarrhea.[52,80] Treatment is based on TMP/SMX.[81]

## Microscopic Diagnosis

Because of their large size, oocysts of *C belli* are usually detected during route O&P examinations. However, because oocysts tend to be shed in small numbers, repeated stool examinations and concentration procedures are recommended. Coccidian-specific stains, such as MAF and safranin, are preferred if permanent stains are used for diagnosis (see **Fig. 1**). As with *C cayetanensis*, screening of wet mounts can be enhanced by using UV microscopy, with both oocyst and sporoblast/sporocyst walls capable of autofluorescence.[7,9,75] There are currently no DFA or molecular procedures approved for routine clinical diagnosis of cystoisosporiasis.

## GIARDIA DUODENALIS
### Biology

The protozoan flagellate parasite *G duodenalis* is a common cause of human diarrheal disease worldwide.[82] It is transmitted through the fecal-oral route, frequently through ingestion of contaminated water and food.[6,76,82] This parasite has a direct life cycle, and the cysts passed in the feces are immediately infectious. These cysts can remain infectious for long periods in moist and cool environments.

### Epidemiology

*Giardia* has a worldwide distribution.[83] It affects people of all ages and has an important impact on public health. In the United States, it is more frequently reported in children aged 1 to 9 years.[84] This parasite has been associated with major outbreaks and can also be present in domestic animals, such as household pets and farm animals. Giardiasis is highly underreported, with data from the United States showing that the number of annually reported cases remained steady for several years at around 20,000, whereas the estimated number of cases was 2 million.[85]

Through molecular genotyping methods, *G duodenalis* has been classified in distinct assemblages or genotypes. Assemblages A and B are the most frequently reported in humans, either in industrialized or nonindustrialized nations. These assemblages have also been reported in cattle, dogs, and cats from different countries around the world. However, other assemblages of *Giardia* have been reported almost exclusively in animal species: assemblages C and D in domestic and wild canids, assemblage F in cats, and assemblage E in ruminants. Therefore, *G duodenalis* is considered a multispecies complex, where assemblages A and B are considered to have broad host specificity and zoonotic potential.[86–89]

## Clinical Manifestations

Approximately 40% of *Giardia* infections may be symptomatic, depending on the population. Symptoms may include diarrhea, cramps, bloating, nausea, and vomiting[6] and may be prolonged. Infections are normally self-limiting, but chronic diarrhea may occur in children[90] and a low proportion of immunocompromised people.[91] There is a report that prolonged giardiasis from early childhood has been associated with poor cognitive function later in life.[92]

Treatment of infections is recommended only when clinical manifestations affect the well-being of the infected person. Drug of choice is metronidazole, although search for alternative therapies is ongoing.[93]

## Diagnostic Testing

### Microscopy

Because cysts are shed sporadically during an infection, detection of *Giardia* may require several stool samples to be examined.[7,9] *Giardia* may be detected by microscopy, immunologic, or molecular methods. *Giardia* cysts and trophozoites can be readily detected via traditional methods such as trichrome staining and FEA concentrations (**Fig. 3**), although microscopy of whole organisms requires trained technicians as well as time to prepare and examine smears. The formalin-ether (Ritchie) concentration method is another common method used for the concentration of stool samples.[55]

### Antigen detection and rapid/point-of-care diagnosis

These assays are standardized and can generate results in a short time. Tests more widely used are antigen detection immunoassays such as DFA tests that detect whole organisms and enzyme immunoassays that detect antigens in stool, which can be completed in 1 to 2 hours. They have been reported to be highly sensitive and specific (see **Table 1B**).[94,95]

PCR assays for *Giardia* have become more common; however, PCR amplification and sequence analysis are more frequently used for genotype/assemblage classification and are not routinely used for diagnosis. The SSU rRNA fragment, commonly amplified by PCR for other enteric parasites, is rich in GC content and thus requires special PCR conditions. Therefore, PCR-based methods have been designed to amplify other informative loci, such as the triose phosphate isomerase, glutamate dehydrogenase, and β-giardin, which are used for the taxonomic or epidemiologic classification into assemblages.[88,89]

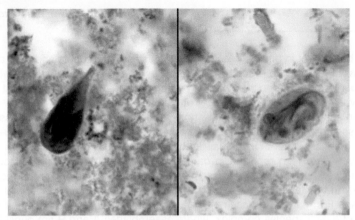

**Fig. 3.** Trophozoite (*left*) and cyst (*right*) of *Giardia duodenalis* (trichrome, original magnification × 1000). (*Courtesy of* DPDx, Centers for Disease Control and Prevention, Atlanta, USA.)

## SUMMARY ON DETECTION OF PARASITES

Microscopy continues to be the primary method for detection of the parasites covered in this review (**Table 2**), highlighting the importance of specimen processing and staining (see **Table 2**) and morphometric characteristics (**Table 3**). Rapid diagnostic assays (lateral flow/immunochromatographic cards) are also available for cryptosporidiosis or giardiasis, including approved devices for their simultaneous detection (see **Table 1**C). At present, there are molecular-based assays for the simultaneous detection of multiple enteric pathogens, which include virus, bacteria, and parasites. Two of these assays have been cleared by FDA and have been reported to have high sensitivity and specificity, including the detection of coinfections (see **Table 1**D).[96,97]

**Table 2**
**Microscopy procedures for detection of *Cryptosporidium* spp, *Cyclospora cayetanensis*, and *Cystoisospora belli***

| Procedure | Parasite | Advantages | Disadvantages |
|---|---|---|---|
| Wet mount (FEA concentrates) | *Cryptosporidium* spp | Concentration allows for better yield<br>FEA concentrate can be used for DFA (see later in the table) | Oocysts may be confused for yeast and other nonparasitic elements<br>Formalin waste |
| | *Cyclospora cayetanensis* | Concentration allows for better yield<br>May be enhanced with differential interference contrast (DIC) or phase microscopy | Oocysts may be confused with nonparasitic elements<br>Formalin waste |
| | *Cystoisospora belli* | Concentration allows for better yield<br>May be enhanced with DIC or phase microscopy | Oocysts shed sporadically so multiple collections should be tested<br>Formalin waste |

(continued on next page)

**Table 2**
*(continued)*

| Procedure | Parasite | Advantages | Disadvantages |
|---|---|---|---|
| Trichrome stain | *Cryptosporidium* spp | Not recommended | Oocysts do not stain well with trichrome; likely to be confused for yeast/fungal elements<br>Specimens in PVA usually not concentrated |
| | *Cyclospora cayetanensis* | Not recommended | Oocysts do not stain well with trichrome<br>Specimens in PVA usually not concentrated |
| | *Cystoisospora belli* | Not recommended | Not readily detected by trichrome<br>Specimens in PVA usually not concentrated |
| Modified Kinyoun acid-fast (MAF) stain | *Cryptosporidium* spp | Uniform staining of oocysts; sporozoites often visible | Oocysts may be confused with yeast and other fungal elements that often stain red to purple with MAF |
| | *Cyclospora cayetanensis* | Oocysts can stain pink to red | Variability in staining; often many oocysts do not stain (ghost forms) and may be overlooked by inexperienced microscopists |
| | *Cystoisospora belli* | Sporoblasts stain red with MAF | Often there is shrinkage of oocyst wall, distorting form of oocysts |
| Hot safranin stain | *Cryptosporidium* spp | Uniform staining of oocysts | Requires heat; messy procedure |
| | *Cyclospora cayetanensis* | More uniform staining of oocysts | Requires heat; messy procedure |
| | *Cystoisospora belli* | Uniform staining of sporoblasts<br>Oocyst wall less likely to collapse than with MAF | Requires heat; messy procedure |
| Ultraviolet microscopy | *Cryptosporidium* spp | Not available | Oocysts do not autofluoresce |
| | *Cyclospora cayetanensis* | Oocyst walls autofluoresce<br>Allows for more rapid screening | Requires special filter with wavelength of 450–490 nm (not routine in most laboratories) |
| | *Cystoisospora belli* | Oocyst and sporoblast walls autofluoresce<br>Allows for more rapid screening | Requires special filter with wavelength of 450–490 nm (not routine in most laboratories) |
| DFA | *Cryptosporidium* spp | Allows for rapid screening of *Cryptosporidium* spp<br>Some allow for simultaneous screening of other organisms (eg, *Giardia*) | Requires microscopy with fluorescence capabilities<br>Could be expensive if not used routinely |
| | *Cyclospora cayetanensis* | None available | None available |
| | *Cystoisospora belli* | None available | None available |

**Table 3**
Comparative morphology of *Giardia duodenalis*, *Cryptosporidium* spp, *Cyclospora cayetanensis*, and *Cystoisospora belli*

| Organism | Size | Other Morphologic Features | Preferred Morphologic Diagnostic Test |
|---|---|---|---|
| *Giardia duodenalis* | Trophozoites, 10–20 μm long Cysts 8.0–10 μm long | Trophozoites: pyriform shape; sucking disk; 2 nuclei; 2 median bodies; 8 flagella (4 lateral, 2 ventral, 2 posterior) Cysts: ovoid shape; 2–4 nuclei; fibrils and median bodies; no flagella | Trophozoites: direct wet mount; trichrome stain Cysts: FEA concentration wet mount; trichrome stain |
| *Cryptosporidium* spp | Oocysts: 4.0–6.0 μm | Oocysts: spherical shape; sporulated in feces (4 sporozoites present) | Modified acid-fast stain; Safranin stain |
| *Cyclospora cayetanensis* | Oocysts: 8.0–10 μm | Oocysts: spherical; unsporulated in fresh feces; refractile globules present | Modified acid-fast stain; Safranin stain; UV microscopy |
| *Cystoisospora belli* | Oocysts: 20–33 μm long | Oocysts: oval to ellipsoidal shape; unsporulated in fresh feces; double-layered hyaline cyst wall; single sporoblast usually present | Modified acid-fast stain; safranin stain; UV microscopy |

## SELF-ASSESSMENT

1. The preferred tests to diagnose *Cyclospora* are
   a. O&P examination using trichrome-stained smears and light microscopy
   b. PCR amplification of the 18s ribosomal rRNA gene
   c. Laboratory-based antigen capture assays approved by FDA
   d. Species-specific point-of-care diagnostic devices
   e. Concentration of stool sample followed by MAF stain, complemented with UV microscopy

2. When there is a potential case of infection with enteric protozoa, it is ideal to request
   a. A single stool sample
   b. Two stool samples collected the same day
   c. Three stool samples collected the same day
   d. The next 3 consecutive stool samples
   e. Three stool samples collected over 7 to 10 days

3. The parasites *Giardia*, *Cyclospora*, *Cryptosporidium*, and *Cystoisospora* may cause similar clinical manifestations. Which tests would be recommended for differential diagnosis of these parasites?
   a. Species-specific antigen detection assays for each parasite
   b. Stool concentration followed by immunofluorescent microscopy
   c. PCR amplification and DNA sequencing of the 18s RNA gene
   d. Stool concentration followed by O&P microscopy (wet mount and trichrome stain) and microscopic examination of acid-fast–stained smear
   e. Species-specific point-of-care diagnostic devices for each parasite

## ANSWERS

Answer 1: E.

Concentration of the sample increases the detection capacity of microscopy, the acid-fast stain drastically helps visualize *Cyclospora*, and UV microscopy allows visualization of the characteristic autofluorescence of oocysts that are 8.0 to 10 μm in diameter.

Answer 2: E.

Parasites may have intermittent shedding, and the sensitivity of coproparasitologic examinations increases by analyzing 3 samples collected over nonconsecutive days.

Answer 3: D.

The concentration of specimens facilitates the detection of enteric protozoa. These parasites can be differentiated based on morphologic (shape and size) and staining characteristics.

## REFERENCES

1. Bern C, Hernandez B, Lopez MB, et al. The contrasting epidemiology of *Cyclospora* and *Cryptosporidium* among outpatients in Guatemala. Am J Trop Med Hyg 2000;63(5–6):231–5.
2. Ortega YR, Sterling CR, Gilman RH, et al. *Cyclospora* species–a new protozoan pathogen of humans. N Engl J Med 1993;328(18):1308–12.
3. Duszynsky DW, Upton SJ, Couch L. The coccidia of the world. Review of coccidia in humans and animals. 2014. Available at: http://biology.unm.edu/biology/coccidia/home.html. Accessed December 8, 2014.
4. Adl SM, Simpson AG, Lane CE, et al. The revised classification of eukaryotes. J Eukaryot Microbiol 2012;59(5):429–93.
5. Wolfe MS. Giardiasis. Clin Microbiol Rev 1992;5(1):93–100.
6. Ortega YR, Adam RD. *Giardia*: overview and update. Clin Infect Dis 1997;25(3): 545–9 [quiz: 550].
7. McHardy IH, Wu M, Shimizu-Cohen R, et al. Detection of intestinal protozoa in the clinical laboratory. J Clin Microbiol 2014;52(3):712–20.
8. Hiatt RA, Markell EK, Ng E. How many stool examinations are necessary to detect pathogenic intestinal protozoa? Am J Trop Med Hyg 1995;53(1):36–9.
9. Garcia L, editor. Diagnostic medical parasitology. 5th edition. Washington, DC: ASM Press; 2007.
10. Pietrzak-Johnston SM, Bishop H, Wahlquist S, et al. Evaluation of commercially available preservatives for laboratory detection of helminths and protozoa in human fecal specimens. J Clin Microbiol 2000;38(5):1959–64.
11. Tyzzer EE. An extracellular coccidium, *Cryptosporidium muris* (Gen. Et Sp. Nov.), of the gastric glands of the common mouse. J Med Res 1910;23(3):487–510.3.
12. Tyzzer EE. *Cryptosporidium parvum* (sp. nov.), a coccidium found in the small intestine of the common mouse. Arch Protistenkunde 1912;26:394–412.
13. Current WL, Reese NC, Ernst JV, et al. Human cryptosporidiosis in immunocompetent and immunodeficient persons. Studies of an outbreak and experimental transmission. N Engl J Med 1983;308(21):1252–7.
14. Malebranche R, Arnoux E, Guerin JM, et al. Acquired immunodeficiency syndrome with severe gastrointestinal manifestations in Haiti. Lancet 1983;2(8355): 873–8.
15. Jonas C, Deprez C, De Maubeuge J, et al. *Cryptosporidium* in patient with acquired immunodeficiency syndrome. Lancet 1983;2(8356):964.

16. Colford JM Jr, Tager IB, Hirozawa AM, et al. Cryptosporidiosis among patients infected with human immunodeficiency virus. Factors related to symptomatic infection and survival. Am J Epidemiol 1996;144(9):807–16.

17. Flanigan T, Whalen C, Turner J, et al. *Cryptosporidium* infection and CD4 counts. Ann Intern Med 1992;116(10):840–2.

18. Navin TR, Weber R, Vugia DJ, et al. Declining CD4+ T-lymphocyte counts are associated with increased risk of enteric parasitosis and chronic diarrhea: results of a 3-year longitudinal study. J Acquir Immune Defic Syndr Hum Retrovirol 1999; 20(2):154–9.

19. Soave R. Waterborne cryptosporidiosis–setting the stage for control of an emerging pathogen. Clin Infect Dis 1995;21(1):63–4.

20. Navin TR, Juranek DD. Cryptosporidiosis: clinical, epidemiologic, and parasitologic review. Rev Infect Dis 1984;6(3):313–27.

21. Ortega YR, Sheehy RR, Cama VA, et al. Restriction fragment length polymorphism analysis of *Cryptosporidium parvum* isolates of bovine and human origin. J protozool 1991;38(6):40S–1S.

22. Sulaiman IM, Xiao L, Yang C, et al. Differentiating human from animal isolates of *Cryptosporidium parvum*. Emerg Infect Dis 1998;4(4):681–5.

23. Peng MM, Xiao L, Freeman AR, et al. Genetic polymorphism among *Cryptosporidium parvum* isolates: evidence of two distinct human transmission cycles. Emerg Infect Dis 1997;3(4):567–73.

24. Xiao L, Sulaiman I, Fayer R, et al. Species and strain-specific typing of *Cryptosporidium* parasites in clinical and environmental samples. Mem Inst Oswaldo Cruz 1998;93(5):687–91.

25. Morgan U, Xiao L, Sulaiman I, et al. Which genotypes/species of *Cryptosporidium* are humans susceptible to? J Eukaryot Microbiol 1999;46(5):42S–3S.

26. Morgan UM, Xiao L, Fayer R, et al. Variation in *Cryptosporidium*: towards a taxonomic revision of the genus. Int J Parasitol 1999;29(11):1733–51.

27. Morgan UM, Xiao L, Fayer R, et al. Epidemiology and strain variation of *Cryptosporidium parvum*. Contrib Microbiol 2000;6:116–39.

28. Xiao L, Morgan UM, Fayer R, et al. *Cryptosporidium* systematics and implications for public health. Parasitol Today 2000;16(7):287–92.

29. Ryan U, Fayer R, Xiao L. *Cryptosporidium* species in humans and animals: current understanding and research needs. Parasitology 2014;141(13):1667–85.

30. Santin M, Trout JM, Xiao L, et al. Prevalence and age-related variation of *Cryptosporidium* species and genotypes in dairy calves. Vet Parasitol 2004;122(2): 103–17.

31. Valenzuela O, Gonzalez-Diaz M, Garibay-Escobar A, et al. Molecular characterization of *Cryptosporidium* spp. in children from Mexico. PLoS One 2014;9(4): e96128.

32. Tzipori S, Widmer G. The biology of *Cryptosporidium*. Contrib Microbiol 2000;6:1–32.

33. Rosales MJ, Cordon GP, Moreno MS, et al. Extracellular like-gregarine stages of *Cryptosporidium parvum*. Acta Trop 2005;95(1):74–8.

34. Petry F. Structural analysis of *Cryptosporidium parvum*. Microsc Microanal 2004; 10(5):586–601.

35. Hijjawi NS, Meloni BP, Ryan UM, et al. Successful in vitro cultivation of *Cryptosporidium andersoni*: evidence for the existence of novel extracellular stages in the life cycle and implications for the classification of *Cryptosporidium*. Int J Parasitol 2002;32(14):1719–26.

36. Fayer R. General biology. In: Fayer R, Xiao L, editors. *Cryptosporidium* and cryptosporidiosis. Boca Raton (FL): CRC press; 2008. p. 1–42.

37. Caccio S, Putignani L. Epidemiology of human cryptosporidiosis. In: Caccio S, Widmer G, editors. *Cryptosporidium* parasite and disease. Wien, Austria: Springer; 2014. p. 43–78.
38. Assessing the public health threat associated with waterborne cryptosporidiosis: report of a workshop. MMWR Recomm Rep 1995;44(RR-6):1–19.
39. Centers for Disease Control and Prevention. Foodborne outbreak of cryptosporidiosis–Spokane, Washington, 1997. MMWR Morb Mortal Wkly Rep 1998; 47(27):565–7.
40. Rose JB, Slifko TR. *Giardia*, *Cryptosporidium*, and *Cyclospora* and their impact on foods: a review. J Food Prot 1999;62(9):1059–70.
41. Ortega YR, Roxas CR, Gilman RH, et al. Isolation of *Cryptosporidium parvum* and *Cyclospora cayetanensis* from vegetables collected in markets of an endemic region in Peru. Am J Trop Med Hyg 1997;57(6):683–6.
42. Koch KL, Phillips DJ, Aber RC, et al. Cryptosporidiosis in hospital personnel. Evidence for person-to-person transmission. Ann Intern Med 1985;102(5): 593–6.
43. Navin TR. Cryptosporidiosis in humans: review of recent epidemiologic studies. Eur J Epidemiol 1985;1(2):77–83.
44. Xiao L, Ryan U. Molecular epidemiology. In: Fayer R, Xiao L, editors. *Cryptosporidium* and cryptosporidiosis. Boca Raton (FL): CRC Press, and IWA Publishing; 2008. p. 119–71.
45. Xiao L. Molecular epidemiology of cryptosporidiosis: an update. Exp Parasitol 2010;124(1):80–9.
46. Yoder JS, Beach MJ, Centers for Disease Control and Prevention, et al. Cryptosporidiosis surveillance–United States, 2003-2005. MMWR Surveill Summ 2007; 56(7):1–10.
47. Yoder JS, Harral C, Beach MJ, et al. Cryptosporidiosis surveillance - United States, 2006-2008. MMWR Surveill Summ 2010;59(6):1–14.
48. Yoder JS, Wallace RM, Collier SA, et al. Cryptosporidiosis surveillance–United States, 2009-2010. MMWR Surveill Summ 2012;61(5):1–12.
49. Ortega Y, Cama V. Foodborne transmission. In: Fayer R, Xiao L, editors. *Cryptosporidium* and cryptosporidiosis. Boca Raton (FL): CRC Press and IWA Publishing; 2008. p. 289–304.
50. Blackburn BG, Mazurek JM, Hlavsa M, et al. Cryptosporidiosis associated with ozonated apple cider. Emerg Infect Dis 2006;12(4):684–6.
51. Cama VA, Bern C, Roberts J, et al. *Cryptosporidium* species and subtypes and clinical manifestations in children, Peru. Emerg Infect Dis 2008;14(10):1567–74.
52. Soave R. Cryptosporidiosis and isosporiasis in patients with AIDS. Infect Dis Clin North Am 1988;2(2):485–93.
53. New drug for parasitic infections in children. FDA Consum 2003;37(3):4.
54. White CA Jr. Nitazoxanide: a new broad spectrum antiparasitic agent. Expert Rev Anti Infect Ther 2004;2(1):43–9.
55. DPDx. DPDx [Web page]. Parasite diagnosis. 2013. Available at: http://www.cdc.gov/dpdx/cryptosporidiosis/dx.html. Accessed December 20, 2014.
56. Catalog of cleared and approved medical device information from FDA. 2014. Database of approved in-vitro diagnostic devices. Available at: http://www.accessdata.fda.gov/scripts/cdrh/devicesatfda/index.cfm. Accessed October 20, 2014.
57. Xiao L, Lal AA, Jiang J. Detection and differentiation of *Cryptosporidium* oocysts in water by PCR-RFLP. Methods Mol Biol 2004;268:163–76.
58. Ashford RW. Occurrence of an undescribed coccidian in man in Papua New Guinea. Ann Trop Med Parasitol 1979;73(5):497–500.

59. Relman DA, Schmidt TM, Gajadhar A, et al. Molecular phylogenetic analysis of *Cyclospora*, the human intestinal pathogen, suggests that it is closely related to *Eimeria* species. J Infect Dis 1996;173(2):440–5.

60. Pieniazek NJ, Herwaldt BL. Reevaluating the molecular taxonomy: is human-associated *Cyclospora* a mammalian *Eimeria* species? Emerg Infect Dis 1997; 3(3):381–3.

61. Franzen C, Muller A, Bialek R, et al. Taxonomic position of the human intestinal protozoan parasite *Isospora belli* as based on ribosomal RNA sequences. Parasitol Res 2000;86(8):669–76.

62. Eberhard ML, Njenga MN, DaSilva AJ, et al. A survey for *Cyclospora* spp. in Kenyan primates, with some notes on its biology. J Parasitol 2001;87(6):1394–7.

63. Eberhard ML, Ortega YR, Hanes DE, et al. Attempts to establish experimental *Cyclospora cayetanensis* infection in laboratory animals. J Parasitol 2000;86(3): 577–82.

64. Ortega YR, Nagle R, Gilman RH, et al. Pathologic and clinical findings in patients with cyclosporiasis and a description of intracellular parasite life-cycle stages. J Infect Dis 1997;176(6):1584–9.

65. Ortega YR, Gilman RH, Sterling CR. A new coccidian parasite (Apicomplexa: Eimeriidae) from humans. J Parasitol 1994;80(4):625–9.

66. Ortega YR, Sterling CR, Gilman RH. Cyclospora cayetanensis. Adv Parasitol 1998;40:399–418.

67. Bern C, Ortega Y, Checkley W, et al. Epidemiologic differences between cyclosporiasis and cryptosporidiosis in Peruvian children. Emerg Infect Dis 2002; 8(6):581–5.

68. Sherchand JB, Cross JH. Emerging pathogen *Cyclospora cayetanensis* infection in Nepal. Southeast Asian J Trop Med Public Health 2001;32(Suppl 2):143–50.

69. Huang P, Weber JT, Sosin DM, et al. The first reported outbreak of diarrheal illness associated with *Cyclospora* in the United States. Ann Intern Med 1995;123(6): 409–14.

70. Torres-Slimming PA, Mundaca CC, Moran M, et al. Outbreak of cyclosporiasis at a naval base in Lima, Peru. Am J Trop Med Hyg 2006;75(3):546–8.

71. Pape JW, Verdier RI, Boncy M, et al. *Cyclospora* infection in adults infected with HIV. Clinical manifestations, treatment, and prophylaxis. Ann Intern Med 1994; 121(9):654–7.

72. Hoge CW, Shlim DR, Ghimire M, et al. Placebo-controlled trial of co-trimoxazole for *Cyclospora* infections among travellers and foreign residents in Nepal. Lancet 1995;345(8951):691–3.

73. Frenkel JK. *Besnoitia wallacei* of cats and rodents: with a reclassification of other cyst-forming isosporoid coccidia. J Parasitol 1977;63(4):611–28.

74. Barta JR, Schrenzel MD, Carreno R, et al. The genus *Atoxoplasma* (Garnham 1950) as a junior objective synonym of the genus *Isospora* (Schneider 1881) species infecting birds and resurrection of *Cystoisospora* (Frenkel 1977) as the correct genus for *Isospora* species infecting mammals. J Parasitol 2005;91(3): 726–7.

75. Lindsay DS, Dubey JP, Blagburn BL. Biology of *Isospora* spp. from humans, nonhuman primates, and domestic animals. Clin Microbiol Rev 1997;10(1):19–34.

76. Marshall MM, Naumovitz D, Ortega Y, et al. Waterborne protozoan pathogens. Clin Microbiol Rev 1997;10(1):67–85.

77. Certad G, Arenas-Pinto A, Pocaterra L, et al. Isosporiasis in Venezuelan adults infected with human immunodeficiency virus: clinical characterization. Am J Trop Med Hyg 2003;69(2):217–22.

78. Cranendonk RJ, Kodde CJ, Chipeta D, et al. *Cryptosporidium parvum* and *Isospora belli* infections among patients with and without diarrhoea. East Afr Med J 2003;80(8):398–401.

79. Sorvillo FJ, Lieb LE, Seidel J, et al. Epidemiology of isosporiasis among persons with acquired immunodeficiency syndrome in Los Angeles County. Am J Trop Med Hyg 1995;53(6):656–9.

80. Modigliani R, Bories C, Le Charpentier Y, et al. Diarrhoea and malabsorption in acquired immune deficiency syndrome: a study of four cases with special emphasis on opportunistic protozoan infestations. Gut 1985;26(2):179–87.

81. Pape JW, Johnson WD Jr. *Isospora belli* infections. Prog Clin Parasitol 1991;2: 119–27.

82. Adam RD. Biology of *Giardia lamblia*. Clin Microbiol Rev 2001;14(3):447–75.

83. Guerrant RL, Hughes JM, Lima NL, et al. Diarrhea in developed and developing countries: magnitude, special settings, and etiologies. Rev Infect Dis 1990; 12(Suppl 1):S41–50.

84. Yoder JS, Gargano JW, Wallace RM, et al. Giardiasis surveillance–United States, 2009-2010. MMWR Surveill Summ 2012;61(5):13–23.

85. Yoder JS, Harral C, Beach MJ, et al. Giardiasis surveillance - United States, 2006-2008. MMWR Surveill Summ 2010;59(6):15–25.

86. Thompson RC, Monis P. *Giardia*–from genome to proteome. Adv Parasitol 2012; 78:57–95.

87. Ryan U, Caccio SM. Zoonotic potential of *Giardia*. Int J Parasitol 2013;43(12–13): 943–56.

88. Feng Y, Xiao L. Zoonotic potential and molecular epidemiology of *Giardia* species and giardiasis. Clin Microbiol Rev 2011;24(1):110–40.

89. Monis PT, Caccio SM, Thompson RC. Variation in *Giardia*: towards a taxonomic revision of the genus. Trends Parasitol 2009;25(2):93–100.

90. Nundy S, Gilman RH, Xiao L, et al. Wealth and its associations with enteric parasitic infections in a low-income community in Peru: use of principal component analysis. Am J Trop Med Hyg 2011;84(1):38–42.

91. Cotte L, Rabodonirina M, Piens MA, et al. Prevalence of intestinal protozoans in French patients infected with HIV. J Acquir Immune Defic Syndr 1993;6(9): 1024–9.

92. Berkman DS, Lescano AG, Gilman RH, et al. Effects of stunting, diarrhoeal disease, and parasitic infection during infancy on cognition in late childhood: a follow-up study. Lancet 2002;359(9306):564–71.

93. Kulakova L, Galkin A, Chen CZ, et al. Discovery of novel antigiardiasis drug candidates. Antimicrob Agents Chemother 2014;58(12):7303–11.

94. Garcia LS, Shimizu RY. Evaluation of nine immunoassay kits (enzyme immunoassay and direct fluorescence) for detection of *Giardia lamblia* and *Cryptosporidium parvum* in human fecal specimens. J Clin Microbiol 1997;35(6): 1526–9.

95. Heyworth MF. Diagnostic testing for *Giardia* infections. Trans R Soc Trop Med Hyg 2014;108(3):123–5.

96. Taniuchi M, Verweij JJ, Sethabutr O, et al. Multiplex polymerase chain reaction method to detect *Cyclospora*, *Cystoisospora*, and *Microsporidia* in stool samples. Diagn Microbiol Infect Dis 2011;71(4):386–90.

97. Khare R, Espy MJ, Cebelinski E, et al. Comparative evaluation of two commercial multiplex panels for detection of gastrointestinal pathogens by use of clinical stool specimens. J Clin Microbiol 2014;52(10):3667–73.

### APPENDIX 1: LABORATORY PROCEDURES FOR THE MICROSCOPIC DETECTION OF COCCIDIAN PARASITES: *CRYPTOSPORIDIUM* SPP, *C CAYETANENSIS*, AND *C BELLI*
#### Modified Kinyoun Acid-Fast Stain

Specimen requirements: unfixed stool or stool preserved in 10% formalin (including FEA concentrates), SAF, or EcoFix.

Procedure
1. Prepare a thin film of stool on a glass microscope slide. Allow to completely air dry (do not use heat blocks to speed up drying).
2. Fix in absolute methanol for 30 seconds.
3. Stain with carbol-fuschin for 1 minute.
4. Rinse and drain with distilled water.
5. Decolorize in 10% sulfuric acid (10 mL sulfuric acid in 90 mL absolute ethanol) for 2 minutes.
6. Rinse quickly and drain with distilled water.
7. Counterstain with 3% malachite green (3 g malachite green in 100 mL distilled water) or methylene blue for 2 minutes.
8. Allow to dry (air dry or on a slide warmer at 60°C).
9. Mount with no. 1 thickness coverslip using Permount (or other sealing reagent).

Procedural notes
- Do not use a slide warmer for the first step (drying of specimen); it cooks the oocysts of *Cryptosporidium*, and they do not retain stain.
- Drain slides between each reagent.
- All reagents should be changed monthly or earlier as needed.

#### Hot Safranin Stain

Specimen requirements: unfixed stool or stool preserved in 10% formalin (including FEA concentrates), SAF, or EcoFix.

Procedure
1. Prepare a thin film of stool on a glass microscope slide. Allow to completely air dry (do not use heat blocks to speed up drying).
2. Fix in acid alcohol (3 mL hydrochloric acid in 97 mL absolute methanol) for 5 minutes.
3. Boil in safranin (1% aqueous solution in distilled water) for 1 minute.
4. Counterstain with 3% malachite green (3 g malachite green in 100 mL distilled water) for 1 minute.
5. Allow to dry (air dry or on a slide warmer at 60°C).
6. Mount with no. 1 thickness coverslip using Permount (or other sealing reagent).

Procedural notes
- Do not use a slide warmer for the first step (drying of specimen); it cooks the oocysts of *Cryptosporidium*, and they do not retain stain.
- Drain slides between each reagent.
- All reagents should be changed monthly or earlier as needed.
- Safranin stain should be boiling when slides are added.

# Intestinal Microsporidiosis

Andrew S. Field, FRCPA, FIAC, DiplomaCytopath(RCPA)[a],
Danny A. Milner Jr, MD, MSc[b],*

## KEYWORDS

- Microsporidium • Enteritis • AIDS • HIV • Immunosuppression • Warthin-Starry
- Diarrhea

## KEY POINTS

- Microsporidia are ubiquitous obligate intracellular parasites most closely related to fungi that are found in a wide range of hosts and have very long environmental survival times.
- Humans become symptomatically infected with 1 of the 14 species causing human disease in the setting of a depressed or failing immune system.
- The diagnosis of microsporidiosis should be attempted by stool examination with special stains and/or tissue biopsy with confirmation by electron microscopy or molecular methods when available.

## EPIDEMIOLOGY AND CLINICAL SPECTRUM OF MICROSPORIDIOSIS

Microsporidia are widespread obligate intracellular parasites. By molecular phylogenetic analysis, they are currently classified as fungi with which they share a common ancestor, but they behave similarly to intestinal protozoa. There are innumerable species of Microsporidium, with only an estimated 2% having proper speciation (~1500). Microsporidia infect a broad range of invertebrates, including fish, mosquitos, and flatworms, as well as vertebrates, and rarely infect humans unless they have an immunocompromised state due to human immunodeficiency virus (HIV) infection, solid organ transplantation,[1,2] chemotherapy, or immune suppression related to chronic autoimmune diseases. There are 14 species infecting humans from 8 genera, with 2 representing the vast majority of infections (**Table 1**). Although the self-limited and almost always asymptomatic infection of immunocompetent hosts is thought to be common, microsporidial diarrheal episodes in patients with AIDS can range from 30% to 70% depending on the series.[3–7] The organisms are most commonly associated with either contaminated unfiltered drinking water or swimming

Disclosures: The authors have no financial disclosures to make.
[a] Department of Anatomical Pathology, St Vincent's Hospital, Notre Dame University Medical School, Victoria Street, Darlinghurst 2010, Sydney, New South Wales, Australia; [b] Brigham and Women's Hospital/Harvard Medical School, 75 Francis Street, Amory 3, Boston, MA 02115, USA
* Corresponding author.
E-mail address: dmilner@partners.org

| Table 1 | | |
|---|---|---|
| **Microsporidium species, diseases, and some reported reservoirs** | | |
| **Species** | **Diseases** | **Environmental Reservoirs** |
| *Anncaliia algerae, Anncaliia connori, Anncaliia vesicularum* | Keratitis, myositis, systemic infection | Unknown |
| *Enterocytozoon bieneusi* | Diarrhea, wasting syndrome, cholangiopathy, cholangitis, acalculous cholecystitis, sinusitis, bronchitis, pneumonitis | Pigs, cattle, chickens, cats, monkeys, dogs |
| *Encephalitozoon cuniculi* | Systemic infection, keratoconjunctivitis, sinusitis, pneumonitis, urinary tract infection, nephritis, hepatitis, peritonitis, seizures, encephalitis | Carnivores, ruminants, primates, rabbits, rodents |
| *Encephalitozoon hellem* | Systemic infection, keratoconjunctivitis, sinusitis, bronchitis, pneumonia, nephritis, ureteritis, cystitis, prostatitis, urethritis | Ostrich, chickens, hummingbirds |
| *Encephalitozoon intestinalis* | Diarrhea, cholangiopathy, cholangitis, acalculous cholecystitis, sinusitis, bronchitis, pneumonitis, urinary tract infection, nephritis, bone lesions; nodular cutaneous lesions | Donkeys, cows, dogs, goats |
| *Microsporidium* spp | Corneal ulcer | Unknown |
| *Nosema ocularum* | Keratitis | Unknown |
| *Pleistophora* spp | Myositis | Fish, crustaceans |
| *Trachipleistophora hominis, Trachipleistophora anthropothera* | Systemic infection, including brain, heart, kidney, eye, myositis, keratoconjunctivitis, sinusitis | Unknown |
| *Vittaforma cornea* | Keratitis, urinary tract infection | Unknown |

*E bieneusi* and *E intestinalis* account for the vast majority of human infections.
*Data from* Refs.[7,26,27]

in lakes, ponds, and rivers in proximity to animal reservoirs.[8] Epidemic outbreaks, such as those seen with *Cryptsporidium*, are rare with none reported in the United States and 1 reported in France with no causal source.[9] The spores of Microsporidium can persist in the environment for 1 to 12 months (or more) depending on the species.

Opportunistic infections by the species *Enterocytozoon bieneusi* and *Encephalitozoon intestinalis* have been reported in patients with heart-lung,[10] renal, and bone marrow transplantation; HIV-positive patients with CD4 counts less than 100 per microliter[11]; and occasionally self-limited transient "traveler's diarrhea" in immune-competent patients.[12] Both species present clinically most commonly with chronic watery diarrhea and malabsorption.[3] Less common presentations of the infection include cholangitis and acalculous cholecystitis with organisms in the biliary and pancreatic tracts, as well as nonspecific sinusitis and rhinitis with organisms in the tracheal, bronchial and nasal epithelium (on biopsy or in washings).[11] In addition, *E intestinalis* can be seen in colonic enterocytes[11,13] and as a disseminated infection in the renal tubular cells. *E bieneusi* had been initially described in a 1985 and was a common infection in patients with AIDS without any effective treatment, whereas the less common *E intestinalis*, first described in patients with AIDS,[3,14,15] could be cleared by albendazole.[13] The incidence of both infections has been greatly reduced by highly active antiretroviral therapy. The route of transmission is thought to be ingestion of spores on food or in water through the fecal-oral or urinary-oral pathways, but direct inoculation into the respiratory epithelium or conjunctiva does occur.[16]

*E bieneusi* is found in pigs, other farm animals, and nonhuman primates, whereas there is a high seroprevalence in the tropics to *E intestinalis* without a known nonhuman host. Other species cause a range of disease in isolated cases and series reported in the literature, but detection methods and diagnostics for all species are similar for clinical purposes.

## DIAGNOSIS BY EXAMINATION OF STOOL

When microsporidial gut infection is suspected, it is appropriate to assess stool and urine samples, but this assessment requires experienced personnel. The diagnosis of microsporidiosis can be made on examination of stools and nasal or bronchial washings, as well as, in the case of *E intestinalis*, on urine, using a modified trichrome stain (the chromotrope 2R) (**Fig. 1**A, B) or fluorescent dye (such as Uvitex 2B), which

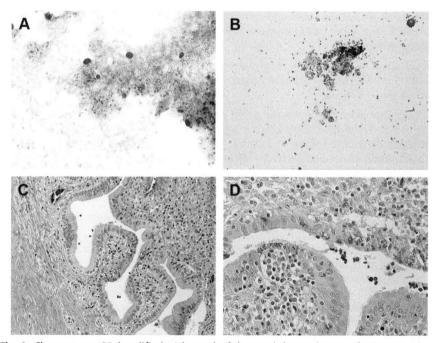

**Fig. 1.** Chromotrope 2R (modified trichrome) of the stool shows clusters of Microsporidium within green counterstained material (original magnification × 400) (*A*). The larger red oval elements are yeast. A similar trichrome stain of stool demonstrates large numbers of clustered and scattered organisms (original magnification × 400) (*B*). Low (original magnification × 200) (*C*) and high (original magnification × 400) (*D*) magnification of a tissue biopsy on trichrome stain show a similar appearance of the organisms within the epithelium of the mucosa. (*Courtesy of* [A] Dr Blaine Mathison, Centers for Disease Control and Prevention; [B–D] Dr Laura Lamps, University of Arkansas.)

stain the chitinous endospore. The accuracy of stool examination for microsporidia is poorly established, but is generally accepted as being high.[17] The actual pattern if any of microsporidial shedding in the infected patient probably relates most to the degree of immune compromise. Stool preparations, urine, sediments of duodenal aspirations, and bile duct aspirations can all be examined for spores, and fixation in formalin, or rinsing in saline or fresh specimens can all yield microsporidial spores, which are robust and highly resistant to manipulation, although drying may reduce infectivity. Stool specimens may benefit from various stool concentration techniques, and polymerase chain reaction (PCR) studies may offer better sensitivity than microscopy.[18] Urine requires high-speed centrifugation.

### Calcofluor Staining of Stools

Smears are prepared from liquid stool diluted in 3 times as much methanol, and air dried. Then 2 drops of a calcofluor solution are applied for 2 to 3 minutes at room temperature, and rinsed under water and counterstained with 0.1% Evans blue in Tris-buffered solution of pH 7.2 for 1 minute. The slides are again rinsed in water, dried, and cover-slipped with Cytoseal60 from Stephens Scientific (Stephens, GA). Microsporidia are seen as bluish white or purple oval halos, which is the chitinous exospore, under an ultraviolet microscope, wavelength 455 nm. The Uvitex 2B, described by vanGool and colleagues in 1993,[19] is no longer available, so Calcofluor White M2R (Sigma Chemical, St Louis, MO) as outlined by Didier and colleagues in 1995[20] is suggested: prepare a 0.5% solution in Tris-buffered saline at pH 7.2. This can be stored at room temperature but has to be centrifuged at 25,000 $g$ for 2 minutes to remove precipitates before use.

## DIAGNOSIS BY EXAMINATION OF TISSUE
### Yield of Tissue Biopsies

The diagnosis of intestinal infections can be made via biopsies of the small intestine, most commonly of the duodenum but also of the terminal ileum,[3] using routine and special histochemical stains, including immunohistochemistry. In the current era of reduced numbers of opportunistic infections passing through the laboratories of developed countries, small-bowel biopsy with or without electron microscopy (EM) and PCR (**Table 2**) may be a reasonable first step rather than stool examination (see **Fig. 1**C, D).

### Morphology

Small-bowel or duodenal biopsies show nonspecific partial villous atrophy, with minimal or no crypt hyperplasia and shortened blunt villi associated with a mild increase in macrophages, lymphocytes, plasma cells, and eosinophils in the lamina propria, and disordering of the superficial enterocytes, particularly over the tips of the villi but not in the crypts (**Fig. 2**A). Degenerate enterocytes become eosinophilic and rounded and are extruded from the epithelium at the villous tips. The round 6-μm plasmodia of *E bieneusi* are seen as small vacuoles in the superficial aspect of the enterocytes (see **Fig. 2**B), indenting the luminal aspect of the nuclei (see **Fig. 2**C), and may show clear slits under high power that may represent polar tubule precursors or endoplasmic reticulum of the plasmodium, and may also show faintly basophilic 1 × 1.5-μm spores that can be very hard to see in the hematoxylin-eosin (H&E) stain even with oil immersion and ×1000 magnification (see **Fig. 2**B–D). Occasionally the spores are seen dispersed on the surface of the epithelium or in the extruded degenerate cells. The spores of *E intestinalis* are larger, 1.0 × 2.2 μm, and easier to see as oval faintly

**Table 2**
**A brief summary of some methods of molecular detection in the literature are shown with species covered**

| Type of Assay | Organisms Detected |
| --- | --- |
| Fluorescent in situ hybridization | Enterocytozoon bieneusi<br>Encephalitozoon hellem |
| Polymerase chain reaction (PCR) with specific primers | Encephalitozoon cuniculi<br>E hellem<br>Encephalitozoon intestinalis<br>E bieneusi<br>Vittaforma corneae |
| PCR (conserved primers) with sequencing | All species (including unknown) |
| Real-time PCR (with probe or melt curve analysis) | E cuniculi<br>E hellem<br>E intestinalis |
| Multiplex PCR | E cuniculi<br>E hellem<br>E intestinalis<br>E bieneusi |
| Oligonucleotide array (with preamplification and species-specific probes) | E cuniculi<br>E hellem<br>E intestinalis<br>E bieneusi |

Adapted from Ghosh K, Weiss LM. Molecular diagnostic tests for microsporidia. Interdiscip Perspect Infect Dis 2009;2009:926521.

birefringent gray-staining spores, filling the larger parasitophorous vacuoles not only in the enterocytes but also in macrophages in the lamina propria (**Fig. 3**A, C). Spores should be differentiated from enterochromaffin granules, which are basal to the nucleus in the surface epithelial cells, and eosinophil granules. The spores occur only on the villous tips and do not occur in crypts where Paneth cell granules occur.

Both E bieneusi and E intestinalis can be found in acalculous cholecystitis in patients with AIDS where the infections will frequently be missed because they are not expected, and in bile duct brushings and washings, where again use of the Warthin-Starry and Giemsa stains will be helpful. Gall stones also may be present. Duodenal biopsies almost always have shown infection at the same time. E intestinalis has rarely been found in colon biopsies (see **Fig. 3**B), and again the use of special stains is required.[11,21] Several cases of granulomatous and suppurative hepatitis have been attributed to microsporidia without actual speciation.

### Special Stains

The spores of microsporidia are stained very distinctly in the Warthin-Starry stain, with a concordance with EM of 100%.[11] The spores stain as honey yellow to bright brown to black distinct oval spores, representing the staining of the spore precursors and spores, which are seen singly or as mulberrylike aggregates, representing the limits of the plasmodium of E bieneusi (see **Fig. 3**C) or the parasitophorous vacuole of E intestinalis (see **Fig. 3**D).[21] It is essential, as with any microbial special stain, that the correct oval cytomorphology of the spores and their correct location within the enterocytes, which is the apical region, should be recognized in the Warthin-Starry stain, as lysosomal and apoptotic debris in enterocytes can mimic the microsporidia,

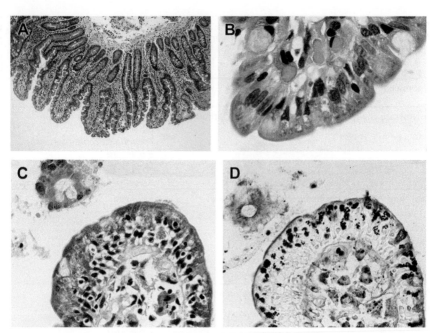

Fig. 2. *E. bieneusi* at low power H&E stain, the duodenal biopsy shows partial villous atrophy and irregularity of villi (original magnification × 100) (*A*). At higher magnification vacuoles can be seen in the superficial cytoplasm of the disordered enterocytes indenting the basal nuclei and containing granules and slits (*B, C*) in the H&E stain (*B*, original magnification × 1000, oil; *C*, original magnification × 400). The larger univacuolar goblet cells are present. The spores and spore precursors can be hard to see in the routine H&E stain (*C*), but are easily seen in the Warthin Starry stain as aggregated dark brown to black spores in the enterocytes (original magnifcation × 400) (*D*). Apoptotic debris can be seen in some enterocytes and lamina propria macrophages (*D*).

especially *E bieneusi* (see **Fig. 3**C). Other stains include the Brown-Brenn and Brown-Hopps modifications of the Gram stain, which stain the mature spores a "gram-positive" violet to purple color and the earlier forms a variable pale red, and the "hot Gram-chromotrope" stain, which combines a modified Gram stain with the Weber chromotrope stain used for stools.[18] The Giemsa stain of nasal and bronchial washes stains the spores a light blue, and in the case of *E intestinalis*, demonstrates a clear posterior vacuole and faint small red punctate dot, possibly the nucleus. The Grocott methenamine silver, Gram, and Periodic acid-Schiff (PAS) with diastase stain are all negative for the spores. The microsporidia can be focal and small in number and the Warthin-Starry stain allows scanning of biopsies. If spores are seen in the lamina propria of small-bowel biopsies in addition to the enterocytes, *E bieneusi* is excluded, and the species-specific diagnosis of *E intestinalis* can be made (see **Fig. 3**D). Similarly, the presence of microsporidia in colonic enterocytes is specific for *E intestinalis*.[11,13]

## WARTHIN-STARRY STAIN FOR SMALL-BOWEL BIOPSIES

Cut sections from paraffin-embedded material on clean slides with no adhesive, such as polylysine or gelatin, are rinsed in distilled water and placed for 30 minutes at

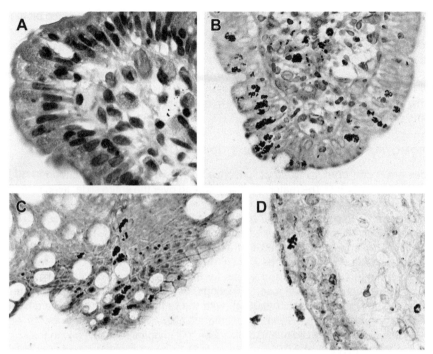

**Fig. 3.** *E intestinalis*: the spores are larger than those of *E bieneusi* and appear as faintly birefringent grey blue granules in vacuoles In the superficial cytoplasm of the duodenal enterocytes and lamina propria macrophages (*A*, original magnification × 1000, oil) in the H&E, and more clearly in the Warthin Starry stain (*B*, original magnification × 400) where the presence of spores in macrophages is diagnostic of *E intestinalis*. *E intestinalis* seen in superficial colonic epithelium (*C*, original magnification × 1000, oil) and respiratory epithelium (*D*, original magnification × 1000, oil) in the Warthin Starry stain at high power.

37°C in 1% silver nitrate, freshly prepared from acidified water pH 4.0 diluting 1:10 a stock 10% silver nitrate solution.[21] After washing the slides in distilled water 3 times, the sections are placed in 15 mL of developing solution (pH 4.0 water, 5% gelatin, mixed and preheated in 60°C water bath, and 1.5 mL 10% silver nitrate and 1.0 mL of 1.5% quinol) in a 60°C water bath until the sections turn a light honey brown. The change from yellow to brown occurs in 2 to 3 minutes and is rapid. The slides are checked, rinsed well in distilled and then hot tap water, repeating the distilled water rinse. The slides are then fixed in 5% sodium thiosulfate for 3 minutes to avoid fading, washed in water for 2 minutes, dehydrated, cleared in xylol, and mounted immediately in a reliable mountant such as Eukitt (O.KindlerGmbH & Co, Freiburg, Germany). The Warthin-Starry stain can have a dirty background if slides treated with an adhesive are used, or glassware is less than clean or rinsed with anything other than distilled water. The working solutions need to be new; especially the quinol (15% hydroxyquinone), which if oxidized produces a yellow-brown background.

## BROWN-BRENN GRAM STAIN FOR TISSUE SECTIONS

Routine 4-μm-thick sections are deparaffinized and rehydrated in distilled water, before being covered in crystal violet for 1 minute, drained, and rinsed with distilled water.[18] Gram iodine solution is then applied for 5 minutes, before rinsing and blotting, and applying decolorizer, such as isopropanol and acetone, rather than absolute alcohol mixed with acetone for approximately 10 seconds until the color stops running, and rinsing again in distilled water. Basic fuchsin rather than safranin O is used for 1 minute, and then the slides are dipped in acetone to start differentiation and immediately into 1% picric acid acetone until the sections are yellowish-pink. Immediately the slides are rinsed quickly in acetone and then in acetone-xylene and then cleared in xylene and mounted.

## CHROMOTROPE STAINING FOR STOOL STUDIES

Slides are made from 10 to 20 μL unconcentrated liquid stool suspended in 30 to 60 mL 10% formalin.[22] The material is thinly spread over the entire slide, fixed in methanol for 5 minutes, and stained for 90 minutes in the chromotrope stain (6 g chromotrope 2R, with 0.15 g fast green, 0.7 g phosphotungstic acid in 3 mL glacial acetic acid; stood for 30 minutes and then mixed with 100 mL distilled water). The slides are then rinsed in acid alcohol (995.5 mL 90% ethyl alcohol with 4.5 mL acetic acid) for 10 seconds, dipped into 95% alcohol as a rinse, dehydrated in 95% alcohol for 5 minutes, 100% alcohol for 10 minutes, and xylene for 5 minutes. The chromotrope blue stain was used by Ryan and colleagues,[18,23] using 0.5 g aniline blue instead of fast green and less phosphotungstic acid (0.25 g), with the remaining staining the same. And Kokoskin and colleagues[24] 1994 suggested staining with the chromotrope for only 10 minutes at 50°C, and Didier and colleagues[18,20] suggested staining with the chromotrope for 30 minutes at 37°C.

### Immunohistochemistry

A number of immunohistochemical stains using various antibodies to either *E bieneusi* or *E intestinalis* have been reported in specialized laboratories, and can be genus or species specific. The commercial availability changes with time. Because *E bieneusi* has been difficult to culture, serology and immunohistochemical stains to detect its infections have been slow to develop. Isolates of the *Encephalitozoon* spp have been cultured.

### Electron Microscopy

EM identifies the unique ultrastructure of the Microsporidium phylum that is the spore with its polar tubule, and can distinguish most of the genera. This technique is considered the gold standard, although it is relatively labor intensive, examines only a small amount of sample, and requires expensive equipment and processes. Exact separation of species traditionally was made by EM, based on the presence or absence of a parasitophorous vacuole and the precise developmental stages, nuclear configuration, and spore characteristics. For example, the *E bieneusi* spore has 5 to 6 coils of the polar tubule in a double, "inner and outer" row, whereas *E intestinalis* has a single row of 5 to 7 coils. But there are limits to the ability of EM to speciate microsporidia, for example, the 3 *Encephalitozoon* spp, *Encephalitozoon cuniculi*, *Encephalitozoon hellem*, and *E intestinalis*, require analysis of the nucleotide sequences of the small subunit rRNA to distinguish them.

In our practice at present, if the light microscopy appearances suggest an opportunistic infection but none can be seen in the H&E and by the special stains described previously, then sections will be cut for specific PCR studies and material will be cut from the paraffin block for EM. There is usually more than one small-bowel or duodenal or terminal ileal biopsy in the block, and a small-bowel biopsy can be cut from the paraffin block, de-paraffinized, postfixed in osmium tetroxide, and processed and embedded in resin, and ultrathin sections cut for toluidine blue staining and examination that may itself be diagnostic (**Fig. 4**D) and EM. If repeat biopsies are performed or stool examination has suggested microsporidial infection, a separate biopsy can be taken at endoscopy, placed in room temperature, not 4°C, glutaraldehyde, and processed directly for EM, which will yield much better preservation of the organism,[15] especially *E bieneusi* and its plasmodia.

The 0.7 to 1.0 × 1.1 to 1.6-μm spores of *E bieneusi* contain the characteristic polar tubule that defines the Microsporidium, which is attached to the anchoring disc at one pole within the outer electron-dense glycoprotein exospore and inner electron-lucent chitinous endospore. The tubule coils around the nucleus, polaroplast, and posterior vacuole, in 2 double coils. At the right pH and calcium milieu in the human small-bowel lumen, the polar tubule unwinds and pops out of the spore, to puncture an enterocyte and inject the sporoplasm into the host cell cytoplasm, creating an uninucleate meront, which has no surrounding parasitophorous vacuole and is in direct contact with enterocyte cytoplasm (see **Fig. 4**B, C). The nucleus of the meront undergoes division to create a multinucleated proliferative plasmodium with cleftlike lucent spaces of

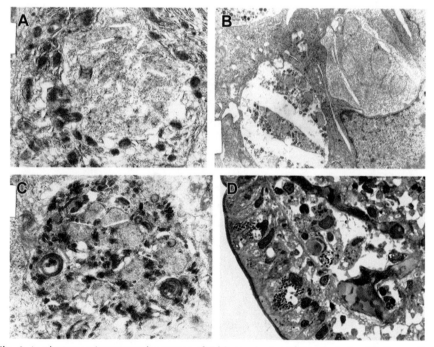

**Fig. 4.** In electron microscopy the stages of *E bieneusi* are pathognomonic with the earliest meront with its plasmodium in direct contact with the cytoplasm of the duodenal enterocyte because there is no parasitophorous vacuole (*A*). The proliferative plasmodium has multiple nuclei and slit like spaces (top right) while the early sporogonial plasmodium has similar multiple nuclei and slit like spaces and in addition the earliest evidence of other organelles (*B*). The later sporogonial plasmodium now has multiple nuclei each associated with the 'stacks of plates' of the early form of the polar tubule, seen in cross section or occasionally longitudinal section (*C*). The toluidine blue resin embedded thick section shows spores of *E intestinalis* in enterocytes and macrophages (*D*).

endoplasmic reticulum (see **Fig. 4**C) and coiled tubule precursors forming a "stack of plates" (see **Fig. 4**C), each of which is associated with a nucleus. Further maturation sees the tubules surround each nucleus in the sporogonial plasmodium, and the membrane of the plasmodium then invaginates pinching off each sporoblast containing a nucleus, polar tubule, and sporoplasm. The exospore then develops around each sporoblast to create the spore. The enterocyte ruptures or is extruded and the spores are released to infect other enterocytes or eventually be found in the stools to contaminate water and surfaces.

*E intestinalis* has a different development. The sporoplasm injected into a host enterocyte from the larger 1.2 × 2.2-μm spore acquires a membrane to form a meront (**Fig. 5**A), which is found attached to a host-derived, membrane-bound parasitophorous vacuole (see **Fig. 5**B). The meront undergoes binary fission (see **Fig. 5**B, C) to create sporonts that undergo tetra sporogony and mature into sporoblasts that are released within the vacuole but are separated by variable amounts of granular material

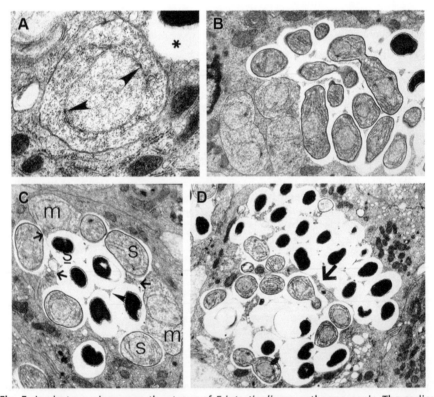

**Fig. 5.** In electron microscopy, the stages of *E intestinalis* are pathognomonic. The earliest meront has a nucleus with membrane (*arrowhead*) and sits within a potential parasitophorous vacuole adjacent a second open vacuole (denoted by *) (*A*). The meront's nucleus divides as do the sporonts as they become enveloped in the open parasitophorous vacuole (*B*). The meronts (m) develop into sporonts (s) and sporoblasts (s̲) with residual enterocyte cytoplasm caught up in the vacuole. Arrowhead indicates septa, arrow short indicates cytoplasmic debris in septa (*C*). Two large parasitophorous vacuoles containing septa, meronts, sporonts and spores coalescing (*arrow*) within an enterocyte (*D*).

secreted by the organisms but also containing some cytoplasmic debris forming incomplete septa (see **Fig. 5**C, D). The sporogonic phases have occasional thin tubular appendages up to 1 mm in length with bulbous bilaminar tips. Sporoblasts mature within the vacuole into spores, each of which contains a nucleus, a tubule with 5 to 7 coils, ribosomes and endoplasmic reticulum, a posterior vacuole, and endospore and exospore (**Fig. 6**A, B). Large parasitophorous vacuoles coalesce within the cytoplasm of enterocytes (**Figs. 5**D and **6**A), and are also seen in lamina propria macrophages as evidence of spore development in macrophages and in very occasional endothelial cells. Spores may be seen free in the background once the host enterocyte ruptures. *E intestinalis* vacuoles with various stages of sporogony have also been seen within colonic epithelium and nasal respiratory epithelium biopsy (see **Fig. 3**C, D) and spores have been demonstrated in a cell block prepared from nasal washings. The microsporidial organisms may be widely spaced and few in number, making EM diagnostic assessment difficult due to the small size of the biopsy.

## Differential Diagnosis and Comorbidities

It is essential that in small-bowel biopsies from immunocompromised patients, particularly those with AIDS, that once a particular infection is found, such as cytomegalovirus (CMV), mycobacteria, cryptosporidia, cyclosporiasis or isosporiasis, leishmaniasis, cryptococcosis, or microsporidiosis, that second and further infections should be routinely sought. For instance, CMV during the AIDS epidemic in Sydney, Australia, was frequently seen as a coinfection with microsporidia and cryptosporidia. The low-power and intermediate-power findings of a mild irregular partial villous atrophy in duodenal or jejunal biopsies are produced by many but not all of these infections (see **Fig. 2**A), and a routine protocol should be followed. Three levels should be cut in the paraffin-embedded biopsies, and levels 1 and 2 stained with the H&E stain, with a Warthin-Starry stain at level 2 specifically for microsporidia along with a CMV immunoperoxidase stain and auramine or other mycobacterial stain at that level. If the lamina propria is expanded, then a PAS with diastase stain should be added to help differentiate the contents of the macrophages present, such as, atypical mycobacteria, cryptococci or leishmania. The differential diagnosis of an organism within the enterocyte includes cyclosporiasis with its elongated larger merozoites with their conus, toxoplasmosis, which has a similar appearance, and *Isospora belli* with its again larger

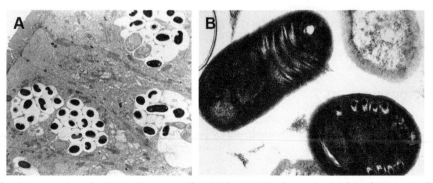

**Fig. 6.** Low power electron microscopy of multiple parasitophorous vacuoles of *E intestinalis* in enterocytes (*A*), and a high power of its spores with a single row of polar tubules wrapping around within the exospore of the spore (*B*).

merozoites with their useful "T-sign" and schizonts.[25] The microsporidial spores are much smaller with a distinctive appearance on the Warthin-Starry stain. The 2-μm to 5-μm maturing trophozoites of *Cryptosporidium parvum*, although present in a parasitophorous vacuole beneath the microvillous membrane of the enterocytes, project into the small-bowel lumen and show some variable basophilic structures representing merozoites to differentiate them from mucin droplets. They are relatively easily diagnosed on H&E, and easily differentiated from the microsporidia. The eventual oocysts that are produced through a sexual cycle involving macro and micro gametocytes are found in the modified Masson trichrome stain in stool preparations.

## DIAGNOSIS BY MOLECULAR METHODS

Although the standard practice in most institutions is a stool examination by microscopy and special stains for clinical diagnosis, molecular testing is possible to detect specific species. Commercial or reference laboratories offering the test do so primarily for the main species of *E bieneusi* or *Encephalitozoon* spp that infect humans, although specialized laboratories may be able to detect any species with expanded primer sets. Published methods are summarized in **Table 2**. The use of molecular tests for confirmation of diagnosis, especially to the species level, can be useful in clinical settings. However, high-throughput screening of stools, especially in settings with a high incidence of HIV, diarrhea, and low medical laboratory resources, must be based on either algorithms or inexpensive prescreens. One of the primary limitations to advanced development of molecular diagnostics for Microsporidium is the lack of genetic sequences from the 14 organisms infecting humans. To date, only *E cuniculi* has been completely sequenced and has contributed the bulk of the 6000 known genes. Although culture methods are available, they are laborious and expensive for many species, and there is no culture system for the most common pathogen, *E bieneusi*, which then would allow sufficient material for genome completion.

## SUMMARY

Microsporidiosis is an opportunistic infection seen mainly in the severely immunosuppressed that presents a diagnostic challenge because of the very small size of the spore, which, however, is ubiquitous and persistent in the environment. Stool examination, and less commonly intestinal biopsy using special stains, remain the most common and widely distributed methods of identification. Although EM has been the definitive diagnostic tool for speciation, genetic sequencing increasingly provides the definitive diagnosis for new species, such as *Anncaliia algerae*. Further genetic sequencing of the common pathogens may allow for the development of advanced molecular diagnostics, providing high diagnostic sensitivity and throughput.

## ACKNOWLEDGMENTS

We would like to dedicate this chapter to Professor Emeritus Elizabeth Canning of the Imperial College London, who mentored Dr Field in his microsporidia work.

## SELF-ASSESSMENT

1. A 37-year-old patient, newly diagnosed as HIV-positive, presented with 4 weeks of copious diarrhea. Which of the following tests is likely to produce a causative pathogen?

a. Stool, fixed in formalin, centrifuged, and prepared with iodine.
b. Small-bowel/colonic biopsies by endoscopy with immunohistochemistry for spirochetes.
c. Stool examination by wet mount, acid-fast stain, and trichrome.
d. Peripheral blood quantitative viral loads.
e. PCR of peripheral blood for a panel of pathogens associated with immunosuppression.

2. Which of the following concepts is most important in determining chronicity of a *Microsporidium* infection?
   a. The polar filament injection system
   b. The environmental survival time
   c. The host immune response
   d. The rate of dissemination to lymph nodes
   e. The quantity of helminth eggs in stool examination

3. Which of the following environmental sources of *Microsporidium* is most important for human disease?
   a. Fish
   b. Donkey
   c. Chicken
   d. Cattle
   e. Crustaceans

ANSWERS

Answer 1: C.
The protozoan parasites that cause watery diarrhea in patients who are HIV-positive include the coccidians and microsporidia. These are best identified using a wet mount, acid-fast stain, and trichrome. Fixed samples in iodine are ideal for larvae and ova of worms. Colonic biopsies for spirochetosis would not detect the most common pathogens in this clinical situation. Peripheral blood assays are of no value, as these infections are not disseminated.

Answer 2: C.
The host immune response is the primary etiology of prolonged microsporidiosis. Polar filaments and environmental survival times do not affect chronicity. The organism does not disseminate. Helminth eggs are not related to *Microsporidium* infection.

Answer 3: D.
Cattle are a common reservoir of both *E intestinalis* and *E bieneusi*, which are the 2 most common causes of microsporidiosis. Donkeys are important for *E intestinalis* and chickens are important for *E bieneusi*. Fish and crustaceans are a source for *Pleistophora*, but this is not a common cause of infection.

**REFERENCES**

1. Sax PE, Rich JD, Pieciak WS, et al. Intestinal microsporidiosis occurring in a liver transplant recipient. Transplantation 1995;60(6):617–8.
2. Rabodonirina M, Bertocchi M, Desportes-Livage I, et al. *Enterocytozoon bieneusi* as a cause of chronic diarrhea in a heart-lung transplant recipient who was seronegative for human immunodeficiency virus. Clin Infect Dis 1996;23(1):114–7.

3. Field AS, Hing MC, Milliken ST, et al. Microsporidia in the small intestine of HIV-infected patients. A new diagnostic technique and a new species. Med J Aust 1993;158(6):390–4.
4. Saigal K, Sharma A, Sehgal R, et al. Intestinal microsporidiosis in India: a two year study. Parasitol Int 2013;62(1):53–6.
5. Wumba R, Longo-Mbenza B, Menotti J, et al. Epidemiology, clinical, immune, and molecular profiles of microsporidiosis and cryptosporidiosis among HIV/AIDS patients. Int J Gen Med 2012;5:603–11.
6. Weiss LM. Microsporidia: emerging pathogenic protists. Acta Trop 2001;78(2):89–102.
7. Wasson K, Peper RL. Mammalian microsporidiosis. Vet Pathol 2000;37(2):113–28.
8. Watson D, Asmuth D, Wanke C. Environmental risk factors for acquisition of microsporidia in HIV-infected persons. Abstract of the 34th Annual IDSA Meeting. Clin Infect Dis 1996;23(903).
9. Cotte L, Rabodonirina M, Chapuis F, et al. Waterborne outbreak of intestinal microsporidiosis in persons with and without human immunodeficiency virus infection. J Infect Dis 1999;180(6):2003–8.
10. Watts MR, Chan RC, Cheong EY, et al. *Anncaliia algerae* microsporidial myositis. Emerg Infect Dis 2014;20(2):185–91.
11. Field AS, Canning EU, Hing MC, et al. Microsporidia in HIV-infected patients in Sydney, Australia: a report of 37 cases, a new diagnostic technique and the light microscopy and ultrastructure of a disseminated species. AIDS 1993;7(Suppl):S27–33.
12. Sandfort J, Hannemann A, Gelderblom H, et al. *Enterocytozoon bieneusi* infection in an immunocompetent patient who had acute diarrhea and who was not infected with the human immunodeficiency virus. Clin Infect Dis 1994;19(3):514–6.
13. Dore GJ, Marriott DJ, Hing MC, et al. Disseminated microsporidiosis due to septata intestinalis in nine patients infected with the human immunodeficiency virus: response to therapy with albendazole. Clin Infect Dis 1995;21(1):70–6.
14. Orenstein JM, Chiang J, Steinberg W, et al. Intestinal microsporidiosis as a cause of diarrhea in human immunodeficiency virus-infected patients: a report of 20 cases. Hum Pathol 1990;21(5):475–81.
15. Canning EU, Field AS, Hing MC, et al. Further observations on the ultrastructure of *Septata intestinalis* Cali, Kotler and Orenstein, 1993. Eur J Protistol 1994;30:414–22.
16. Didier ES, Stovall ME, Green LC, et al. Epidemiology of microsporidiosis: sources and modes of transmission. Vet Parasitol 2004;126(1–2):145–66.
17. Didier ES, Weiss LM. Microsporidiosis: Current Status. Curr Opin in Infect Dis 2006;19(5):485–92.
18. Weber R, Deplazes P, Schwartz D. Diagnosis and clinical aspects of human microsporidiosis. Contrib Microbiol 2000;6:166–92.
19. van Gool T, Snijders F, Reiss P, et al. Diagnosis of intestinal and disseminated microsporidial infections in patients with HIV by a new rapid fluorescence technique. J Clin Pathol 1993;46(8):694–9.
20. Didier ES, Orenstein JM, Aldras A, et al. Comparison of three staining methods for detecting microsporidia in fluids. J Clin Microbiol 1995;33(12):3138–45.
21. Field AS, Marriott DJ, Hing MC. The Warthin-Starry stain in the diagnosis of small intestinal microsporidiosis in HIV-infected patients. Folia Parasitol (Praha) 1993;40(4):261–6.

22. Weber R, Bryan RT, Owen R, et al. Improved light-microscopical detection of microsporidia spores in stool and duodenal aspirates. The Enteric Opportunistic Infections Working Group. N Engl J Med 1992;326(3):161–6.

23. Ryan NJ, Sutherland G, Coughlan K, et al. A new trichrome-blue stain for detection of microsporidial species in urine, stool, and nasopharyngeal specimens. J Clin Microbiol 1993;31(12):3264–9.

24. Kokoskin E, Gyorkos TW, Camus A, et al. Modified technique for efficient detection of microsporidia. J Clin Microbiol. 1994;32(4):1074–5.

25. Field AS. Light microscopic and electron microscopic diagnosis of gastrointestinal opportunistic infections in HIV-positive patients. Pathology 2002;34(1):21–35.

26. Chapter 181. In: Cohen J, Powderly WG, Opal SM, editors. Infectious diseases. 3rd edition. China: Mosby Elsevier; 2010.

27. Cotruvo JA, Dufour A, Rees G, et al. Waterborne Zoonoses. WHO; 2001. Chapter 16.

# Multiplex Polymerase Chain Reaction Tests for Detection of Pathogens Associated with Gastroenteritis

Hongwei Zhang, MD, PhD[a], Scott Morrison, MSc[a],
Yi-Wei Tang, MD, PhD[b],*

## KEYWORDS

- Gastroenteritis • Multiplex PCR • Laboratory-developed test

## KEY POINTS

- Conventional laboratory diagnostic techniques are time consuming and often lack sensitivity and specificity in detecting the causes of infectious gastroenteritis.
- Multiplex polymerase chain reaction (PCR)–based tests have been used in gastroenterology diagnostics in recent years because of their high sensitivities and specificities, as well as their versatility.
- Numerous laboratory-developed multiplex PCR tests have been reported for detection and identification of microbial pathogens in stool and, recently, 2 multiplex tests, the Luminex xTAG Gastrointestinal Pathogen Panel and BioFire FilmArray GI test, have been approved by the US Food and Drug Administration for use in clinical practice.
- The clinical relevance of the multiplex PCR tests remains to be determined in the diagnosis of infectious gastroenteritis.

## INTRODUCTION

Infectious gastroenteritis is a worldwide health problem with an estimated 2 billion cases of diarrhea that occur yearly and causes more than 2 million deaths every

Funding: This study was supported in part by a clinical trial contract between the Vanderbilt University Medical Center and the Luminex Corporation (VUMC 38228) as well as a research agreement between the Memorial Sloan-Kettering Cancer Center and the Luminex Corporation (SK2013-0929) awarded to Y.-W. Tang.
Disclosure: H. Zhang and S. Morrison are employees of Luminex Corporation, the commercial manufacturer of the xTAG Gastrointestinal Pathogen Panel.
[a] Luminex Corporation, 12212 Technology Boulevard, Austin, TX 78727, USA; [b] Clinical Microbiology Service, Memorial Sloan-Kettering Cancer Center, Weill Cornell Medical College, Cornell University, 1275 York Avenue, S428, New York, NY 10065, USA
* Corresponding author.
*E-mail address:* tangy@mskcc.org

year.[1–4] For children less than 5 years of age, infectious gastroenteritis or diarrhea is the leading cause of death worldwide, with an estimated 1.9 million children dying every year.[1,5,6] In 2010, there were an estimated 1.731 billion episodes of diarrhea (36 million of which progressed to severe episodes).[7] In the United States, acute gastroenteritis is a major cause of illness with an estimated 179 million episodes annually.[8] A report from Lucado and colleagues[9] on infectious enteritis and food-borne illness in the United States during 2010 found that nearly 1.3 million inpatient hospital stays had diagnoses of enteritis or gastrointestinal symptoms.

A wide range of enteric pathogens cause infectious gastroenteritis. Common causative agents include bacteria such as *Campylobacter*, *Salmonella*, *Shigella*, *Clostridium difficile*, and pathogenic *Escherichia coli*[10,11]; viruses such as norovirus, rotavirus, and adenovirus serotypes 40 and 41[12–14]; and parasites such as *Giardia*, *Entamoeba histolytica*, and *Cryptosporidium*.[15,16] Early identification of the causative pathogen is still a challenge in the clinical laboratory. Stool culture is the primary diagnostic tool for suspected bacterial infection. Selective agars and subsequent morphologic, biochemical, and serologic testing are usually required in order to identify and confirm the suspected culture isolate. Stool culture–based diagnosis is time consuming, labor intensive, and costly on a per-positive-culture basis.[17–21] In addition to this low culture-positive yield, there is a significant variability between physicians in requesting a stool culture for a given patient.[22] Inconsistent testing leads in part to inconsistent treatment, such as the use of antimicrobial therapy. Rapid and accurate identification of the infectious agent allows clinicians to choose the appropriate antimicrobials if needed, or to avoid them if they are not indicated.

Most viruses that cause infectious gastroenteritis cannot be cultured. Methods such as electron microscopy (EM) examination and immunoassay have been used for viruses such as norovirus, rotavirus, and adenovirus. These methods require significant expertise, are labor intensive, and can be subjective in interpretation. Microscopic examination is still routinely used for parasite identification. An ova and parasite examination requires a well-trained technologist to examine the prepared specimen. Because the examination is mainly focused on morphology, the interpretation is subjective. Furthermore, in some cases the clinician cannot distinguish different species; for example *E histolytica* (pathogenic) and *Entamoeba dispar* (nonpathogenic).[23] Rapid and accurate diagnostic tools are needed for infectious gastroenteritis.

## EMERGING MOLECULAR DIAGNOSTIC TOOLS

Emerging diagnostic assays have started to be used in microbiology, virology, and parasitology laboratories in gastroenterology. These tests address limitations of conventional diagnostics by taking advantage of technological advances.

Molecular tests for various enteric bacterial pathogens have been developed and are sold by several companies. The evolution of molecular diagnostic assays for detection of toxigenic *C difficile* shows the availability of different molecular technologies and the adoption of molecular testing for a gastrointestinal pathogen. In January 2009, the US Food and Drug Administration (FDA) approved several in vitro diagnostic (IVD) molecular assays for detection of toxigenic *C difficile*. Most of these assays offer rapid turnaround times (<2 hours) with minimal hands-on time, and high sensitivity and specificity compared with toxigenic culture. Key features and applications of the *C difficile* assays are provided by Svensson and LaSala[24] and Dunbar and colleagues.[25]

New diagnostic tools such as enzyme immunoassay (EIA) and molecular tests have shown higher positive rates of campylobacter infection than are found by culture.[26] Most laboratories use selective culture techniques for isolation of *Campylobacter jejuni* and *Campylobacter coli*, which suggested that they are the primary species associated with gastroenteritis. Platts-Mills and colleagues[27] used EIA and polymerase chain reaction (PCR) tests for campylobacter infection in children with diarrhea in the developing world. The investigators showed a higher rate of campylobacter infection using these methods.

Molecular diagnostic tools for detection of gastrointestinal viruses, such as norovirus, are emerging rapidly. In April 2014 Cepheid Xpert Norovirus was marketed as a Conformité Européenne (CE) IVD product under the European directive on in vitro diagnostic medical devices. Cepheid Xpert Norovirus is a qualitative test for rapid identification and differentiation of noroviruses genogroup I (GI) and genogroup II (GII). The assay is claimed to provide high sensitivity (100% for GI and GII) and high specificity (99.5% GI and 98.9% GII) with a total turnaround time of less than 1 hour.[28] A PCR-based diagnostic test for norovirus was used for a study on global prevalence of norovirus in gastroenteritis.[29] The study showed that norovirus is a key gastroenteritis pathogen associated with almost a fifth of all cases of acute gastroenteritis. In addition, noroviruses are a major cause of closure of hospital wards, and are associated with increased hospitalization and mortality among the elderly. Transplant patients have significant risk of acquiring persistent norovirus gastroenteritis. The emerging molecular tests for Noroviruses have led to the increased recognition of its significance in gastroenteritis and to calls for antiviral treatment and prophylaxis of norovirus infections, and possibly vaccination.[30]

## DETECTION AND IDENTIFICATION OF GASTROINTESTINAL PATHOGENS IN A MULTIPLEX FORMAT

The most promising emerging technologies are using multiplex molecular assays or pathogen class–specific multiplex molecular assays for comprehensive syndromic gastrointestinal pathogen detection. In the past few years, with the advances in molecular technologies along with the improved technologies for sample preparation and nucleic acid extraction/purification, multiplex reverse transcriptase (RT) PCR–based detection has gradually been introduced into diagnostic laboratories.

The advantages of testing 1 sample for multiple common pathogens using a single test are (1) to reduce the turnaround time for accurate results, (2) to identify coinfections, (3) to use the high negative predictive value of a multiplex assay to avoid unneeded infection control precautions, (4) to benefit from the high sensitivity and specificity that most molecular testing offers, and (5) to help health care providers provide better care to patients.

Multiplex molecular detection of respiratory virus nucleic acid has revolutionized the routine laboratory diagnosis of viral infections since the first multiplex testing for respiratory viruses, xTAG Respiratory Virus Panel (RVP) (Luminex Corporation, United States) received FDA clearance in January 2008. Over the past 6 years, there have been more than 9 commercial molecular diagnostic assays for the detection of respiratory viruses. The utility of such assays and their advantages and disadvantages have been studied and reviewed extensively.[31–36] With the promise shown in respiratory multiplex testing, efforts have been made to show the utility of multiplex molecular testing in gastrointestinal infections.

In the recent study by Liu and colleagues[37] the performance and benefit of 3 multiplex molecular platforms for the detection of 15 enteropathogens were evaluated against conventional comparator methods (bacterial culture, enzyme-linked immunosorbent assay [ELISA], and PCR) using more than 1500 clinical samples across 5 laboratories worldwide. Laboratory-developed PCR-Luminex assay, multiplex real-time

PCR, and TaqMan array card assays cost US$25 to $60 per sample. When using 7 ELISA kits, from different companies, 3 types of culture media, and various biochemical reagents in order to test different enteropathogens, the total reagent cost per sample was about $200. In addition to the cost savings from multiplex molecular testing, the turnaround time for multiplex syndromic panel testing takes hours or days for testing 100 samples instead of weeks for conventional comparator methods.[37,38]

There are 2 main categories of multiplex molecular testing. One category is known as syndromic panels. A multiplex syndromic panel usually includes most common pathogens responsible for a particular array of symptoms. For example, a multiplex panel for diarrhea may test for the most common causative agents from various pathogen classes such as bacteria, viruses, and parasites. Luminex xTAG Gastrointestinal Pathogen Panel (GPP) and BioFire's FilmArray Gastrointestinal Panel are such syndromic panels. The other category of multiplex molecular assays includes a class of pathogens in a multiplex panel. Becton Dickinson's BD MAX System has 3 products for enteric pathogens, (BD Max System Enteric Bacterial Panel, Parasite Panel, and Viral Panel) and each panel targets 1 class of pathogen.

Multiplex testing for gastroenteritis is still in its infancy compared with multiplex testing for respiratory tract infection. Using multiplex detection and identification of gastrointestinal pathogens has made notable progress in the past couple of years. It is anticipated that multiplex testing will increase diagnostic positivity, identify coinfections, improve turnaround times, and may reduce the use of antibiotics. There are multiplex RT-PCR–based laboratory-developed tests (LDTs) and commercial assays (mostly not yet FDA approved) available for gastrointestinal pathogen testing.[25,39] As more multiplex testing becomes available, the value of using such a test will be assessed and recognized. Evaluations of xTAG GPP by Wessels and colleagues[40] showed the added value of this multiplex test in terms of the increased positivity rate, 1 test with multiple answers, and providing results within 1 day. Current gastrointestinal research multiplex assays and commercial multiplex assays are discussed later.

## CURRENT MULTIPLEX GASTROINTESTINAL RESEARCH ASSAYS

Research-developed assays have been in the forefront in the application of advanced molecular detection technology for research and/or diagnostic use in laboratories. LDTs that use multiplex molecular testing for gastroenteric pathogens are listed in **Table 1** with the relevant institutions and the pathogens that these tests detect.

Milwaukee Health Department Laboratory developed and validated a 19-plex GPP using Luminex xTAG analyte-specific reagents (ASRs).[41] This LDT can simultaneously screen for diarrhea-causing pathogens, including 9 bacteria (C jejuni, Salmonella spp, Shigella spp, enterotoxigenic E coli [ETEC], Shiga toxin–producing E coli [STEC], E coli O157:H7, Vibrio cholerae, Yersinia enterocolitica, and toxigenic C difficile), 3 parasites (Giardia lamblia, Cryptosporidium spp, and E histolytica), and 4 viruses (norovirus GI and GII, adenovirus 40/41, and rotavirus A) directly from fecal specimens. The evaluation study of this multiplex LDT included 48 reference isolates and 254 clinical specimens. The overall comparative performance of the multiplex test with conventional methods in clinical samples was 94.5% (range, 90%–97%), with 99% specificity. The study indicated that this multiplex assay enables sensitive and specific screening and identification of the major acute diarrheal pathogens.

Another Luminex platform–based multiplex PCR assay was developed by Liu and colleagues[37] from the Division of Infectious Diseases and International Health, University of Virginia. The multiplex RT-PCR assay detects 15 common enteropathogens, including 5 viruses (adenovirus, astrovirus, norovirus GII, rotavirus, and sapovirus), 7

**Table 1**
Recently published multiplex research assays for the syndromic identification of gastroenteritis-causing agents

| Research Assay Development Site/Institute/ Laboratory | Pathogen Targeted in the Multiplex Assay | Sample Type and Nucleic Acid Amplification/ Detection Method | Performance | References |
|---|---|---|---|---|
| Milwaukee Health Department Laboratory | Total 19 targets: C jejuni, Salmonella, Shigella, ETEC, STEC, E coli O157:H7, Vibrio cholerae, Yersinia enterocolitica, and toxigenic Clostridium difficile), Giardia lamblia, Cryptosporidium, E histolytica, norovirus GI/ GII, adenovirus 40/41 and rotavirus A | Stool, multiplex RT-PCR; Luminex microsphere detection | Sensitivity: 94.5% (90%–97%) Specificity: 99% | Navidad,[41] 2013 |
| Division of Infectious Diseases and International Health, University of Virginia | Total 15 pathogens: Adenovirus, astrovirus, norovirus GII, rotavirus, sapovirus, Campylobacter, Salmonella, V cholerae, EAEC, ETEC, EPEC, Cryptosporidium, G lamblia, and E histolytica | Multiplex RT-PCR-Luminex microsphere detection | Sensitivity: 86.2% (median) Specificity: ≥95% | Liu,[37] 2014 |

(continued on next page)

**Table 1**
*(continued)*

| Research Assay Development Site/Institute/Laboratory | Pathogen Targeted in the Multiplex Assay | Sample Type and Nucleic Acid Amplification/Detection Method | Performance | References |
|---|---|---|---|---|
| Department of Pediatrics, McMaster University, Hamilton, ON, Canada | Total 16 pathogens: EHEC (stx1/stx2), E coli O157, Salmonella, Shigella, Campylobacter, Yersinia entercolitica, C difficile, C difficile tcd B, Listeria monocytogenes, Vibrio parahaemolyticus, norovirus GI/GII, rotaviruses, astroviruses, adenoviruses 40/41, sapovirus, G lamblia, and Cryptosporidium | Nanoliter real-time PCR panel | Cryptosporidium sensitivity greater than microscopy or EIA | Goldfarb,[42] 2013 |
| Department of Microbiology, Faculty of Medicine, Chiang Mai University, Chiang Mai, Thailand | Total 10 viruses: Rotavirus (A/C), adenovirus, norovirus GI/GII, sapovirus, astrovirus, Aichi virus, Parechovirus, and Enterovirus | Multiplex RT-PCR | 47.2% positivity rate on infants and children with acute gastroenteritis | Khamrin et al,[43] 2011 |
| Provincial Laboratory for Public Health, Edmonton, Alberta, Canada | Total 5 viruses: Rotavirus, norovirus, sapovirus, astrovirus, and adenovirus | Stool, real-time PCR | Higher positivity rate than with microscopy | Pang et al,[44] 2014 |
| Regional Virus Laboratory, Royal Victoria Hospital, Belfast, Northern Ireland, United Kingdom | Total 4 viruses: Rotavirus, norovirus, astrovirus, and adenoviruses 40/41 | Stool, real-time (TaqMan) | Sensitivity: 95%–99% Specificity: 95%–100% | Feeney,[45] 2011 |

| Department of Microbiology and Immunology, Weill Medical College of Cornell University | Total 7 bacteria: Campylobacter, Vibrio, Shigella, Salmonella, L monocytogenes, Y enterocolitica, and diarrheagenic E coli | Stool, multiplex PCR/LDR assay | Sensitivity: 91%–100% Specificity: 98%–100% | Rundell,[46] 2014 |
|---|---|---|---|---|
| Laboratory Medical Science Cluster, UiTM, Malaysia | Total 4 bacteria: Salmonella, Shigella, EHEC, and Campylobacter | Stool, multiplex PCR | Contrived sample sensitivity and specificity: 100%. LoD 1 × 10$^3$ CFU/mL | Al-Talib,[47] 2014 |
| Department of Biology, Faculty of Science, Mahidol University, Bangkok 10,400, Thailand | Total 4 toxin genes of C difficile: tcdA, tcdB, cdtA, and cdtB | Stool multiplex PCR | Sensitivity and specificity: 100%. LoD: ~22 copies | Chankhamhaengdecha,[48] 2013 |

Abbreviations: CFU, colony-forming units; EAEC, enteroaggregative E coli; EHEC, enterohemorrhagic E coli; EPEC, enteropathogenic E coli; ETEC, enterotoxigenic E coli; LDR, ligation detection reaction; LoD, limit of detection; STEC, Shiga toxin–producing E col; UiTM, Universiti Teknologi MARA.
Data from Refs.[37,41–48]

bacteria (*C jejuni/C coli*, *Salmonella* spp, *V cholerae*, enteroaggregative *E coli* [EAEC], ETEC, enteropathogenic *E coli* [EPEC], and enteroinvasive *E coli* [EIEC]), and 3 parasites (*Cryptosporidium* spp, *Giardia* spp, and *E histolytica*). The assay was used in a multicenter study that showed that molecular tests can be deployed successfully in different parts of the world, detect enteropathogens with high sensitivity and specificity, and identify mixed infections.[37]

Nanoliter real-time PCR panel is another novel technology that allows users to perform multitarget panels using very low volumes. This technology is a high-throughput quantitative real-time RT-PCR platform that can perform more than 3000 separate PCR reactions in parallel in 33-nL volumes in through holes (similar to wells on a microtiter plate). A multiple-target nanoliter real-time PCR panel was developed for 16 major diarrheal pathogens by Goldfarb and colleagues.[42] This panel detects:

Eight bacteria:
1. Enterohemorrhagic *E coli* (EHEC), via detection of *stx* 1, *stx* 2, *E coli* O157
2. *Salmonella* spp
3. *Shigella* spp
4. *Campylobacter* spp
5. *Yersinia entercolitica*
6. *C difficile, C difficile tcd* B
7. *Listeria monocytogenes*
8. *Vibrio parahaemolyticus*

Six viruses:
1. Norovirus group 1
2. Norovirus group 2
3. Rotaviruses
4. Astroviruses
5. Adenoviruses 40/41
6. Sapoviruses

Two parasites:
1. *G lamblia*
2. *Cryptosporidium* spp

This nanoliter real-time PCR panel was used to test stool samples collected from Canada's Arctic region, Qikiqtani (Baffin Island) Region of Nunavut. This PCR-based assay detected *Cryptosporidium* spp that were missed by microscopy or EIA.

Several multiplex molecular LDTs have been developed for the detection of gastrointestinal viruses over the years. Khamrin and colleagues[43] from the Department of Microbiology, Faculty of Medicine, Chiang Mai University, Thailand, developed a single-tube multiplex PCR for the detection of 10 viruses, including rotaviruses group A and C, adenovirus, norovirus GI, norovirus GII, sapovirus, astrovirus, Aichi virus, parechovirus, and enterovirus. On evaluation of this novel 10-multiplex viral panel against a total of 235 stool samples collected from infants and children with acute gastroenteritis, 111 of the 235 (47.2%) stool samples were positive for a pathogen. The study suggested that this multiplex PCR is useful as a rapid and cost-effective diagnostic tool for the detection of major pathogenic viruses causing diarrhea.[43]

Similarly, Pang and colleagues[44] from the Provincial Laboratory for Public Health, Edmonton, Alberta, Canada, developed a Enteric Virus testing Panel using real-time PCR that simultaneously detects 5 enteric viruses (EVs), including rotavirus, norovirus, sapovirus, astrovirus, and enteric adenovirus, in stool samples. In the study reported by Pang and colleagues,[44] a total of 2486 sporadic gastroenteritis samples submitted for EV testing using EM between July 2008 and July 2009 were tested with this EVPrtPCR panel. The real-time assay detected 30% more viruses than were identified by EM.

In 2011, the Regional Virus Laboratory of Royal Victoria Hospital, Belfast, United Kingdom developed and validated a multiplex TaqMan assay for the detection of viral gastroenteritis.[45] The assay probes for 4 different viruses: rotavirus, norovirus (genogroups I and II), astrovirus, and adenovirus (serotypes 40 and 41). In a validation study using 137 specimens, the assay showed sensitivity for adenovirus of 97.3%, for rotavirus of 100%, and for norovirus of 95.1%; and specificity for adenovirus of 99%, for rotavirus of 100%, and for adenovirus 97.9%. Astrovirus gave 100% sensitivity and specificity with the samples tested. The assay has been successfully used in routine diagnostic services.

Multiplex LDT for the detection of various bacterial enteric pathogens has been developed by various laboratories. A multiplex PCR/ligation detection reaction (LDR) assay was developed by Rundell and colleagues[46] for the detection of bacterial pathogens from stool specimens. The panel targets 7 bacterial pathogens: *Campylobacter* spp, *Vibrio* spp, *Shigella* spp, *Salmonella* spp, *L monocytogenes*, *Y enterocolitica*, and diarrheagenic *E coli*. The sensitivity and specificity of the assay were assessed using primarily contrived samples (cultured-negative stool specimens spiked with known isolates) and a small number of clinical specimens from Haiti. The overall sensitivity ranged from 91% to 100% and the overall specificity ranged from 98% to 100% depending on the species. The study showed that it is feasible to use a PCR/LDR multiplex assay for the detection of a panel of enteric bacterial pathogens.

A 5-gene panel was recently developed by Al-Talib and colleagues[47] for the identification of the common hemorrhagic bacteria in stool samples. Specific primer sets were designed for ompC of *Salmonella* genus, virA gene for *Shigella* genus, eaeA gene for EHEC, 16S ribosomal RNA (rRNA) for *Campylobacter* genus, and hemA for an internal control. This 1-tube multiplex PCR assay had a limit of detection of 1 $\times$ $10^3$ colony-forming units (CFU) at the bacterial cell level and 100 pg at the genomic DNA level. Evaluation with 223 bacterium-spiked stool specimens showed 100% sensitivity and specificity. The assay has a 4-hour turnaround time for the identification of hemorrhagic bacteria.

Multiplex molecular testing not only applies to detecting multiple different pathogens, it is also used to detect and distinguish different subtypes for a given organism. A multiplex PCR assay was developed by Chankhamhaengdecha and colleagues[48] to detect various *C difficile* ribotypes, other *Clostridium* spp, and non-*Clostridium* strains by targeting different toxin genes: tcdA, tcdB, cdtA, and cdtB. The study showed 100% specificity with the ability to detect as low as ~22 genomic copy numbers per PCR reaction.

Research laboratory–developed multiplex assays have been used in other applications. For example, Heidary and colleagues[49] developed a multiplex PCR assay for the detection of antibiotic resistance genes for diarrheagenic *E coli*. Wang and colleagues[50] explored a multiplex PCR approach for detecting 6 non-O157 STEC virulence genes and showed that the multiplex PCR tests had comparable results with serologic testing. In summary, research or laboratory-developed multiplex molecular tests have been used for gastroenteritis research and clinical diagnostics in certain institutions. The laboratory-developed multiplex tests mentioned and listed in this article (see **Table 1**) are examples of the advancement of molecular testing in gastroenterology and there may be many other similar molecular tests developed by various laboratories over the years.

## CURRENT ENTERIC MULTIPLEX COMMERCIAL ASSAYS

The review of Gastrointestinal multiplex commercial assays has 2 parts. First is an overview of currently available Gastrointestinal multiplex commercial assays, and second is a detailed discussion on the 2 FDA-approved syndromic multiplex assays: Luminex xTAG GPP and BioFire FilmArray Gastrointestinal Panel. **Table 2** provides a detailed breakdown of these commercial multiplex assays: manufacture, test name, US IVD (FDA approved) or CE IVD, number of Gastrointestinal pathogens detected, time to result, throughput, sample processing/extraction, specimen type, assay technology, specialized equipment requirement, and assay complexity. **Table 3** lists pathogens that are detected by each of these multiplex assays.

### Overview of Multiplex Commercial Assays

Over the past few years the gastroenterology diagnostic market has witnessed a surge of commercial multiplex diagnostic assays for the detection of various gastroenteric pathogens. These multiplex commercial assays differ in many aspects, including the number of different pathogens that the assay detects, throughput of the assay, overall time to results, regulatory status, and the complexity of the assay. Of the commercial multiplex assays, only four assays are considered as comprehensive syndromic (virus, bacteria, and parasite) multiplex RT-PCR–based assays. The other commercial assays are multiplex assays that allow detection of members of a specific class of pathogens.

Luminex's xTAG GPP was the first syndromic GI multiplex assay that received FDA clearance[51] and was CE marked in May 2011. xTAG GPP is based on multiplex RT-PCR for target amplification and detection using Luminex microsphere xMAP and xTAG technologies. The assay is approved for the detection of 14 pathogens (8 bacteria, 3 viruses, and 3 parasites).[52]

The FilmArray Gastrointestinal Panel produced by BioFire is a self-contained system using PCR with melt analysis of the PCR product for analyte detection. The FilmArray Gastrointestinal Panel received FDA clearance for the detection of 20 pathogens (11 bacteria, 5 viruses, and 4 parasites).[53] Both xTAG GPP and FilmArray Gastrointestinal Panel are discussed later.

The GastroFinder Smart 17 Fast, produced by PathoFinder, is a non–FDA-approved but CE-marked real-time PCR-based multiplex GI assay that allows the detection of 17 pathogens (9 bacteria, 4 viruses, and 4 parasites). The assay does not require specialized equipment. Sample preparation is performed using standard commercially available nucleic acid purification techniques and RT-PCR/detection is achieved using a standard real-time thermal cycler. The high level of multiplexing on a standard real-time thermal cycler is achieved using PathoFinder's SmartFinder technology, in which hybridization probes are ligated together to create amplimers of varying length that can be differentiated by melt-curve analysis. Limited performance data are available for the GastroFinder assay. One study of 120 retrospective clinical samples found that the sensitivity ranged from 60% to 100%; specificity information was not provided.[54]

Another comprehensive syndromic multiplex assay is the BioCode 3000 Gastrointestinal Pathogen Panel recently developed and launched by Applied BioCode, Inc. (Santa Fe Springs, CA). The assay utilizes proprietary barcoded magnetic beads and integrates amplification, hybridization and detection processes to cover 18 bacteria (*Campylobacter, Clostridium difficile* toxin A/B, *Salmonella, Shigella,* enteroinvasive *E coli,* enteroaggregative *E coli,* enteropathogenic *E coli,* enterotoxigenic *E coli,* shiga toxin-producing *E coli, E coli* O157, *Aeromonas, Vibrio, Y enterocolitica*), viruses

**Table 2**
Commercial multiplex assays available for syndromic identification of gastroenteritis-causing agents

| Manufacture – Test Name | US IVD | CE IVD | Number Pathogens Detected | Time to Result (h) | Throughput | Sample Preprocessing | Stool Source | Technology | Specialized Equipment Required | Complexity |
|---|---|---|---|---|---|---|---|---|---|---|
| Luminex xTAG GPP | Yes | Yes | 14 | 5 | 96 | Yes | Raw, Cary-Blair | Multiplex end point RT-PCR, hybridization | Yes | High |
| BioFire FilmArray Gastrointestinal | Yes | No | 22 | 1 | 1 | No | Cary-Blair | Multiplex RT-PCR, melt analysis | Yes | Low |
| Applied BioCode GI Panel | No | No | 19 (B=12, V=3, P=3) | 5 (estimated) | 96 | Yes | Raw, Cary-Blair | Multiplex PCR, target capture | Yes (BioCode MDx 3000) | High |
| BD MAX Enteric Bacterial Panel | Yes | Yes | 4 | 4 | 24 | No | Raw, Cary-Blair | Microfluidic real-time PCR | Yes | Low |
| BD MAX Enteric Virus | No | Yes | 2 | 4 | 24 | No | Raw | Microfluidic real-time PCR | Yes | Low |
| BD MAX Enteric Parasite | No | Yes | 3 | 4 | 24 | No | Raw, formalin fixed | Microfluidic real-time PCR | Yes | Low |
| Nanosphere Verigene Enteric Pathogen | Yes | Yes | 8 | 2 | 1 | No | Cary-Blair | Microarray | Yes | Low |
| Hologic (Gen-Probe) ProGastro SSCS | Yes | Yes | 4[b] | 4 | 96[a] | Yes | Cary-Blair | Multiplex real-time PCR | No | Medium |
| PathoFinder GastroFinder Smart 17 Fast | No | Yes | 17 | 5 | 96 | Yes | Not specified | Multiplex RT-PCR, ligation probe melt analysis | No | High |
| r-Biopharm Rida Gene HS, BS, VS, PS | No | Yes | HS = 3, BS = 3, VS = 4, PS = 4 | 2 | 96[a] | Yes | Raw | Multiplex real-time PCR | No | Medium |

(continued on next page)

**Table 2**
*(continued)*

| Manufacture – Test Name | US IVD | CE IVD | Number Pathogens Detected | Time to Result (h) | Throughput | Sample Preprocessing | Stool Source | Technology | Specialized Equipment Required | Complexity |
|---|---|---|---|---|---|---|---|---|---|---|
| Seegene Seeplex Diarrhea ACE V, B1, and B2 | No | Yes | V = 4 B1 = 5 B2 = 5 | 9–10 | 96[a] | Yes | Raw, Cary-Blair, rectal swabs | Multiplex PCR, capillary electrophoresis | No | High |
| Serosep EntericBio Gastro Panel 1 (P1) and 2 (P2) | No | Yes | P1 = 4 P2 = 6 | 3 | 96[a] | No | Not specified | Multiplex real-time PCR | No | Low |
| Fast-Track Diagnostics FTD stool P, EPA, B, V | No | Yes | P = 3 EPA = 3 B = 6[b] V = 5[b] | 6 | 96 B = 48 V = 48 | Yes | Not specified | Multiplex real-time PCR, RT-PCR | No | Medium |
| Diagenode- G-DiaBact (B), G-DiaNota (V), G-Diapara (P) | No | Yes | B = 2 V = 3 P = 3 | 4 | 96 | Yes | Raw | Multiplex real-time PCR, RT-PCR | No | Medium |
| Genetic Signatures EasyScreen enteric B, V, protozoan | No | Yes | B = 9[c] V = 8[c] P = 5[b] | 5 | B = 32 V = 32 P = 48 | Yes | Not specified | Multiplex real-time PCR, RT-PCR | No | Medium |
| AusDiagnostics fecal B, gastrointestinal parasites | No | No | B = 5 P = 4 | 3 | B = 12 P = 14 | Yes | Not specified | Multiplex tandem real-time RT-PCR | Yes | Low |
| Genomica CLART EnteroBac | No | Yes | 7[b] | 5 | 48 | Yes | Raw | Multiplex PCR, microarray | Yes | High |

*Abbreviations:* B, bacterial stool; BS, bacterial stool; EPA, Enterovirus, Parechovirus, Adenovirus; HS, hospital stool; P, parasites and protozoan; PS, parasitic stool; V, viral; VS, viral stool.

[a] When running 1 panel.
[b] Two tubes per wells required for coverage.
[c] Three tubes per well required for coverage.

# Table 3
## Gastroenteritis-causing pathogens detected by commercially available syndromic multiplex assays

| Manufacture/Assay | Aeromonas | Campylobacter | C difficile | Clostridium perfringens | EAEC | EPEC | ETEC lt/st | STEC stx1/stx2 | E coli O157 | L monocytogenes | Plesiomonas shigelloides | Salmonella | Shigella | Vibrio | V cholerae | Y enterocolitica | Adenovirus F40/41 | Astrovirus | Enterovirus | Norovirus GI/GII | Rotavirus A | Sapovirus | Cryptosporidium | Cyclospora cayetanensis | Blastocystis hominis | Dientamoeba fragilis | E histolytica | G lamblia |
|---|---|---|---|---|---|---|---|---|---|---|---|---|---|---|---|---|---|---|---|---|---|---|---|---|---|---|---|---|
| Luminex xTAG GPP | — | ✔ᵃ | ✔ | — | — | — | ✔ | ✔ | ✔ | — | — | ✔ | ✔ | — | ✔ | ✔ | ✔ | — | — | ✔ | ✔ | — | ✔ | — | — | — | ✔ | ✔ |
| BioFire FilmArray Gastrointestinal | ✔ᵃ | ✔ | ✔ | — | ✔ | ✔ | ✔ | ✔ | ✔ | — | ✔ | ✔ | ✔ | ✔ | ✔ | ✔ | ✔ | ✔ | — | ✔ | ✔ | ✔ | ✔ | ✔ | — | — | ✔ | ✔ |
| BD MAX Enteric B, V,ª parasiteª | — | ✔ B | — | — | — | — | ✔ B | ✔ B | ✔ | — | — | ✔ B | ✔ B | — | — | ✔ B | — | — | — | ✔ V | ✔ V | ✔ P | ✔ P | — | — | — | ✔ P | ✔ P |
| Nanosphere Verigene Enteric Pathogen | — | ✔ | — | — | — | — | ✔ | ✔ | ✔ | — | — | ✔ | ✔ | ✔ | — | ✔ | — | — | — | ✔ | ✔ | — | — | — | — | — | — | — |
| Hologic (Gen-Probe) ProGastro SSCS | — | ✔ | — | — | — | — | — | ✔ | ✔ | — | — | ✔ | ✔ | — | — | — | — | — | — | — | — | — | — | — | — | — | — | — |
| PathoFinder GastroFinder Smart 17 Fast | ✔ | ✔ | ✔ | — | — | — | ✔ | ✔ | ✔ | — | — | ✔ | ✔ | — | — | ✔ | ✔ | ✔ | — | ✔ | ✔ | ✔ | ✔ | — | — | — | ✔ | ✔ |
| r-Biopharm Rida Gene HS, BS, VS, PS | — | ✔ B | ✔ HS | — | — | — | — | — | — | — | — | ✔ B | — | — | — | ✔ B | ✔ V2 | ✔ V2 | — | ✔ V2 | ✔ V2 | ✔ P | ✔ P | — | — | ✔ P | ✔ P | ✔ P |
| Seegene Seeplex Diarrhea ACE V, Ba and 2 Bb | ✔ Bb | ✔ Ba | ✔ Ba | ✔ Bb | — | — | ✔ Bb | ✔ Bb | — | — | — | ✔ Ba | ✔ Ba | ✔ Ba | — | ✔ Ba | ✔ V2 | ✔ V | ✔ V | ✔ V | ✔ V | ✔ P | — | — | — | — | — | ✔ |
| Serosep EntericBio Gastro P1 and P2 | ✔ | ✔ | — | — | — | — | ✔ | ✔ | ✔ | — | — | ✔ | ✔ | — | — | ✔ | — | — | — | ✔ | ✔ | ✔ | ✔ | — | — | — | ✔ | ✔ |
| Fast-Track Diagnostics FTD stool P, EPA, B, V | — | ✔ B2 | ✔ B2 | — | — | — | ✔ B2 | ✔ B2 | — | — | — | ✔ B2 | ✔ B2 | — | — | ✔ B2 | ✔ V3 | ✔ V3 | ✔ V3 | ✔ V3 | ✔ V3 | ✔ V3 | ✔ P | — | — | — | ✔ P | ✔ P |
| Diagenode- G-DiaBact (B), G-DiaNota (V), G-Diapara (P) | — | ✔ B | — | — | — | — | — | — | — | — | — | ✔ B | — | — | — | ✔ B | — | — | — | ✔ V3 | ✔ V3 | ✔ V3 | ✔ P | — | — | — | — | ✔ P |
| Genetic Signatures EasyScreen Enteric B, V, protozoan | ✔ P3 | ✔ P3 | ✔ P3 | — | — | — | ✔ P3 | ✔ P3 | — | ✔ P3 | — | ✔ P3 | ✔ P3 | — | — | ✔ P3 | ✔ V3 | ✔ V3 | ✔ V3 | ✔ V3 | ✔ V3 | ✔ P2 | ✔ P2 | — | ✔ P2 | ✔ P2 | ✔ P2 | ✔ P2 |
| AusDiagnostics fecal B, gastrointestinal parasites | — | ✔ B | ✔ B | — | — | — | — | — | — | — | — | ✔ B | ✔ B | — | — | ✔ B | — | — | — | — | — | ✔ P | ✔ P | — | ✔ | ✔ P | ✔ P | ✔ P |
| Genomica – CLART EnteroBac | ✔ | ✔ | ✔ | ✔ | Undifferentiated | | ✔ | ✔ | — | ✔ | ✔ | ✔ | ✔ | — | ✔ | ✔ | — | — | — | — | — | — | — | — | — | — | — | — |

Numbers indicate the number of tubes per wells required for each test or subpanel.

*Abbreviations:* Ba, bacterial 1; Bb, bacterial 2; P1, panel 1; P2, panel 2.

ᵃ Test/analyte not included in IVD version.

(norovirus group I/II, adenovirus F, rotavirus A), and parasites (*Cryptosporidium, E histolytica, G lamblia*) causing diarrhea (Michael Aye, personal communication) (see **Table 2**).

Of the rest commercial multiplex assays for specific pathogen classes, 3 assays have received FDA clearance: the Nanosphere Verigene Enteric Pathogen test (June 2014 clearance), the BD MAX Enteric Bacterial assays (May 2014 clearance), and the Hologic ProGastro SSCS (January 2013 clearance). The Nanosphere Verigene Enteric Pathogen test is a 2-step automated platform covering 6 bacterial and 2 viral targets. A Cary-Blair stool sample is loaded into a cartridge on a sample processing unit that extracts and amplifies the target nucleic acid. The amplified nucleic acid is automatically transferred to a microarray that uses gold nanoparticle probes and a silver staining process to generate signal. The microarray is then analyzed using the Verigene reader system. The sensitivity for the Verigene system for prospectively collected sample evaluation ranged from 67% to 100%, whereas the specificity ranged from 99% to 100%.[55]

The BD MAX Enteric Bacterial Panel received FDA clearance for detecting 4 bacterial targets from raw stool or stool in Cary-Blair transport medium. The assay runs on the BD MAX microfluidic automation platform, which incorporates sample preparation and microfluidic real-time PCR detection into 1 system. The system can simultaneously process up to 24 samples in 4 hours. Based on an FDA 510(k) summary, the sensitivity of the BD MAX Enteric Bacterial Panel ranged from 85% to 100%, whereas the specificity ranged from 98% to 99% when tested with 3457 samples from patients suspected of having acute bacterial gastroenteritis, enteritis, or colitis.[56] BD has also developed an enteric parasite panel that detects 3 parasitic targets from raw stool or formalin-fixed stool. At the time of this review the BD Enteric Parasite panel is CE IVD (May 2014) but not FDA approved. A unique aspect of the BD MAX system is that it is an open platform, which allows other assay manufactures or laboratories to develop assays to run on the platform.

The third FDA-approved panel for the detection of bacterial pathogens is the Hologic ProGastro SSCS panel. The assay detects 4 bacterial pathogens from stool in Cary-Blair transport medium in a 2-tube TaqMan-based real-time PCR assay. The ProGastro SSCS assay runs on a standard real-time thermal cycler (eg, Cepheid SmartCycler). Nucleic acid from Cary-Blair stool samples can be extracted and purified using the bioMerieux NucliSENS easyMAG extractor. The sensitivity of the assay ranged from 95% to100% with a specificity of 99% as reported in the 510(k) summary.[57] In a separate study the ProGastro SSCS assay was compared with culture for the identification of *Campylobacter* spp (*C jejuni* and *C coli*), *Salmonella* spp, and *Shigella* spp, and with broth enrichment followed by an FDA-approved EIA for the identification of STEC isolates in stool specimens. When results based on the ProGastro SSCS assay and bidirectional sequencing for discrepancy analysis were compared with conventional testing, the sensitivity of the ProGastro SSCS assay was 100% for all pathogens, and the specificities ranged from 99.4% to 100%.[58]

The rest of the 7 multiplex assays have not received FDA clearance. These assays detect for 2 to 4 pathogen targets (low/moderate plex) per reaction well. Although these assays do not provide the same level of multiplexing as some of the other GI diagnostics, they typically provide the user with more choice in terms of the pathogens they wish to test for. Usually the low-plex/medium-plex assay manufacturers create several assays, some of which can be run concurrently. Most of the low-plex/medium-plex assays are based on multiplex real-time PCR detection, but some of these assays differ in sample preparation/extraction step, assay reagents, and signal detection mechanisms.

Serosep's EntericBio Gastro Panel is unique in that it does not require traditional nucleic acid purification; instead, the stool samples are incubated with a sample preparation buffer followed by heating at 97°C for 30 minutes to release bacterial DNA. The cooled sample is then added directly to lyophilized PCR reagents. The sample processing and PCR setup of the Serosep assay can be performed with an epMotion liquid handler, which results in very little hands-on time.[59] The EntericBio real-time Gastro Panel I for simultaneous detection of *C jejuni*, *C coli*, and *Campylobacter lari*, STEC, *Salmonella* spp, and *Shigella* spp was evaluated by Koziel and colleagues[60] with a total of 528 prospectively collected samples from patients with acute gastroenteritis. The assay reported 84 positive results, including *Campylobacter* spp (n = 44), 35 Stx1/Stx2 (n = 35), *Shigella* spp (n = 3), and *Salmonella* spp (n = 6). Comparing with a previous version of this assay and culture results from retrospective samples, the sensitivity and specificity of the assay were reported as 100% and 97.8% respectively.

The sample preparation is also unique for Genetic Signature's EasyScreen Enteric assays (Sydney, Australia), which use the company's 3base technology to convert all cytosine bases in the starting nucleic acid sample to thymine. The resulting reduction in sequence variation allows a higher number of multiplex targets to be run under similar conditions.[61] This universal sample processing technology was evaluated by Siah and colleagues[62] with 487 characterized stool samples positive for bacteria, viruses, protozoa, and *C difficile*. The processed samples were subsequently tested using 4 multiplexed real-time PCR panels. The study suggested that these multiplex real-time PCR panels with universal sample preparation generated results that were comparable with conventional methods, but with the added advantage of streamlined and rapid diagnosis of gastrointestinal pathogens.[62] One study was reported on the EasyScreen Enteric Parasite Detection Kit for the identification of 5 common enteric parasites: *Blastocystis* spp, *Cryptosporidium* spp, *Dientamoeba fragilis*, *Entamoeba* complex, and *Giardia intestinalis* in human clinical samples. Compared with real-time PCR and microscopy, the EasyScreen Enteric Parasite Detection Kit showed 92% to 100% sensitivity and 100% specificity on testing a total of 358 stool samples.[63]

The workflows for R-BioPharma AG (Darmstadt, Germany), Fast-Track Diagnostics (Sliema, Malta) and Diagenode assays all follow the tradition real-time PCR workflow of nucleic acid purification, PCR setup, and amplification/detection.[64–66] Similarly, these companies offer specific pathogen panels of low/moderate plex capacity per panel. A recent study by Biswas and colleagues[67] evaluated and compared the diagnostic accuracy, turnaround time, and ease of use of 3 multiplex molecular panels: the RIDAGENE Bacterial Stool and EHEC/EPEC Panels, the FTD Bacterial Gastroenteritis, and the BD MAX Enteric Bacterial Panel. The study tested the 3 panels with 116 retrospective samples and 318 prospective stool samples. Conventional culture-based techniques and consensus among molecular assays were used as the gold standards. A positive test was based on either a positive culture or agreement in 2 of the 3 molecular panels. The 3 multiplex molecular panels were more sensitive than culture for most of the targets, detecting an additional 13 cases that were culture negative. All 3 molecular panels gave much faster turnaround time than culture: less than 3 hours versus 66.5 hours for culture. The BD MAX panel was the fastest, easiest to use, and most flexible.[67]

Genomica has developed the 2-tube CLART EnteroBac panel, which detects 7 analytes. The assay follows the traditional molecular workflow for sample extraction and amplification; however, detection is performed on a low-density microarray that is analyzed by the company's clinical array reader. A unique feature of the CLART EnteroBac panel is that it differentiates some of the *Campylobacter* and *Yersinia* species.[68]

AusDiagnostics Faecal Bacteria and Gastrointestinal Parasites panels deviate from the traditional real-time PCR workflow with their multiplex tandem PCR technology. In this PCR system, extracted nucleic acid is preamplified in a single-well multiplex PCR reaction, then several aliquots of the preamplification material are transferred into a single-plex intercalating dye real-time PCR reaction where amplification and melt-curve analysis are used to detect the present targets.[69] This multiplex tandem PCR (MT-PCR)–based assay was developed for the detection of 4 protozoan parasites (*Cryptosporidium* spp, *D fragilis*, *E histolytica*, and *G intestinalis*). This 4-plex assay was evaluated with 472 fecal samples. When using single-plex real-time PCR as comparator, this 4-plex MT-PCR assay had 100% sensitivity and specificity. The traditional microscopy examination only gave a sensitivity of approximately 38% to 56%, highlighting the superior sensitivity of molecular testing.[70]

Seegene's Seeplex Diarrhea ACE assays use the company's dual priming oligonucleotide technology to provide increased specificity during PCR amplification. The dual priming oligonucleotide technology is based on placing a polydeoxyinosine linker near the 3′ end of the primer, which slightly destabilizes it, reducing the chance of nonspecific priming. The Seeplex Diarrhea assay also differs from the other assays in that it uses auto–capillary electrophoresis for detection of the amplified products.[71] There are 2 patient cohort–based evaluation studies on Seeplex Diarrhea ACE assays. One study was by Coupland and colleagues[72] to evaluate Seeplex Diarrhea ACE multiplex detection for 4 viruses and/or 10 bacteria with 223 patients' samples. Compared with conventional methods and norovirus-specific RT-PCR, Seeplex Diarrhea ACE panels showed 100% positive concordance for adenovirus, norovirus, *Campylobacter* spp, *E coli* O157, *Shigella* spp, or *Vibrio* spp. The ACE panels missed 12.5% of rotavirus, 50% of *C difficile* toxin B, and 15.8% of *Salmonella* spp of the positive samples. The second study was conducted with 245 pediatric patients using Seeplex Diarrhea ACE assays (ACE-Bacteria 1, Bacteria 2, and Viral assays) collectively detecting 15 enteric pathogens, including *Salmonella* spp, *Shigella* spp, *Vibrio* spp, toxin B–producer *C difficile*, *Campylobacter* spp, *Clostridium perfringens*, *Y enterocolitica*, *Aeromonas* spp, *E coli* O157:H7, verocytotoxin-producing *E coli*, adenovirus, group A rotavirus, norovirus GI and GII, and astrovirus.[73] This study showed better sensitivity for multiplex PCR than routine methods, except for *Salmonella* spp and toxigenic *C difficile*.

### United States Food and Drug Administration–Approved Syndromic Multiplex Assays: Luminex xTAG Gastrointestinal Pathogen Panel and BioFire FilmArray Gastrointestinal Panel

#### Luminex xTAG Gastrointestinal Pathogen Panel

Luminex's xTAG GPP assay was the first large multiplex syndromic panel that received FDA 510(k) clearance (January 2013) for the detection of gastroenteritis-causing pathogens including bacteria, viruses, and parasites. With the recent September 2014 clearance, xTAG GPP can be used to detect 14 most common pathogens (8 bacterial, 3 viral, and 3 parasitic pathogens) from a single sample in both raw stool specimens and stool in Cary-Blair media. The assay is based on Luminex's xTAG and xMAP technologies. The workflow of the assay starts with a sample pretreatment step with bead beating in order to break the cell wall of parasitic pathogen followed by nucleic acid extraction/purification, and a single multiplex RT-PCR followed by bead hybridization and detection.

The bead beating step in the pretreatment is required for any lysis-resistant parasites, such as *Cryptosporidium* oocysts. This step is performed by adding ~100 mg of stool, 100 μL of liquid stool, or 400 μL of stool in Cary-Blair medium to a Bertin

SK38 bead tube to which NucliSENS easyMAG lysis buffer and the internal control (xTAG MS2) are also added. The bead tube is then vortexed for 5 minutes and incubated at room temperature for 10 minutes, followed by a brief centrifugation. The volumes of input stool vary between plain stool and stool in Cary-Blair because of the dilution factor that occurs when a stool sample is placed in Cary-Blair medium. To minimize PCR inhibition, an appropriate amount of stool input is important (ie, not to add too much stool specimen). Wessels and colleagues[40] noted that reducing the amount of stool input into the assay reduced the PCR inhibition rate from 7.6% to 2.3%. The overall rate of PCR inhibition (as determined by an internal control failure) ranges from as high as between14% and 16%[52] to between ~2.3% and 7.7%.[40,74] Note that when the internal control is inhibited a positive analyte finding can still be made if an analyte produces a positive signal; however, the analytes cannot be identified as negative if no internal control signal is obtained. It is recommended that the purified nucleic acid from inhibited samples be diluted 1:10 and the assay rerun. This dilution procedure has been shown to recover greater than 80% of inhibited samples.[40,75]

The xTAG GPP US IVD product insert recommends that nucleic acid extraction be performed using a bioMerieux NucliSENS easyMAG running the specific A 1.0.2 protocol. Under this protocol, 200 μL of pretreated material are used with an elution volume of 70 μL of purified nucleic acid (the extraction run takes approximately 55 minutes). However, the xTAG GPP CE IVD product insert also states that the QIAamp MinElute Virus Spin Kit by Qiagen can be used. In addition to the 2 recommended nucleic acid extraction/purification platforms, end users have applied other extraction methods and platforms with xTAG GPP. Other extraction platforms include Roche's MagNA Pure.[75] Qiagens EZ1 virus mini kit,[76] Qiagen's QIAsymphony,[40] and the Abbott m2000sp instrument.[77]

The multiplex RT-PCR setup for the Luminex xTAG GPP assay follows a standard molecular workflow. It is recommended that all RT-PCR reaction setups be performed on cold blocks or PCR coolers, to prevent nonspecific activity of the RT. Ten microliters of purified nucleic acid are added to the reaction and it is placed on a standard end point thermal cycler. The thermal cycling takes approximately 2 hours and 10 minutes. In the product insert Luminex highlights the importance of maintaining a clean pre-PCR area. Because the xTAG GPP assay is an open system that requires handling of amplified material in the hybridization step, the risk of contamination should be noted.

The xTAG GPP hybridization and detection reaction is a liquid phase reaction in which amplified RT-PCR product is combined with the xTAG GPP bead mix and the fluorescent reporter streptavidin r-phycoerythrin (SAPE). During the hybridization reaction, tags on the amplified RT-PCR product hybridize with their complement tag on the Luminex microspheres and the SAPE reporter binds to the biotin on the amplified product. The signal detection and data acquisition are obtained by a Luminex 100, Luminex 200, or MAGPIX instrument in which the sample is read. Data analysis is performed by the xTAG GPP TDAS (xTAG Data Analysis Software) software. The TDAS software provides the result and reports with one of 3 outcomes for each sample: POS (positive), NEG (negative), or No Call. The No Call result is given when one of the assay parameter is not met or there is an internal control failure. An important aspect of the TDAS software is that it allows flexibility for end users to only select the analytes that they wish to detect, which in turn masks those results that the end users do not wish to see.

The FDA 510(k) clinical study of xTAG GPP reports an overall sensitivity of 80.0% to 100.0% for all analytes with the exception of ETEC. The sensitivity for ETEC was 25.0% (2 of 8); the 6 ETEC samples that were reported as false-negative by xTAG

GPP were tested using 4 other well-characterized nucleic acid amplification tests (NAATs), only 1 of the 4 NAATs determined that the 6 samples were positive. The specificity of the xTAG GPP assay ranged from 89.8% to 99.9%, with a negative predictive value of greater than 99%. Despite this high level of specificity, the FDA placed a presumptive positive warning on the xTAG GPP assay, requiring confirmation of positive results by another FDA-approved method.[52] Zboromyrska and colleagues[76] found that the sensitivity of ETEC heat-stable/heat-labile (ST/LT) in xTAG GPP was superior to their multiplex PCR used for routine testing.

Since xTAG GPP was made commercially available (first through CE IVD in May 2011, then FDA clearance in January 2013, and extended approval in September 2014), several studies have reported on the xTAG GPP assay's clinical utility, overall performance, and potential benefit in outbreak situation.

During the 2011 outbreak of a new aggressive EHEC strain in Germany, in order to manage the exponential increase of suspected cases, xTAG GPP was used by Kliniken der Stadt Köln gGmbH, Cologne, as a prescreening tool, partially because of its high throughput (up to 96 samples per batch). More importantly, the assay discriminates STEC from a broad panel of pathogens that are implicated in infectious diarrhea, providing the dual benefit of rapid time to result and high throughput.[78]

The reported clinical utility and overall performance of xTAG GPP varies from study to study, perhaps because of the inconsistency of sample populations, sample types (eg, fresh or frozen), sample processing, and extraction methods used, and most importantly because of comparator methods used for the studies. In a study by Beckmann and colleagues,[77] 2 study populations were used: 312 consecutive stool samples from 127 pediatric patients with gastroenteritis and 185 adult travelers with suspected parasitic infections. Multiplex xTAG GPP was evaluated against a combination of comparator methods: direct antigen detection, bacterial culture, and microscopy. Rotavirus (27%) was the most prevalent in pediatric population, whereas in adult traveler ETEC (4%) was the predominant pathogen identified by xTAG GPP. However, microscopic examination reported 23% *Blastocystis hominis* in adult travelers, which is not covered by the xTAG GPP. All positive results by xTAG GPP for adenovirus, rotavirus, *C difficile*, and *Cryptosporidium* were confirmed, but not all positive results for norovirus and *Giardia* were confirmed.[77] In the study by Claas and colleagues[79] the norovirus performance of xTAG GPP was comparable with real-time PCR, with 100% sensitivity and specificity for norovirus GI and 92.5% sensitivity and 97.6% specificity for norovirus GII. Giardia was reported to be detected with 100% sensitivity and 98.9% specificity when using real-time PCR as comparator. Similarly, in the same study, the positive agreement for adenovirus 40/41 was 20% (4 of 20) when using real-time PCR as comparator but 100% (9 of 9) using bidirectional sequencing.

The overall sensitivity of xTAG GPP in detecting bacterial pathogens is comparable with bacterial culture. The different results from studies for *Salmonella* are worth noting. Compared with culture, *Salmonella* sensitivity was reported as 100% (10 of 10) and specificity 98.4% (1143 of 1161) in the xTAG GPP FDA study; similarly 100% sensitivity (11 of 11) and 97.4% specificity (1349 of 1385) were observed for *Salmonella* by Halligan and colleagues.[80] However, in the study published by Mengelle and colleagues,[74] the sensitivity of *Salmonella* was 77.8% (7 of 9) and specificity was 96.2% (356 of 370).

### BioFire's FilmArray Gastrointestinal Panel

BioFire's FilmArray Gastrointestinal Panel runs on the company's automated FilmArray instrument. The US IVD version of the FilmArray gastrointestinal assay simultaneously detects the nucleic acid from 13 bacterial, 5 viral, and 4 parasites responsible for causing gastroenteritis in about 1 hour (see **Table 3**).[53] The FilmArray gastrointestinal assay is completely automated, with nucleic acid extraction, amplification, and detection all occurring within the assay pouch. The hands-on preparation takes approximately 5 minutes and involves adding rehydration solutions to the assay pouch and loading the Cary-Blair stool sample, which is achieved with a provided consumable.[81] Once the sample is loaded the FilmArray instrument subjects the sample to bead beating followed by nucleic acid extraction. The extracted nucleic acid is then amplified in a nested multiplex RT-PCR reaction to enrich the target sequences; after the initial PCR step is complete the amplified material is moved to the second PCR step, which occurs on the film array where several single-plex PCR reactions occur. Detection of analytes is achieved by using end point melt-curve analysis. The FilmArray gastrointestinal assay returns 1 of 4 results: Detected, Not Detected, N/A, and Invalid. The N/A result occurs when E coli O157 is detected but stx1/stx2 is not detected, or when EPEC is detected with stx1/stx2. The Invalid results can be caused by instrument or software failure or internal control failure.[53]

The result from the clinical trial with 1556 patients was that the sensitivity of the FilmArray ranged from 94.5% to 100% and the specificity ranged from 97.1% to 100% depending on the target.[53] The overall assay success rate for samples in the prospective clinical trial was 99.4% for the initial testing and 99.9% on repeat testing. It is unclear whether this success rate includes invalid results caused by PCR inhibition.

Care must be taken when comparing the published performance characteristics (sensitivity and specificity) of syndromic panels. Different comparator methods have often been used to establish the assay's performance characteristics. For example, microscopy was used for establishing the performance of the parasitic targets in the xTAG GPP assay, whereas an NAAT, bidirectional sequencing, was used to establish the performance of the same targets in the FilmArray gastrointestinal assay. Although the NAATs used were independent of the assay they are still molecular-based assays, which may provide a higher degree of concordance with a molecular test than microscopy would.

To date only 1 independent cohort study has been published using the BioFire FilmArray Gastrointestinal Panel. The study compares the performances of the BioFire FilmArray gastrointestinal assay and the Luminex xTAG GPP assay.[81] The study included 230 prospectively collected stool samples in Cary-Blair medium and retrospective testing of 270 stool samples in Cary-Blair medium. The Investigation Use Only (IUO) version of the BioFire assay was used, whereas the Research Use Only (RUO) version of the xTAG GPP assay was used. The IUO/RUO versions of the assays used in this study differ from the IVD version in that the IVD FilmArray Gastrointestinal does not have a claim for *Aeromonas* and the xTAG GPP IVD does not have a claim for *Y enterocolitica*. Khare and colleagues[81] found that both assays had high sensitivity and specificity (>90%) for the targets included in the IVD versions of the assays; **Table 4** provides a summary of these results. In the prospective arm of this study the sensitivities of the BioFire and Luminex assays were nearly equivalent; *C difficile* and norovirus were the only 2 targets with differences in sensitivity between the assays. BioFire was more sensitive for *C difficile* (100% vs 95.8% for GPP), whereas Luminex was more sensitive for norovirus (100% vs 91.7%). In the retrospective arm of the study, BioFire's sensitivity was higher than that of Luminex. Khare and colleagues[81] noted that this difference in sensitivity may be related to using only 100 µL of Cary-Blair stool for the extraction, which is 4-fold less than is used for xTAG GPP.

The specificity of the xTAG GPP assay was nearly identical (within 1%) to the FilmArray Gastrointestinal Panel. Norovirus GI/GII was the only target in the xTAG GPP assay that showed a significant difference in specificity (GPP, 88.3%; FilmArray,

**Table 4**
A summary of Khare and colleagues'[61] results for the sensitivity and specificity of the BioFire FilmArray gastrointestinal assay (IUO) and the Luminex xTAG GPP assay (RUO) in a 230-sample prospective and 270-sample retrospective study

| Target | Prospective | | | | Retrospective | | | | Combined | | | |
|---|---|---|---|---|---|---|---|---|---|---|---|---|
| | FilmArray | | xTAG GPP | | FilmArray | | xTAG GPP | | FilmArray | | xTAG GPP | |
| | Sensitivity (%) | Specificity (%) | Sensitivity (%)ᵃ | Specificity (%)ᵃ | Sensitivity (%) | Specificity (%) | Sensitivity (%)ᵃ | Specificity (%)ᵃ | Sensitivity (%) | Specificity (%) | Sensitivity (%)ᵃ | Specificity (%)ᵃ |
| *Aeromonas* spp | 100 | 100 | — | — | 23.8 | 100 | 23.8 | — | 27.3 | 100 | — | — |
| *Campylobacter* | 100 | 100 | 100 | 100 | 96.6 | 99.6 | 79.3 | 100 | 96.9 | 99.8 | 81.3 | 100 |
| *C difficile* toxin A/B | 100 | 96.6 | 95.8 | 97.2 | 91.7 | 97.9 | 91.7 | 98.3 | 95.0 | 97.3 | 93.3 | 99.1 |
| *P shigelloides* | ND | 100 | — | — | 100 | 100 | 100 | — | 100 | 100 | — | — |
| *Salmonella* spp | 100 | 99.6 | 100 | 100 | 100 | 100 | 83.3 | 100 | 100 | 99.8 | 84.0 | 100 |
| *Y enterocolitica* | ND | 100 | ND | 100 | 100 | 99.6 | 48.1 | 100 | 100 | 99.8 | 48.1 | 100 |
| *Vibrio* spp | ND | 100 | — | — | ND | ND | — | — | ND | 100 | — | — |
| *V cholerae* | ND | 100 | ND | 100 | ND | ND | ND | ND | ND | 100 | ND | 100 |
| EAEC | ND | ND | — | — | ND | ND | — | — | ND | 100 | — | — |
| EPEC | ND | ND | — | — | ND | ND | — | — | ND | 100 | — | — |
| ETEC | 100 | 100 | 100 | 100 | ND | ND | ND | ND | 100 | 100 | 100 | 100 |
| STEC | ND | 100 | ND | 100 | 100 | 99.2 | 96.4 | 99.6 | 100 | 99.4 | 96.4 | 99.8 |
| *E coli* O157 | ND | 100 | ND | 100 | 100 | 100 | 90.9 | 99.6 | 100 | 100 | 90.9 | 99.8 |
| *Shigella*/EIEC | 100 | 99.6 | 100 | 99.5 | 90.9 | 99.6 | 81.8 | ND | 92.3 | 99.6 | 84.6 | 100 |
| *Cryptosporidium* | 100 | 100 | 100 | 100 | 100 | 100 | 100 | 100 | 100 | 100 | 100 | 100 |
| *C cayetanensis* | ND | 100 | — | — | ND | ND | — | — | ND | 100 | — | — |
| *E histolytica* | ND | 100 | ND | 100 | 0 | 100 | 100 | 100 | 0.0 | 100 | 100 | 100 |
| *G lamblia* | 100 | 100 | 100 | 100 | 100 | 100 | 100 | 100 | 100 | 100 | 100 | 100 |
| Adenovirus 40/41 | 100 | 99.2 | 100 | 100 | 90 | 99.2 | 80 | 100 | 90.9 | 99.4 | 81.8 | 100 |
| Norovirus GI/GII | 91.7 | 99.5 | 100 | 90.8 | 93.2 | 100 | 93.2 | 85.8/99.5ᵇ | 92.9 | 99.6 | 94.6 | 88.3/95.3ᵇ |
| Rotavirus A | ND | 99.6 | ND | 99.1 | 100 | 99.6 | 92.9 | 99.6 | 100 | 99.2 | 92.9 | 99.4 |
| Sapovirus | 100 | ND | — | — | 90.3 | 100 | — | — | 93.2 | 100 | — | — |
| Astrovirus | 100 | ND | — | — | 100 | 100 | — | — | 100 | 100 | — | — |

*Abbreviation:* —, analyte not included in the xTAG GPP assay; ND, not determined.

ᵃ 100-μL Cary-Blair stool input used; Luminex recommends 400 μL of Cary-Blair stool in the US IVD version of the xTAG GPP package insert.

ᵇ Retrospective false-positives for norovirus GII were retested with a new lot of xTAG GPP; 31 of 32 false-positives were resolved with retesting.

*Data* from Khare R, Espy MJ, Cebelinski E, et al. Comparative evaluation of two commercial multiplex panels for detection of gastrointestinal pathogens by use of clinical stool specimens. J Clin Microbiol 2014;52(10):3667–73.

99.7%). Khare and colleagues[81] showed that this discrepancy may have been linked to a specific reagent lot, because on retesting with a new lot of reagents the xTAG GPP specificity for norovirus GII was 99.5%.

In terms of workflow and turnaround time, Khare and colleagues[81] found that the FilmArray gastrointestinal assay required approximately 5 minutes of hands-on time and a time to result of about 1 hour, whereas the xTAG GPP assay required approximately 60 minutes of hands-on time and had a time to result of 5 to 6 hours. The throughput that could be obtained in a normal 8-hour shift with the FilmArray gastrointestinal assay was 7 to 8 samples, whereas the xTAG GPP assay could produce results for 96 samples within 1 shift.[81]

## CLINICAL RELEVANCE OF THE MULTIPLEX ASSAYS

Development and implementation of molecular techniques, especially those in multiplex formats, have significantly improved workflow and diagnostic output in diagnosis of GI infections. However, the clinical utility of multiplex assays is still to be established. Earlier adopters and studies of these multiplex assays have indicated that multiplex assays could save time to detect a specific infectious organism. This advantage is important because specific therapy could be initiated in case of bacterial infection. The clinical relevance of a multiplex assay also lies in its negative predictive value. A negative result could mean deisolating a patient and saving the unnecessary burden that would otherwise result. Kahlau and colleagues[82] showed that the xTAG GPP assay provided same-day results, whereas conventional methods took about 3 days. Multiplex assays also gave 19 (of 104 total) positive results that were not requested by ordering physicians.

The performance characteristics and limitations of the multiplex molecular tests must be clearly understood by both laboratory personnel and clinicians to ensure proper use and interpretation. As techniques continue to advance, more and more microorganisms will be detected simultaneously from fecal specimens; whether from microbial contamination, colonization, infection, or disease merits further investigation. For example, a study of a 19-plex LDT performed by Navidad and colleagues[41] showed that a multiplex assay could be suitable as a primary screening tool for enteric bacteria, viruses, and parasites. Additional extensive studies are needed to further investigate the clinical relevance of multiplex molecular assays in the diagnosis of gastrointestinal infections. Prompt exchange of relevant information between clinicians and laboratories is essential for the reliable molecular diagnosis of infectious gastroenteritis.

## SELF-ASSESSMENT

1. An investigator has designed 1 primer set that targets the conserved regions of the bacterial 16S rRNA gene to detect a panel of common bacterial pathogens. This set is considered as:
   a. Real-time PCR
   b. Broad-range PCR
   c. Multiplex PCR
   d. Random PCR
   e. Nested PCR
2. Which of the following microbial agents is least likely to be a cause of infectious gastroenteritis?
   a. E coli
   b. Rotavirus

c. *Salmonella*
d. *Campylobacter*
e. *E histolytica*

3. Which of the following pathogens requires an additional sample preprocessing step, such as bead beating, before routine nucleic acid extraction?
   a. *Campylobacter* spp
   b. *Y enterocolitica*
   c. Norovirus
   d. *C difficile*
   e. *Cryptosporidium* spp

Answers

Answer 1: (b)

Broad-range PCR is different from the multiplex PCR described in the article, which involves the use of multiple sets of primers to target several loci.

Answer 2: (a)

Nonpathogenic *E coli* in gut is part of normal flora and should not be considered as a pathogen causing diarrhea. None of the other organisms are considered to be normal flora.

Answer 3: (e)

Bead beating helps to crack open lysis-resistant parasitic cysts (such as *Cryptosporidium* oocysts) to ensure the efficiency of the subsequent nucleic acid extraction (this applies to *Giardia* as well).

**REFERENCES**

1. Farthing M, Salam MA, Lindberg G, et al. Acute diarrhea in adults and children: a global perspective. J Clin Gastroenterol 2013;47(1):12–20.
2. Kosek M, Bern C, Guerrant RL. The global burden of diarrhoeal disease, as estimated from studies published between 1992 and 2000. Bull World Health Organ 2003;81(3):197–204.
3. Thielman NM, Guerrant RL. Clinical practice. Acute infectious diarrhea. N Engl J Med 2004;350(1):38–47.
4. Bresee JS, Marcus R, Venezia RA, et al. The etiology of severe acute gastroenteritis among adults visiting emergency departments in the United States. J Infect Dis 2012;205(9):1374–81.
5. Guerrant RL, Kosek M, Moore S, et al. Magnitude and impact of diarrheal diseases. Arch Med Res 2002;33(4):351–5.
6. Liu L, Johnson HL, Cousens S, et al. Global, regional, and national causes of child mortality: an updated systematic analysis for 2010 with time trends since 2000. Lancet 2012;379(9832):2151–61.
7. Walker CL, Rudan I, Liu L, et al. Global burden of childhood pneumonia and diarrhoea. Lancet 2013;381(9875):1405–16.
8. Wikswo ME, Hall AJ. Outbreaks of acute gastroenteritis transmitted by person-to-person contact–United States, 2009-2010. MMWR Surveill Summ 2012;61(9):1–12.
9. Lucado J, Mohamoud S, Zhao L, et al. Infectious enteritis and foodborne illness in the United States, 2010 statistical brief #150. Healthcare Cost and Utilization Project (HCUP) statistical briefs [Internet]. Rockville (MD): Agency for Health Care Policy and Research (US); 2013. Available at: http://www.ncbi.nlm.nih.gov/books/NBK137749/?report=printable. Accessed November 1, 2014.

10. Hofreuter D. Defining the metabolic requirements for the growth and colonization capacity of *Campylobacter jejuni*. Front Cell Infect Microbiol 2014;4:137.
11. Chen HM, Wang Y, Su LH, et al. Nontyphoid salmonella infection: microbiology, clinical features, and antimicrobial therapy. Pediatr Neonatol 2013;54(3): 147–52.
12. Blanton LH, Adams SM, Beard RS, et al. Molecular and epidemiologic trends of caliciviruses associated with outbreaks of acute gastroenteritis in the United States, 2000-2004. J Infect Dis 2006;193(3):413–21.
13. de Wit MA, Koopmans MP, van Duynhoven YT. Risk factors for norovirus, Sapporo-like virus, and group A rotavirus gastroenteritis. Emerg Infect Dis 2003;9(12):1563–70.
14. Bok K, Green KY. Norovirus gastroenteritis in immunocompromised patients. N Engl J Med 2012;367(22):2126–32.
15. Katz DE, Taylor DN. Parasitic infections of the gastrointestinal tract. Gastroenterol Clin North Am 2001;30(3):797–815.
16. Mehta S, Fantry L. Gastrointestinal infections in the immunocompromised host. Curr Opin Gastroenterol 2005;21(1):39–43.
17. Dusch H, Altwegg M. Evaluation of five new plating media for isolation of Salmonella species. J Clin Microbiol 1995;33(4):802–4.
18. Perez JM, Cavalli P, Roure C, et al. Comparison of four chromogenic media and Hektoen agar for detection and presumptive identification of *Salmonella* strains in human stools. J Clin Microbiol 2003;41(3):1130–4.
19. Perry JD, Ford M, Taylor J, et al. ABC medium, a new chromogenic agar for selective isolation of Salmonella spp. J Clin Microbiol 1999;37(3):766–8.
20. Bennett WE Jr, Tarr PI. Enteric infections and diagnostic testing. Curr Opin Gastroenterol 2009;25(1):1–7.
21. Gaillot O, di Camillo P, Berche P, et al. Comparison of CHROMagar *Salmonella* medium and Hektoen enteric agar for isolation of salmonellae from stool samples. J Clin Microbiol 1999;37(3):762–5.
22. Guerrant RL, Van Gilder T, Steiner TS, et al. Practice guidelines for the management of infectious diarrhea. Clin Infect Dis 2001;32(3):331–51.
23. Kebede A, Verweij JJ, Petros B, et al. Short communication: Misleading microscopy in amoebiasis. Trop Med Int Health 2004;9(5):651–2.
24. Svensson AM, LaSala PR. Pathology consultation on detection of *Clostridium difficile*. Am J Clin Pathol 2012;137(1):10–5.
25. Dunbar SA, Zhang H, Tang YW. Advanced techniques for detection and identification of microbial agents of gastroenteritis. Clin Lab Med 2013;33(3):527–52.
26. Platts-Mills JA, Kosek M. Update on the burden of Campylobacter in developing countries. Curr Opin Infect Dis 2014;27(5):444–50.
27. Platts-Mills JA, Liu J, Gratz J, et al. Detection of *Campylobacter* in stool and determination of significance by culture, enzyme immunoassay, and PCR in developing countries. J Clin Microbiol 2014;52(4):1074–80.
28. Cepheid Xpert Norovirus assay. Available at: http://www.cepheid.com/administrator/components/com_productcatalog/library-files/f5e5a03863c93410f24f504b8aafa955-Xpert-Norovirus-Brochure-EU-3013-04.pdf. Accessed November 1, 2014.
29. Ahmed SM, Hall AJ, Robinson AE, et al. Global prevalence of norovirus in cases of gastroenteritis: a systematic review and meta-analysis. Lancet Infect Dis 2014; 14(8):725–30.
30. Rocha-Pereira J, Neyts J, Jochmans D. Norovirus: targets and tools in antiviral drug discovery. Biochem Pharmacol 2014;91(1):1–11.

31. Mahony JB, Blackhouse G, Babwah J, et al. Cost analysis of multiplex PCR testing for diagnosing respiratory virus infections. J Clin Microbiol 2009;47(9): 2812–7.

32. Wu W, Tang YW. Emerging molecular assays for detection and characterization of respiratory viruses. Clin Lab Med 2009;29(4):673–93.

33. Yan Y, Zhang S, Tang YW. Molecular assays for the detection and characterization of respiratory viruses. Semin Respir Crit Care Med 2011;32(4):512–26.

34. Ginocchio CC, Zhang F, Manji R, et al. Evaluation of multiple test methods for the detection of the novel 2009 influenza A (H1N1) during the New York City outbreak. J Clin Virol 2009;45(3):191–5.

35. Pierce VM, Hodinka RL. Comparison of the GenMark Diagnostics eSensor respiratory viral panel to real-time PCR for detection of respiratory viruses in children. J Clin Microbiol 2012;50(11):3458–65.

36. Buller RS. Molecular detection of respiratory viruses. Clin Lab Med 2013;33(3): 439–60.

37. Liu J, Kabir F, Manneh J, et al. Development and assessment of molecular diagnostic tests for 15 enteropathogens causing childhood diarrhoea: a multicentre study. Lancet Infect Dis 2014;14(8):716–24.

38. Houpt E, Gratz J, Kosek M, et al. Microbiologic methods utilized in the MAL-ED cohort study. Clin Infect Dis 2014;59(Suppl 4):S225–32.

39. Gray J, Coupland LJ. The increasing application of multiplex nucleic acid detection tests to the diagnosis of syndromic infections. Epidemiol Infect 2014;142(1):1–11.

40. Wessels E, Rusman LG, van Bussel MJ, et al. Added value of multiplex Luminex Gastrointestinal Pathogen Panel (xTAG® GPP) testing in the diagnosis of infectious gastroenteritis. Clin Microbiol Infect 2014;20(3):O182–7.

41. Navidad JF, Griswold DJ, Gradus MS. Evaluation of Luminex xTAG gastrointestinal pathogen analyte-specific reagents for high-throughput, simultaneous detection of bacteria, viruses, and parasites of clinical and public health importance. J Clin Microbiol 2013;51(9):3018–24.

42. Goldfarb DM, Dixon B, Moldovan I, et al. Nanolitre real-time PCR detection of bacterial, parasitic, and viral agents from patients with diarrhoea in Nunavut, Canada. Int J Circumpolar Health 2013;72:19903.

43. Khamrin P, Okame M, Thongprachum A, et al. A single-tube multiplex PCR for rapid detection in feces of 10 viruses causing diarrhea. J Virol Methods 2011; 173(2):390–3.

44. Pang XL, Preiksaitis JK, Lee BE. Enhanced enteric virus detection in sporadic gastroenteritis using a multi-target real-time PCR panel: a one-year study. J Med Virol 2014;86(3):1594–601.

45. Feeney SA, Armstrong VJ, Mitchell SJ, et al. Development and clinical validation of multiplex TaqMan® assays for rapid diagnosis of viral gastroenteritis. J Med Virol 2011;83(9):1650–6.

46. Rundell MS, Pingle M, Das S, et al. A multiplex PCR/LDR assay for simultaneous detection and identification of the NIAID category B bacterial food and waterborne pathogens. Diagn Microbiol Infect Dis 2014;79(2):135–40.

47. Al-Talib H, Latif B, Mohd-Zain Z. Pentaplex PCR assay for detection of hemorrhagic bacteria from stool samples. J Clin Microbiol 2014;52(9):3244–9.

48. Chankhamhaengdecha S, Hadpanus P, Aroonnual A, et al. Evaluation of multiplex PCR with enhanced spore germination for detection of Clostridium difficile from stool samples of the hospitalized patients. Biomed Res Int 2013;2013: 875437.

49. Heidary M, Momtaz H, Madani M. Characterization of diarrheagenic antimicrobial resistant *Escherichia coli* isolated from pediatric patients in Tehran, Iran. Iran Red Crescent Med J 2014;16(4):e12329.
50. Wang XG, Zhang YH, Wang P, et al. Establishment and application of multiplex PCR for non-O157 H7 STEC virulence genes detection. Zhonghua Shi Yan He Lin Chuang Bing Du Xue Za Zhi 2013;27(50):388–91.
51. Luminex xTAG GPP K121894. 2013. Available at: http://www.accessdata.fda.gov/cdrh_docs/reviews/K121894.pdf. Accessed November 1, 2014.
52. Luminex xTAG GPP K140377. 2014. Available at: http://www.accessdata.fda.gov/cdrh_docs/reviews/k140377.pdf. Accessed November 1, 2014.
53. BioFire's FilmArray GI panel K140407. 2014. Available at: http://www.accessdata.fda.gov/cdrh_docs/reviews/k140407.pdf. Accessed November 1, 2014.
54. PathoFinder's GastroFinder Smart 17 Fast. 2013. Available at: http://www.pathofinder.com/products/smartfinder/gastrofinder-smart-17-fast. Accessed November 1, 2014.
55. Verigene® Enteric Pathogens Nucleic Acid Test (EP) K140083. 2014. Available at: http://www.accessdata.fda.gov/cdrh_docs/pdf14/K140083.pdf. Accessed November 1, 2014.
56. BD MAX Enteric Bacterial Panel K140111. 2014. Available at: http://www.accessdata.fda.gov/cdrh_docs/pdf14/K140111.pdf. Accessed November 1, 2014.
57. Hologic (Gen-Probe) ProGastro SSCS Assay K123274. 2013. Available at: http://www.accessdata.fda.gov/cdrh_docs/pdf12/K123274.pdf. Accessed November 1, 2014.
58. Buchan BW, Olson WJ, Pezewski M, et al. Clinical evaluation of a real-time PCR assay for identification of *Salmonella*, *Shigella*, *Campylobacter* (*Campylobacter jejuni* and *C. coli*), and Shiga toxin-producing *Escherichia coli* isolates in stool specimens. J Clin Microbiol 2013;51(12):4001–7.
59. Serosep. Available at: http://www.entericbio.com. Accessed November 1, 2014.
60. Koziel M, Kiely R, Blake L, et al. Improved detection of bacterial pathogens in patients presenting with gastroenteritis by use of the EntericBio real-time Gastro Panel I assay. J Clin Microbiol 2013;51(18):2679–85.
61. Genetic Signature. Available at: http://geneticsignatures.com/infectious-pathogen-detection/easyscreen-3base-technology/. Accessed November 1, 2014.
62. Siah SP, Merif J, Kaur K, et al. Improved detection of gastrointestinal pathogens using generalised sample processing and amplification panels. Pathology 2014;46(1):53–9.
63. Stark D, Roberts T, Ellis JT, et al. Evaluation of the EasyScreen™ enteric parasite detection kit for the detection of *Blastocystis* spp., *Cryptosporidium* spp., *Dientamoeba fragilis*, *Entamoeba* complex, and *Giardia intestinalis* from clinical stool samples. Diagn Microbiol Infect Dis 2014;78(2):149–52.
64. R-Biopharma Web site. Available at: http://www.r-biopharm.com/products/clinical-diagnostics/molecular-diagnostics. Accessed November 1, 2014.
65. Fast-track Diagnostics. Available at: http://www.fast-trackdiagnostics.com/products/. Accessed November 1, 2014.
66. Diagenode Diagnostics. Available at: http://www.diagenodediagnostics.com/en/list-products-2.php. Accessed November 1, 2014.
67. Biswas JS, Al-Ali A, Rajput P, et al. A parallel diagnostic accuracy study of three molecular panels for the detection of bacterial gastroenteritis. Eur J Clin Microbiol Infect Dis 2014;33(11):2075–81.

68. Genomica. Available at: http://www.genomica.es/en/in_vitro_diagnostics_clart_enterobac.cfm. Accessed November 1, 2014.
69. AusDiagnostics. Available at: http://www.ausdiagnostics.com/qilan/ADMain GeneList.jsp?ProductID=1142&CatNo=6509001. Accessed November 1, 2014.
70. Stark D, Al-Qassab SE, Barratt JL, et al. *Cryptosporidium* spp., *Dientamoeba fragilis*, *Entamoeba histolytica*, and *Giardia intestinalis* in clinical stool samples. J Clin Microbiol 2011;49(1):257–62.
71. Seegene. Available at: http://www.seegene.com/neo/en/introduction/core_dpo. php. Accessed November 1, 2014.
72. Coupland LJ, McElarney I, Meader E, et al. Simultaneous detection of viral and bacterial enteric pathogens using the Seeplex® Diarrhea ACE detection system. Epidemiol Infect 2013;141(10):2111–21.
73. Onori M, Coltella L, Mancinelli L, et al. Evaluation of a multiplex PCR assay for simultaneous detection of bacterial and viral enteropathogens in stool samples of paediatric patients. Diagn Microbiol Infect Dis 2014;79(2):149–54.
74. Mengelle C, Mansuy J, Prere M, et al. Simultaneous detection of gastrointestinal pathogens with a multiplex Luminex-based molecular assay in stool samples from diarrhoeic patients. Clin Microbiol Infect 2013;19(10):E458–65.
75. Patel A, Navidad J, Bhattacharyya S. Site-specific clinical evaluation of the Luminex xTAG gastrointestinal pathogen panel for detection of infectious gastroenteritis in fecal specimens. J Clin Microbiol 2014;52(8):3068–71.
76. Zboromyrska Y, Hurtado J, Salvador P, et al. Aetiology of traveller's diarrhoea: evaluation of a multiplex PCR tool to detect different enteropathogens. Clin Microbiol Infect 2014;20(10):O753–9.
77. Beckmann C, Heininger U, Marti H, et al. Gastrointestinal pathogens detected by multiplex nucleic acid amplification testing in stools of pediatric patients and patients returning from the tropics. Infection 2014;42(6):961–70.
78. Malecki M, Schildgen V, Kamm M, et al. Rapid screening method for multiple gastroenteric pathogens also detects novel enterohemorrhagic *Escherichia coli* O104:H4. Am J Infect Control 2012;40(1):82–3.
79. Claas EC, Burnham CA, Mazzulli T, et al. Performance of the xTAG® gastrointestinal pathogen panel, a multiplex molecular assay for simultaneous detection of bacterial, viral, and parasitic causes of infectious gastroenteritis. J Microbiol Biotechnol 2013;23(7):1041–5.
80. Halligan E, Edgeworth J, Bisnauthsing K, et al. Multiplex molecular testing for management of infectious gastroenteritis in a hospital setting: a comparative diagnostic and clinical utility study. Clin Microbiol Infect 2014;20(8):O460–7.
81. Khare R, Espy MJ, Cebelinski E, et al. Comparative evaluation of two commercial multiplex panels for detection of gastrointestinal pathogens by use of clinical stool specimens. J Clin Microbiol 2014;52(10):3667–73.
82. Kahlau P, Malecki M, Schildgen V, et al. Utility of two novel multiplexing assays for the detection of gastrointestinal pathogens - a first experience. Springerplus 2013;2(1):106.

# Moving?

## Make sure your subscription moves with you!

To notify us of your new address, find your **Clinics Account Number** (located on your mailing label above your name), and contact customer service at:

**Email: journalscustomerservice-usa@elsevier.com**

**800-654-2452** (subscribers in the U.S. & Canada)
**314-447-8871** (subscribers outside of the U.S. & Canada)

**Fax number: 314-447-8029**

**Elsevier Health Sciences Division**
**Subscription Customer Service**
**3251 Riverport Lane**
**Maryland Heights, MO 63043**

*To ensure uninterrupted delivery of your subscription, please notify us at least 4 weeks in advance of move.

Printed and bound by CPI Group (UK) Ltd, Croydon, CR0 4YY

03/10/2024

01040496-0009